take heart

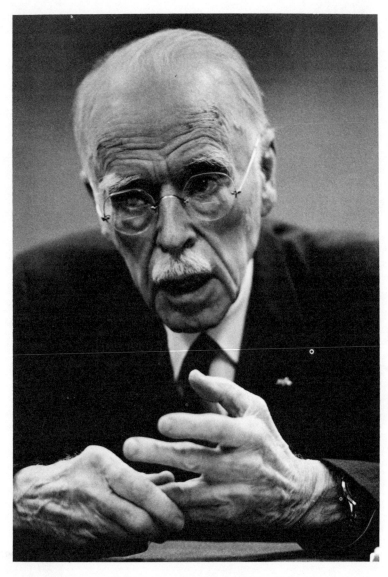

Dr. Paul D. White at the Japan Heart Institute, May 6, 1970.

take heart

the life and prescription for living of
Dr. Paul Dudley White

OGLESBY PAUL

Distributed by

The Harvard University Press

for

The Francis A. Countway

Library of Medicine

Boston: 1986

Library of Congress Cataloging-in-Publication Data

Paul, Oglesby, 1916–
  Take heart.

  Bibliography: p.
  Includes index.
  1. White, Paul Dudley, 1886–1973
2. Cardiologists—Massachusetts—Biography.   I. Title.
RC666.72.W47P38   1986   616.1′2′00924   [B]   86-3170
ISBN 0-674-86745-9

To two great ladies
with appreciation for
their encouragement and support

Ina Reid White
Jean Lithgow Paul

Contents

List of Illustrations

Preface

There are few, if any, practicing doctors whose lives have had a profound influence on millions of people. Dr. Paul Dudley White was a heart specialist who was such a one. He was the world's leading authority on the heart. When he spoke, people listened because he was honest and direct, because he was experienced and wise, and because what he said made sense. His prescription for life was designed to help people keep well and prevent disease by emphasizing three things—optimism, regular physical activity, and productive work. The current popularity of physical exercise stems in good part from his teaching over 50 years. He showed how this could be done regularly, safely, pleasurably, and inexpensively. He was a champion as well as a personal example of how, despite increasing age, one should have active interests and some useful role to play in the world, no matter how modest. He believed profoundly that the individual should not become worn down and depressed and ineffective by the tragedies and the problems around him or her, but try to appreciate and enjoy the good things that happen just as often and are frequently overlooked.

His philosophy was meant for everyone, but being a noted heart specialist, he framed it particularly for the hundreds of thousands of people with heart disease. It was Paul White more than anyone else who helped many of the men and women who had experienced heart attacks to resume their normal activity and get back to work. His role as a widely-quoted consultant in caring for President Eisenhower at the time of his heart attack dramatized to the world his belief that such a person need not be treated as some frail and delicate object but could continue as President of the United States, run for office again, play golf, and expect years of useful life. His advice, characterized by optimism and confidence, was ahead of his time and was confirmed by the course of events.

The putting-down on paper of the thoughts and style and events in the life of this remarkable man brings out other sides of his character. He was an admirable model for anyone in the health field, especially physicians and students. His warm interest in patients, regardless of their station in life, his astute analysis of human illnesses, his energy and hard work, his lack of interest in financial gain, and his generosity toward students are useful reminders of qualities every physician should hope to possess. His success shows that these attributes do indeed make a difference. His remarkable contributions to new knowledge in medical science began in 1913 and continued almost to his death in 1973.

A warm appreciation of these qualities was written by Dr. Samuel A. Levine, himself an outstanding heart specialist and close friend of Paul White, at the time of Paul White's 60th birthday in 1946. It is an excellent sketch to introduce his biography:

> He is first a physician. Thousands of individuals rich and poor will ever remain grateful and indebted to him for wise counsel and care when they were in ill health. Many are aware that they owe their very lives to his medical wisdom. Secondly, he is a teacher. Hundreds of students and physicians from our own country and all parts of the world have come and remained with him to study and learn from his experience. He never was too busy (though he had sufficient reason to be) to give valuable time to anyone who wished to work and learn. His clinic has become the "mecca" of the world for those interested in cardiology. Apart from this, there is hardly a community of importance here and abroad to which he has not traveled to lecture and share the knowledge that he has acquired. Thirdly, he is a clinical investigator. Through these past thirty odd years he has continued to work arduously and intelligently in search of knowledge, making careful detailed observations, and constantly discovering new useful medical truths. His innumerable medical publications and books form a source from which the entire medical profession draws guidance and valuable aid in the treatment of their patients. Finally, he is a humanitarian. Medical history, books and works of the past, that form the handsome eternal framework of our venerable profession and culture, interest him greatly. Also his time, his energy and even his purse are not spared in behalf of social and communal responsibilities. In his quiet way he does not neglect the duty of an enlightened and liberal minded citizen.

Recognized early as a leader, he also contributed enormously to the founding and the success of many organizations, including the American Heart Association, the National Heart Institute, and various international bodies. Linked with the Harvard Medical School and the Massachusetts General Hospital, his life work added distinction and lustre to these institutions. Paul White was unique in the trust he inspired throughout the world. Truly an international figure, he was the most widely recognized and esteemed heart specialist; and he used his authority throughout the six continents not solely for the sake of science, but also in the quest for world peace through the ways of science.

The writing of this biography of Paul White has been both easy and difficult. Easy because I have been fortunate in having an admirable and dynamic subject whom I personally knew well, in having the complete cooperation of his family, professional colleagues, former secretaries, patients and friends, and in having access to a large volume of correspondence and manuscripts. Difficult because in 87 years, Paul White was extraordinarily active and involved, and to recount or even summarize all that transpired in his life would be to prepare an encyclopedia. It has therefore been necessary to be highly selective. Preparation of the biography at this time was stimulated both by the wish to take advantage of the dwindling number of his contemporaries and the larger group of his near-contemporaries who could provide their reminiscences; and by the opportunity to have such a volume on hand for the World Congress of Cardiology to be held in Washington, DC in September 1986 and dedicated to the memory of Paul Dudley White.

In many instances I have quoted from Paul White's associates, students, and friends. I have chosen not to identify my own observations since they relate intimately to so many aspects of the biography; to state my personal relation to each circumstance and situation would be unduly repetitious and I believe not helpful. However, to provide for the record a few facts, I shall cite the following. I first met Dr. Paul White when I was a third year student at the Harvard Medical School 1940–1941 assigned to medicine at the Massachusetts General Hospital. He was one of my teachers on the wards. Then when I was an intern at the Massachusetts General Hospital during the war years of 1942–1943, he was my attending physician for two months on the West Medical service. On returning to the Hospital over three years later from active duty as a doctor in the Navy, I held the appointment of Resident in Cardiology under him for a year followed by another year in which I helped him in the care of his private patients, was in charge of his post-graduate course, worked with him in the clinics, and wrote with him four medical papers. In 1948, I moved to Chicago and from that time until his death in 1973, I saw him in various other roles. As a Council chairman and later President of the American Heart Association, I attended meetings of the Strain and Trauma Committee of which he was the leader and I also saw him in relation to other Heart Association activities. I served on the Board of Directors of the International Cardiology Foundation of which he was the President and attended meetings of that organization in New York, Boston, Chicago, Houston, Mexico City, Tel Aviv and London. For many years, the Council on Epidemiology of the American Heart Association had its annual meetings in Chicago under my aegis and Dr. Paul White used to join us for these scientific occasions, often staying with us. In my teaching role at the Presbyterian-St. Lukes Hospital and later at the Passavant Memorial Hospital, both in Chicago, I invited him to lecture and make clinical rounds with us and he also assisted on occasion in furthering the work of the Chicago Heart Association. I last saw him in August 1973 two months before his death when he joined me and others involved in the Multiple Risk Factor Intervention Trial for lunch at the Harvard School of Public Health in Boston.

Profound thanks are due first to the White family. Paul White's widow, Mrs. Ina Reid White, has been helpful throughout, has talked freely and on many occasions about their life together, has read the manuscript, and has offered suggestions many of which have been adopted. Her total support has been most deeply appreciated. I am grateful also to their daughter, Penelope White Kincaid, to Paul White's nephew, J. Warren White of Columbia, SC and his wife Corelli, and to his nieces Barbara Faden Thomas of Marblehead, MA and Dorothy Faden Ellis of Weston, MA for their willingness to talk with me and review their own family records. Paul White's cousin, H. Bowen White, also was most kind in discussing the genealogy of the White family.

I have interviewed many who have been his associates or students (a designation used broadly) at the Massachusetts General Hospital. They have provided a wealth of background information which I gratefully acknowledge. Some are quoted in one or more chapters; others who do not find their names mentioned will understand, I trust. Their recollections were invaluable not only for one or more anecdotes but for filling in gaps and reinforcing emphases in a total picture. These physicians whom I had the pleasure of talking with include Edward F. Bland, Francis L. Chamberlain, Mandel E. Cohen, Richard S. Cosby, Lewis Dexter, Allan L. Friedlich, Edgar Haber, J. Willis Hurst, Benedict F. Massell, Gordon S. Myers, Edward S. Orgain, Reno R. Porter, John J. Sampson, Royal S. Schaaf, Harold N. Segall, William Paul Thompson, Edwin O. Wheeler, Conger Williams, and William J. Zukel.

I wish particularly to express my indebtedness to Dr. Thomas W. Mattingly who not only talked with me at length but also provided me with invaluable data regarding the illnesses of President Eisenhower. Dr. Ashton Graybiel and I were unable to get together but he very helpfully sent me a large amount of correspondence. Dr. Ernest Craige and Dr. E. Grey Dimond both sent me fine tapes recording phases of their associations with Paul White. Dr. Gardner Middlebrook called to relate a most characteristic episode, and Dr. Harry Bliss generously wrote me of his recollections. I have also taken advantage of the papers of the late Dr. Howard B. Sprague which have been deposited with the Countway Library. Miss Louise Wheeler, Miss Helen Donovan, her sister Mrs. Agnes Donovan Walsh, and George Shallcross gave me tremendous assistance in regard to Paul White's office and the operation of the cardiac laboratory at the Massachusetts General Hospital. Other information regarding the Massachusetts General Hospital, and photographs, were kindly given to me by Mr. Martin Bander, Dr. John D. Stoeckle, and Mr. Joseph Stukas. Dr. Florence Avitabile was a source of a vast amount of information both of the 264 Beacon Street office and of the problems surrounding the International Cardiology Foundation. Mrs. Margaret Thayer was also most helpful about the former.

Many others have contributed greatly to my store of knowledge by generously agreeing to lengthy interviews and being helpful with specific

areas. I wish to thank them for their courtesy. The list includes Norman
Cousins, John D. Eisenhower, Dr. Lewis January, Mary Lasker, Lady
Lewis, Dr. Victor W. Sidel, Dr. Joseph W. Volker, and Dr. James Watt.

I have bothered to a variable degree and received information from
many others and wish to express my appreciation to them also by iden-
tifying them here: Albert M. Baer, Griffing Bancroft, Dr. Leo Blacklow,
Alton L. Blakeslee, Dr. David H. Clement, Dr. J. Worth Estes, Dr. Laur-
ence B. Ellis, Dr. David G. Freiman, the late Senator Jacob K. Javits, the
late James L. Jenks, Jr., Dr. Ancel Keys, Emily Kimbrough, Dr. Robert
L. King, Dr. Theodore G. Klumpp, Natalie Kreisle, Salvatore Leto, Sonya
Loew, Stefan Lorant, Dr. Bernard Lown, Prof. Paul Lukl, Sir John and
Lady McMichael, Dr. and Mrs. David C. Miller, Dr. Irvine H. Page, Prof.
Alwin M. Pappenheimer, Jr., Dr. Jean Jones Perdue, the late Dr. David
D. Rutstein, Dr. James A. Shannon, Dr. Steven S. Spencer, Dr. Jeremiah
Stamler, Dr. Frederick J. Stare, Prof. Tao Shou-chi, Dr. Joseph B.
VanderVeer, the late Dr. Joseph T. Wearn, and Dr. Irving S. Wright.

Mr. Walter Lord was most kind in showing me how he as a fine professional writer organized his material. Mr. Jacques Barzun took a generous
interest in my project. Mr. Richard J. Wolfe, Curator of Rare Books at
the Countway Library of Medicine at the Harvard Medical School and
his staff have been patient and understanding during the many months
of my labors. The same is true for the staff of the Word Processing Center
of the Medical School which has accepted my many revisions with tolerance and good humor, and for Diane Q. Forti who has made excellent
editorial suggestions. David Ford provided the fine design.

The onerous task of organizing and preparing an inventory of the vo-
luminous files containing the Paul D. White papers has been and is being
accomplished successively by two fine research librarians, Mrs. Judith H.
Goetzl and Mrs. Elizabeth Cherniack, aided for some months by Vivian
Yee. Without their great assistance, writing this biography would have
been an impossibility.

I wish to thank the Rockefeller University Library for permission to
quote from the letter from Paul White to Alfred E. Cohn dated January
16, 1916; the *National Geographic Magazine* to quote from "Hunt-

ing the Heartbeat of a Whale" by Paul Dudley White and Samuel W. Matthews published in its issue of July 1956; Doubleday and Company, Inc. to quote from *The White House Years: Mandate for Change 1953–1956* by Dwight D. Eisenhower, and from *The Drama of Albert Einstein* by Antonina Vallentin; Alfred A. Knopf Inc. to quote from *Sketches in the Sand* by James Reston; Random House Inc. to quote from *The Faulkner Reader* by William Faulkner; Norman Cousins to quote from *Dr. Schweitzer of Lambaréné* published by Harper and Row; Harvard University Press to quote from *The Inquisitive Physician* by Francis M. Rackemann; Macmillan and Co. Ltd. to quote from *Gitanjali* by Rabindranath Tagore; and Harper and Row to quote from *Firsthand Report* by Sherman Adams. The excellent photograph of Paul White walking along the bank of the Charles River holding an umbrella was taken by Theodore Polumbaum. The cartoon by Jim Dobbins entitled *Last House Call* is reprinted with permission of the *Boston Herald.*

My gratitude is of course also due to those whose financial support paid for the larger portion of the work of the research librarians. These donors include the National Heart, Lung and Blood Institute, The American Heart Association, The Markell Foundation, Mr. Ronald Williams, and Dr. and Mrs. Bernard J. Walsh. I especially wish to thank Mr. Robert P. Gwinn whose several contributions have been of inestimable assistance.

It is very probable that I have failed to acknowledge the contributions of some whose kindness and goodwill should be recognized. My apologies to them and my hope that they will feel sufficiently rewarded by the appearance of the biography. Needless to say, any omissions, errors in statement, or other aberrations must be laid solely at my door.

Oglesby Paul, M.D.
Professor of Medicine, Harvard Medical School
Senior Physician, Brigham and Women's Hospital
Boston

Chronology

Paul Dudley White born Roxbury, Massachusetts, June 6, 1886

Roxbury Latin School, 1898–1904

Harvard College, 1904–1907

Harvard Medical School, 1907–1911

House officer, Massachusetts General Hospital, 1911–1913

First publication of clinical research, 1913

Study with Sir Thomas Lewis, London, 1913–1914

House physician, Massachusetts General Hospital, 1914–1916

Paul White starts Cardiac Outpatient Clinic, Massachusetts General Hospital, 1916

Volunteer medical officer, British Expeditionary Force, Camiers, France, 1916

Medical officer, Massachusetts General Hospital, Base Hospital No. 6, Talence, France, 1917–1919

Relief service, American Red Cross, Eastern Macedonia, 1919

Start of private practice, Massachusetts General Hospital, 1919

Instructor in medicine, Harvard Medical School, 1921

Publication with M. M. Myers of "The Classification of Cardiac Diagnosis," 1921

Marriage to Ina Helen Reid, 1924

Member founding group, American Heart Association, 1924

Description of Wolff-Parkinson-White Syndrome, 1930

First edition of "Heart Disease," 1931

Adoption, Penelope Dudley White, 1936; Alexander Warren White, 1939

President, American Heart Association, 1941–1943

Clinical professor of medicine, Harvard Medical School, 1946

Chairman, Unitarian Service Committee medical teaching mission to Czechoslovakia, 1946

Founding member, International Council of Cardiology, 1946

Executive Director, National Advisory Heart Council, 1948–1957

Attempts to obtain electrocardiogram of a whale, 1952, 1953, 1954, 1956, 1957

President, World Congress of Cardiology, Washington, D.C., 1954

President, International Society of Cardiology, 1954–1958

First visit to U.S.S.R., 1956

Founder with Louis N. Katz, International Society of Cardiology Foundation,
   1957
First U.S. member of Academy of Medical Sciences of U.S.S.R., 1961
Heart attack, 1970
Visit to People's Republic of China, 1971
Died, Boston, Massachusetts, October 31, 1973

take heart

Take heart, fair days will shine

THE PIRATES OF PENZANCE, W. S. GILBERT

CHAPTER ONE

The Beginnings

"The next day, we were flown to Canton and a member of the Chinese Medical Association flew with us to escort us, and he escorted us right to the border and put us on the train. On the train, Paul immediately sat down and got out a notebook and began writing a press release; and he and I crossed out words and rewrote and redrafted, and he prepared a good, brief press release. He did it in two copies—one he could keep and one he could hand them. When we got to Sheung Shui, which is the border, we got off and had to walk across, and our luggage was toted by porters. We got another train for Hong Kong, and it immediately started out. When we got to the first stop—there were about five or six stops on that train—reporters started climbing in the windows. It was an amazing sight. They were literally coming in like the lemmings leaving on their way to the sea. They were coming in over the seats, they were coming in down the aisles, coming through the windows, television cameras were stuck at us, microphones held against us, and I don't mean five or ten, but I mean twenty or thirty. Dr. White and I were interviewed; our wives were interviewed. It turned out that the story was that we were there because Mao had had a heart attack, and we just simply had to assure them that we knew nothing about it. They didn't believe us in the least. They thought we were not telling the truth. We went on to our hotel where another press interview was held. Paul, as soon as he got his luggage and got his interviews over, was on his way to a plane for Rome. The old gentleman was full of energy and enthusiasm and didn't have a single sign of fatigue. The last I saw of him, he was heading for the plane for Rome, with that little pigeon-toed walk of his, that quick

1

little way of walking along with the brim of his hat turned up, laughing and waving at the reporters."

Such was Dr. E. Grey Dimond's description of Paul Dudley White in the final hours of his trip to the People's Republic of China in September 1971. The invitation had come at last, after many years of frustrated attempts. The trip, which was the first visit of a group of doctors from the United States to China in twenty years, had been exhilarating and successful. Paul White was received everywhere as the senior and most eminent member of the delegation. The press conferences after crossing the border, with their hectic disorganized atmosphere, had been a good measure of the importance the world media were to attach to the whole undertaking. What an appropriate way for this 85-year-old Boston physician to close a long, illustrious career! But it does not appear that he looked upon himself as finished with productive work. He would keep on, or at least try to, for it had always been his philosophy that at every age and particularly as the years advanced, it was keeping active and keeping active usefully that made life matter. For him, achievements had come not just with the energies and discoveries of youth or the maturity and intellectual strength of middle age but also with the experience and poise he brought to his sixties and seventies and eighties. That Paul White could accomplish so much usefully for so long and with such enjoyment was—as with most other human attributes—a reflection of both genetic and acquired influences.

The ancestors of Paul Dudley White on his father's side were solid, decent residents of Massachusetts. Apparently content with the environment they found on settling just south of Boston, they stayed there within a radius of no more than 20 miles for 300 years. Whatever restlessness made the first White cross the Atlantic seems to have been thoroughly extinguished in that ordeal. The first member of the family to reach North America was Thomas White who became a freeman in Weymouth in 1635, was a land-owner and selectman there and Deputy to the General Court of the Colony, and died in 1679 at the age of 80. Fifth in direct descent from Thomas was Micah White (1758–1841), a selectman in Randolph where he was a member of the North Baptist Church. It is apparent that he served during the Revolution as a private in Captain Silas Wild's company of Minutemen from Braintree, enlisting April 28, 1775 and mustering out October 6, 1775. Probably from respect for this military experience and for Revolutionary heroes, when a son was born to Micah and his wife Sarah Mann White on July 12, 1801, they named him Warren for Major General Joseph Warren, the famous physician who was killed at the Battle of Bunker Hill on June 17, 1775. This Warren White (1801–1878) married his first cousin Lorena Mann, lived in Randolph, Cambridge and Boston Highlands, and was one of the owners of the Blue Hill Turnpike.

Their son Ephraim Mann White (1830–1869) of Randolph was Paul Dudley White's grandfather. He and his first wife, Mary Frances Niles, set up housekeeping in Charlestown on the slope of historic Bunker Hill, and it was there on November 12, 1858 that their only child, Herbert Warren White, was born. The young mother tragically died of cholera at the age of 23, less than a year after the birth of her son; and in 1861, Ephraim married again and unhappily to Carrie E. Richards, a marriage which ended in divorce.

Ephraim was one of those who traveled to California briefly at the time of the Gold Rush. He later served in the Union Army in 1862 and 1863, mainly in Louisiana, being attached to Company E of the 47th Regiment of the Massachusetts volunteer infantry, a company numbering 103 men, all but 16 of whom came from Charlestown, Massachusetts. His older brother, Charles Warren White, had meanwhile started a small business in Boston making trusses for the treatment of hernias. The youngest brother Elisha Mann White, who had studied at the Harvard Medical School for two years, had acquired experience as a hospital steward in the Army, and then went on to obtain an M.D. in 1864 from Jefferson Medical College. In 1865, all three brothers, Ephraim, Charles, and Elisha, joined in establishing in Boston C.W. White and Company which sold trusses, crutches, and orthopedic equipment—evidently very successfully. Ephraim's affiliation with his two brothers was, however, destined to be brief, as he died from tuberculosis aged only 39 in September 1869 in Randolph.

Herbert Warren White, Ephraim's son and Paul Dudley White's father, wrote a diary in 1876 when he was 16 years of age; the first pages contained a poignant recollection of his early years with his father and stepmother.

> I cannot write much for each day as the space is very limited, yet not to [sic] much so for my calm life. Since no great events have ever happened to me—but I stop when I look back over my life for there are some things that have happened which do not now seem great yet are not in every life. Let me look over them; the early death of my mother, but since I never knew a mother's care, I do not miss it (I was but nine months old); by my father's second marriage I came in possession of a French step-mother, who used me not with care since she did not like me. She was so brutal in her treatment of me that father dared not to leave me with her so he removed me to Grandpa Niles in the country. This harsh usage I remember but little of since I was about three or four years old at the time so it does not seem of much consequence.
>
> About the first fright that I had was several months after I came out here. My step-mother came out here to claim me (she had now parted from my father) by force. I have never been so much scared since, I believe. I went to school then. Father came out here quite often (nearly every Saturday) and at last health began to give way and he went out West to Winnona, Minn. Sept 65. He grew better but one time he caught a severe cold from which he never recovered. He spit blood and the physicians told him to go home as he must die. He came home. Then I first made a real acquaintance with my father. He used to talk a great deal to me, telling me his great desire to have me grow up a good honorable man rather than to be rich and dishonorable. He grew weaker and weaker until on the fourth of July 1869 he died after he had been home about six months.

In an autobiographical sketch Herbert Warren White prepared in 1928, he further recalled an episode involving "my dad's morning devotionals. Stepmother was angry and voluble, saucy, overflowing with taunting words. Father read aloud a few lines from the Bible, Marm White sputtering all the while. Before we knelt for the morning prayer, my dad, quite sudden, took madam firmly by the fold of her garments, run her into the kitchen, turned key in the door, then knelt down beside me and offered his morning prayer to the racket of thumping and kicking and scolding going on behind that kitchen door. He took his time. I could not hear what he said for the noise."

Herbert Warren White thus had a rocky start in life, losing his mother before he was a year old, acquiring the classic nasty stepmother, and then losing his father when he was only 10. It was fortunate that his mother's parents, who lived on a farm located in both Randolph and Braintree, took him in and evidently cared for him well. H. Warren White (which he preferred to Herbert Warren White) started in school at the Charlestown public school at the age of 4 and transferred two years later when he was living with his grandparents to grammar school in Randolph. He graduated from the Braintree High School at the age of 18.

He decided that he needed some classical study if he was to enter college, and so moved to Boston where, living with an uncle, he spent a year at the Boston Latin School. At this point, he was decisively influenced by his father's brothers in selecting a career. Both Uncles Charles Warren White and Elisha Mann White, doing well in their medical supply business, encouraged their nephew to go into medicine, hopefully into the new field of orthopedic surgery which would clearly be an asset to the family enterprise. Entrance into medical school was not difficult then for an intelligent applicant with a favorable high school preparation, and it was not until 1901 that the Harvard Medical School made a bachelor's degree a requirement for admission. He therefore went from the one year at the Boston Latin School directly into the Harvard Medical School without a full college preparation and graduated in 1880 after only three years of study. A four-year course of study was not to be required for another 8 years.

His formal education thus completed in a relatively brief period, H. Warren White and a medical school classmate, Godfrey Ryder, then spent a year abroad in travel and study in Berlin, Dresden, Vienna, and Paris. In Paris in February 1881, he was exposed to smallpox while on hospital rounds with Professor Parrot, but was unconcerned because he had been supposedly successfully vaccinated at least twice. However, the presumed protection proved a failure. A few days later in London, he became very ill, walked a mile to the London Fever Hospital, and after two days was diagnosed as a case of smallpox. He was therefore transferred to the Highgate Small-Pox Hospital by ambulance. He later (January 25, 1894) published an account of his illness in the *Boston Medical and Surgical Journal* in which he wrote:

> I remember that ride very well. The small-pox ambulance was constructed something like an American hearse. The patient was wrapped in blankets, shoved in, and the doors shut. It was like attending your own funeral.

The first night in the hospital was a frightful experience:

> I arrived late and was put into the centre of a long ward with 20 or 30 others. A howling snow-storm outside. There were large ventilators over each bed (like those in dissecting-rooms), and they were so wide open I felt the snow sift in upon my face during the night. The patient in the bed to my right was in a howling delirium all night long, but quieted down and died about daylight. Another died across the room, three beds away, on my left. There were no screens to put around them.

He made a slow recovery and stayed in London for a time making rounds at King's College Hospital with the famed Joseph Lister, whose research and teaching on antisepsis were revolutionizing surgery, and then visited Edinburgh. The trip abroad was followed by several months of additional study in New York at the Postgraduate School. With his education completed, he returned to Boston to start a general practice— not to go into orthopedics as his uncles had wished.

On June 6, 1882, H. Warren White married Elizabeth Abigail Dudley of Boston whom he had first met in the Harvard Street Church where she sang in the choir and was a Sunday school teacher. Elizabeth Abigail was the daughter of Barzillia Dudley, born in 1808 in Windham, Vermont, and his wife Caroline A. King, born in 1821, whose father Henry King came from St. John, New Brunswick and whose mother, Abigail Stairs, was a native of Philadelphia. Barzillia Dudley, who was the son of John and Betsey Dudley, is listed in Windham, Vermont in the 1830 federal census. He was working in Memphis, Tennessee as an engineer in the waterworks when his daughter Elizabeth Abigail Dudley was born September 19, 1859. With the start of the Civil War, he and his family returned north to Massachusetts. He must have had some musical talent as the roster of soldiers in the Civil War from Massachusetts lists Barzilla Dudley, aged 50 and residing in Somerville, as serving as a musician in Company K, 20th Regiment, Massachusetts volunteer infantry from December 28, 1861 until February 25, 1863 when he was discharged for disability. He died in Boston from a fall April 28, 1874, but his wife survived until 1912, dying at the age of 90 years and 8 months.

H. Warren White and his wife lived from 1882 to 1888 at 294 Dudley Street in the Roxbury section of the near south side of Boston where, for $300 a year, he had both a home and office. He later wrote how he and his wife "started very modestly on a cash basis and aided by her thrift and watchfulness, we were able to make both ends meet." It was at this address that their first child Miriam was born March 29, 1884, followed by Paul Dudley White born June 6, 1886. On March 29, 1962, Paul Dudley White in a letter to the *New England Journal of Medicine* mentioned that he had been named for Chief Justice Paul Dudley.* That H. Warren White of Roxbury and his wife chose to name their first son Paul Dudley White probably reflects chiefly the local distinction in Roxbury of this important colonial gentleman. The H. Warren White family in 1888 moved a short distance to 161 Warren Street, and in 1899 they bought a new house at 151 Humboldt Avenue also in Roxbury where they lived and reared their children and in which Dr. H. Warren White had his office for 27 years. Two more children, Joseph Warren White and Dorothy Quincy White, were born in 1892 and 1899.

H. Warren White accepted many kinds of cases in his practice. For example, his patients in January 1883 had problems which included infected fingers, asthma, tuberculosis, erysipelas, meningitis, measles, and cholera. He helped with and on his own performed deliveries, and also

---

* This eminent jurist was the grandson of Thomas Dudley, the second governor of Massachusetts, and the son of Joseph Dudley, who also was a governor. Born in Roxbury September 3, 1675, he graduated from Harvard College at the age of 14, after studying law was Attorney General of the colony for 16 years, and then was Chief Justice of the colony's highest court, the Superior Court. Judge Paul Dudley died on January 25, 1751 and was buried in Roxbury. His five children all died very young, and thus Paul Dudley White cannot be a direct descendant, although he may possibly have descended along a collateral line.

performed autopsies. It does not appear that he did any major surgery, but he did accept patients with fractures, might assist in operations, and administered anaesthesia with ether. On one occasion after assisting with a very bloody amputation, he wrote ruefully that he was sorry that he had worn his best pants. By 1896, his practice was clearly growing as he

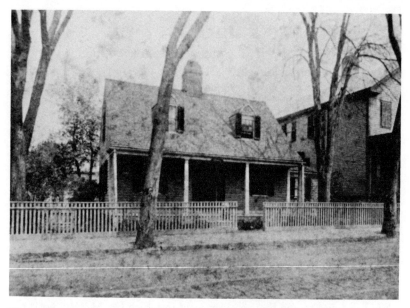

House at 294 Dudley Street, Roxbury, birthplace of Paul Dudley White.

was seeing 8 to 14 patients a day. Thereafter he maintained a busy office and home practice until his death on November 21, 1929; indeed he died of a heart attack on his way to make a house call.

In the latter half of the 19th century, Boston was becoming crowded with immigrants, especially from Ireland, and to help provide free care to these often impoverished people, Dr. Francis F. Whittier and Dr. H. Warren White established in October 1886 a dispensary in an unused room in a building provided by the adjacent Ruggles Street Baptist Church. By 1892, these two doctors with three other physicians were providing without charge professional care to over 2500 people a year. Because of the evident need and the success of this venture, the Boston

Baptist Hospital was incorporated in 1893 with Dr. White as one of the signers of the Agreement of Association, and a year later new quarters with 15 beds were provided in the Longwood area where the New England Deaconess Hospital is now situated, although the dispensary continued to provide outpatient care. Because of neighborhood opposition to having a hospital in that location, it was moved to the Parker Mansion on Parker Hill shortly thereafter and was renamed the New England Baptist Hospital. As such, it continues to this day. Dr. White was President of the hospital staff in 1894, was Medical Director 1903 to 1905, and was a member of the Board of Trustees for more than 20 years.

H. Warren White was also a physician at St. Elizabeth's Hospital in Boston and taught at Tufts Medical School where he was Lecturer and later Professor of the Theory and Practice of Medicine, a role which he particularly enjoyed. For over 40 years, he was also a director of the Roxbury Charitable Society which contributed about $12,000 annually to help the poor and needy in the Roxbury area, and was a long-time member of the Roxbury Society for Medical Improvement. In 1928, he wrote: "How I did all this, kept up a steady obstetric work and general practice, is to me now astonishing and unbelievable. I only had one horse and never stood up in my Goddard buggy and galloped around 'for effect' as some country doctors I've seen do."

He was a devout Baptist. His 1876 diary states: "The greatest event that has happened was when I professed religion and joined the church." All his life he was a regular church-goer, taught Sunday school for many years, and on January 25, 1901, was chosen to be a deacon of the Dudley Street Baptist Church, a position he held until his death. An example of his piety was his Thanksgiving Day prayer dated November 26, 1925:

Oh Heavenly Father: We thank Thee as the years roll around for the return of this festival of Thanksgiving! It is a reminder of the long line of Pilgrim Fathers preceding us. It's a reminder that all we have in such abundance comes to us from Thy hand that too often we take it all without a thought from whence it came. Fill us now with a true gratitude that may be pleasing to Thee, and that may have a thought for the less fortunate around about us and may we never forget that "all the world is Kin." We thank Thee today for each other, and as a family we would be truly helpful and a blessing to each other, and rejoice in Thy kind dealings with us. That we gather here all in so much health and strength, so much of work to do, and so much hopeful interest in each other's welfare. Be Thou especially with the absent ones today, as we all think of them, make more sure and more real, that final *grand reunion* of all God's children in their Heavenly Father's house above! Humbly we pray all this in Jesus' name! Amen!

H. Warren White seems to have been decidedly astute in the area of finances. "I made the discovery that it didn't much matter how much one earned but it mattered a whole lot how much one spent," he wrote at the end of his life. His practice brought in a steady income and he was

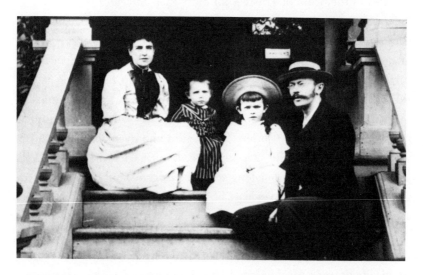

White family on front steps, probably at 161 Warren Street, Roxbury, about 1888–1889.
Left to Right: Mrs. Elizabeth Abigail Dudley White, Paul White's mother; Paul Dudley White; Miriam White, Paul White's elder sister; Dr. H. Warren White, Paul White's father.

fortunate in his investments in the stock market. He was able to take the family away regularly in the summers, usually for a month, and most often to Maine or New Hampshire but at times to Martha's Vineyard. He and his wife—whom he always referred to as "Lad" (from Elizabeth Abigail Dudley)—also took extended winter trips each year including to California, Italy, Bermuda, the British Isles, Israel, and North Africa. He scorned an interest in possessions and said that investments in books and travel and the church paid him his biggest dividends. While the family did not live in an atmosphere of luxury, they seem to have always had two servants to do the cooking and the housework. In those days with the flood of young women reaching Boston from Ireland, domestic help was extremely cheap.

With his reading and his several visits about the United States and overseas, he was not just a limited general practitioner but was unusually and broadly informed and took a keen interest in the world around him.

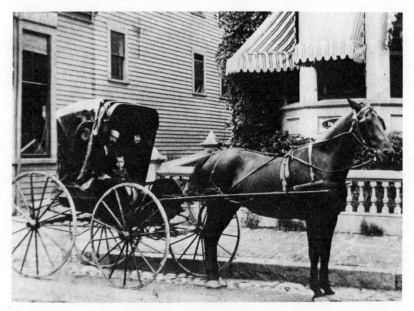

Dr. H. Warren White and son Paul, about 1890.

He was also with his community activities a fine citizen, devoting time and energy to helping others.

H. Warren White's granddaughter remembers going at Thanksgiving and Christmas to 151 Humboldt Avenue—a good-sized Victorian house painted gray situated on about a half-acre of land, with a plaque bearing the words "H. Warren White, M.D." near the front door. There was a big entrance, Dr. White's office was on the right as one entered, and there was a stairway in the middle. Her grandfather showed her that in his office were two big jars of pills, one of which he explained was full of sugar pills which he used as a placebo for patients whose symptoms he suspected to be neurotic. He had the unusual routine of weighing everyone before and after the big festive meals on Thanksgiving and Christmas and of keeping a written record of the results. He evidently enjoyed a huge, old-fashioned meal himself and recorded the weights with a twinkle in his eye to see who had gained the most.

As in many physicians' families, the four White children found that their father, being a hard-working and dedicated family physician, had relatively little time for his offspring. His son Paul did get some early limited exposure to medicine through his father, going with him on house calls, but not always with a positive response as shown by an entry in his diary of September 26, 1904: "Went out riding with pa on his round of calls. Not very exciting, but then—." He at times made out his father's bills; thus he recorded earning $2.00 for this task for the month of December 1904. Later in his last year of medical school, he might see a few of his father's patients when his father was ill, as on January 29, 1911 when H. Warren White had "la grippe" and his son saw four patients for him. On the whole, the influence of the father on the selection of a career by his son seems to have been far more through propinquity and example than through any deliberate attempt by the parent to expose him to and stimulate him in medicine. Indeed, writing in 1967 in response to an inquiring letter, Paul White said that he and his brother "expressed a strong desire to avoid the profession when we were young." Doubtless a constraint to a warm and relaxed family atmosphere was the pervasive influence of Dr. H. Warren White's religion. The family's social life revolved around the affairs of the Dudley Street Baptist Church. No alcohol was served or seen in the White home, and playing cards and going to the theater were not encouraged. There was to be no smoking before the age of 20. Dancing or attendance at concerts was frowned upon unless they had religious or patriotic content. It was characteristic that when Paul White was studying at Harvard College, his father seems to have visited him only when there was a lecture on a religious topic or to go to chapel services.

Paul White clearly had great admiration for his father, but the relationship between the two does not seem to have been a close one. When H. Warren White died in 1929, his son Paul wrote a tribute to him which was published in the *New England Journal of Medicine* on January 9, 1930. It eloquently recognized his father's role as a doctor, counselor, and friend to many, described his life with comments from his father's writings, and said almost nothing about him as a husband and father. While some of this omission may have represented a New England distaste for a display of emotion, it is likely that it also signaled a more respectful than affectionate relationship. His daughter-in-law recalls Dr. H. Warren White as a fine person who lived a life of great moral integrity and was the dominating figure of the family. His grandson recalls him also with great respect and as a person with considerable reserve; but his granddaughter emphasized that despite his strong attachment to the Baptist Church, he was not sanctimonious and could be fun.

H. Warren White's wife, Elizabeth Abigail, was a quiet, gentle person, short in stature like her son Paul, quite formal in manner and devoted to her husband and children. She did not have the breadth of interest of her husband but enjoyed her home and subordinated her whole life to the needs of her family. On her death at the age of 88, her son Paul wrote a stirring tribute to her and to all wives and mothers of physicians which was published in the *Boston Herald* of July 27, 1948. This said in part:

> I would like to pay a tribute to the wives and mothers of physicians, for my late mother was both. Their lives of service, sacrifice, and devotion are perforce dedicated not only to their families, but generally to the demands of suffering humanity. It is a double task and privilege which the world at large often fails to recognize, but which is heroically borne by hundreds of thousands of women the world-over. And in my travels I have found the same self-sacrifice everywhere.
>
> The physician himself may have the constant care of his many patients who, although usually very considerate, may require his presence in the dead of night or in the midst of a dinner party or of a play or a concert or as he is about to set on some long-planned and eagerly anticipated holiday or vacation. Many

a time as a boy did I see this happen when father, who was a family doctor, was so summoned. Courage of the mother then was needed to conquer the disappointments of the whole family and such was gently shown on many an occasion by my mother.

Paul White's childhood lacks the vivid colors of precocity, abnormal behavior, grievous illness or family disaster. The second child in a good Christian home, he seems to have had normal activities and happy relations with his brother, two sisters, and playmates, and few escapades. In August 1890 at the age of four years, he was away with his mother and sister Miriam at the seashore, and his mother wrote to his father: "Paul has been getting up after bed time and cutting up at a great rate. He powdered his hair so thoroughly that his head has looked white for two or three days. We found the soap stuck full of pins and as a finale the same night he cut his hair, and it was not an even cut I can assure you. I suppose the children feel so well that they have some superfluous spirit that has to be worked off in some way." She concluded the letter with "Paul is a miserable looking fellow with his hair gouged out in one place. Please tell me what to do. I am a little blue this P.M. though I am perfectly well. With my best love as always, Lad." That Paul had superfluous energy at the age of four seems to have been a harbinger of what was to characterize his adult life.

A remarkable event took place when he was still a small boy, on the occasion of being taken to see the new Christian Science Church in Boston. There, he later recounted, he met its founder, Mary Baker Eddy, who placed her hand on his head and pronounced with startling accuracy that he would grow up to be a great man. Perhaps she did this with all little boys as a matter of good public policy. Since the White family lacked any ties to Mrs. Eddy or her church, and since she only very rarely visited the building and never held public receptions there, this episode appears all the more an extraordinary chance encounter.*

Paul White was entered by his parents in the lower school of the Roxbury Latin School in September 1898 when he was twelve years old. This

---

* Mary Baker Eddy visited the original church which was opened in 1894 only three times: April 1, 1895, May 26, 1895 and January 5, 1896. She never visited the new church which was completed in 1906.

was, and is, a distinguished private school, founded in 1645 by John Eliot, pastor of the church in Roxbury 1631–1690 and the leading missionary influence among the Indians. The School numbered among its graduates the same Chief Justice Paul Dudley after whom Paul White was named, as well as the eminent doctors John and Joseph Warren for the latter of whom Paul White's great grandfather and brother were named. It was only for boys and had no boarding pupils, so the class was composed of students mostly residing in the Boston area. Paul White was to stay there for six years including one extra year beyond graduation. In that period, he had a strong classical education that included six years of Latin, three years of Greek, four years of French, four years of German, five years of English, and courses in mathematics, history and science.

He began a diary in 1901 that made frequent references to his lessons and mentions sports including ball-playing and fencing. It also mentioned going to church which he seems to have done faithfully every Sunday as well as to the Junior Christian Endeavor Society every Monday night, and he mentions reading the Bible every night. He was appointed President of the Junior Christian Endeavor Society in March 1903. His tolerance of religious subjects was not always great as one entry of January 18, 1902 indicates attendance at a prayer meeting with a subject of "How to Resist Temptation"; Paul White's comment in his diary was "I choke on it." Another entry of August 28, 1904 was "Went to the Baptist church with Dorothy. Best of the sermon was its brevity."

His diary also contained varied statistics including his height, weight, hat, shoe and collar sizes, Victor bicycle number, and watch case and works numbers. This was the start of a life-long habit of a meticulous recording of names, dates, places and facts of interest. His note on his 17th birthday June 6, 1903 revealed an unsophisticated 17-year-old: "Gracious! how ancient I am. For today is my birth day and I am 17 years old. Just think of it!" A week later he got long trousers and two weeks later graduated from Roxbury Latin School cum laude and also won the Latin Prize. He was also admitted to Harvard College that same month. However, on account of his age and size, as he wrote in his diary, he stayed the additional year beyond graduation taking more English, German, advanced mathematics, physics and chemistry—and these were nine-month courses—and also being Editor of the school paper the *Tri-pod*. William C. Collar, one of his teachers, in composing a reference for him in 1905 wrote: "Scholarship, character, industry of a very high order. Most deserving in all ways."

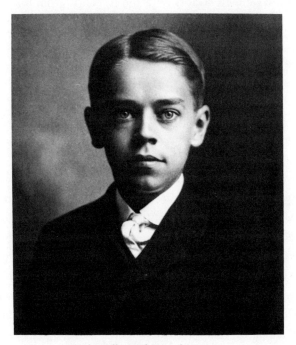

Paul Dudley White in his teens.

Paul White's years at Roxbury Latin School seem to have been very happy ones, and later in life he looked back on them with gratitude and a pleasant nostalgia. In 1957 he addressed the graduating class of the school presenting the kind of personal testimonial which headmasters, faculty, alumni, families, and hopefully students particularly like to hear each spring. After referring to his good fortune in having had some of the finest teachers in the country he went on to say:

Two results of this program of study which would seem to be 'stiff' in many prep schools today have been of inestimable value to me all my life. The first was the obligation, early imposed and early accepted, of learning how to study and especially how to concentrate. Happily we had no radio, television, or jalopies to distract us then. When on many occasions during the years that have followed, it has been necessary to burn the midnight oil to get essential work done, both in war and in peace, those early years at the Roxbury Latin School proved of enormous importance; in fact, without them my life might well have been worse than humdrum.

A second invaluable result for me in later life was the grounding I received in history and the languages, indeed in the entire program. For later writing, drill in English grammar and composition was fundamental. I still shudder, probably excessively, when I hear or read a split infinitive. French and German have been of great importance to me as a physician in my study of the great medical contributions of the past and in my visit to clinics on the European continent throughout the years.

In 1967, in an article written for the *Saturday Review*, he called particular attention to one of his teachers at the School:

There was one very special subject—Greek—routinely taught at the Roxbury Latin School which, by chance, altered my life. We boys were exposed to a remarkable teacher—Clarence Gleason—who was so stimulating that I learned the language well enough to simplify later my translation of the scientific anatomical terms during my first year in medical school; to induce me to begin my medical missionary work in Macedonia in 1919; and to decipher some of the Russian words to which I have been exposed in recent years.

In September 1904 he enrolled as a freshman at Harvard College in a class numbering 700. This first year he continued to live at home in Roxbury, at times walking the five miles to Harvard Square in as short a time as an hour and five minutes. His course work included English, history, Greek, German and zoology. His comment in his diary on December 8, 1904 "The skeleton and the heart-system in zoology—very interesting" is the first clue of a possible tilt toward science. He had a daily English theme—"good practice but a bore"—had good but not outstanding grades, went to the varsity games, and recorded considerable bicycling as on April 19, 1905: "Rode my wheel out nearly to Framingham (just beyond Natick) & then on the way home followed the leading Marathon runners into Boston (all the way). Rode in all 35 miles." Here too was early evidence of his enthusiasm for walking and bicycling, forms of exercise particularly suitable for his slender physique. In May of 1905, in an application for a scholarship the following year, he responded to a query as to occupation in view after graduation with "probably teaching."

The summer of 1905 was the first of four in which he was to serve for a little over a month as a counselor at Camp Becket. Camp Becket, located on a 200-acre farm near Becket in the Berkshires in western Massachusetts, was operated by the YMCA. It accepted 150 boys 12 years of age or older at a charge of $4.50 a week. Here Paul White was one of the group leaders, played baseball with the campers, went swimming and hiking, built a tennis court, did farm chores and led in various social activities. His brother Warren also went to the camp and it was clearly a very rewarding experience for both of them. Paul White all his life looked back upon these summers as eminently worthwhile in helping to give boys, some of whom were underprivileged, a healthy relaxed outdoor environment and an exposure to fine but not oppressive moral standards.

The rustic surroundings and simple life in July and early August 1905 were followed by a two-week visit to the home of a college classmate, Harold B. Platt, at Shelter Island Heights near the tip of Long Island. This appears to have been his baptism in a more fashionable and affluent world, a baptism which did not lead then or later to admiration for this style of living: "Gee-whiz. What a style. And they call this a country town. Best of clothes, collars, crowds of fashionable people, delicacies on the table—that's all—rotten!!! I detest the place and will be glad to get back to a sensible home." His initial negativism was somewhat tempered by a successful visit to Manhattan where in addition to a dinner at the Hardware Club he saw Times Square, the Metropolitan Museum, Grant's Tomb and went out to the Bronx Botanical Garden and the New York Zoological Park. His father had to send him some money for the trip back to Boston evidently chiding him in the accompanying letter for being prodigal.

The summer of 1905 and the autumn which followed in which he began his sophomore year at Harvard brought a major change in Paul White's life. For the first time, he began to separate himself from the closeness and the life-style of his home and family. The experience at Camp Becket, in which he and Warren were away from their parents, was a successful one, and the journey to New York opened his eyes to very different surroundings from 151 Humboldt Avenue, Roxbury. On returning to college, he and Harold Platt moved into the Harvard Yard into a room in Thayer Hall, a room which lacked any central heating, so they had to order in coal and wood. He began eating at Memorial Hall. He was also awarded a $200 Burr Scholarship. Briefly, with the lack of familiar inducements to study, his grades suffered and he received only a C+ in History 16A, a D on a Government I test, and even an E on an economics paper.

Perhaps it was these academic problems which made him see an ophthalmologist who found that he needed glasses which he was to wear thereafter for the rest of his life. His final grades for the year were good with three A's, one A −, three B's, one B −, and one C + (in Government I, given by A. Lawrence Lowell, the future President of the University). He heard a "fine talk" by President Charles William Eliot and noted that he had seen Houdini perform some of his marvelous tricks at the Harvard Union. The change in his life seems to have been really accomplished when his diary recorded that on May 10, 1906 he played poker and won and the next month he even took a girl to the Wellesley Float with tepid results—"Fair time" was the verdict. In May of 1906 he also obtained a live frog for his room for experiments. He obtained an A in Zoology 2 and that summer while again at Camp Becket wrote in his diary that he dissected two snakes and a turtle.

In June of 1906 he visited with his father the five handsome new Harvard Medical School buildings forming a quadrangle facing Longwood Avenue in Boston where the American Medical Association was then having its annual meeting. He was clearly much impressed. Indeed, he returned to the School the next day to spend more time viewing the exhibits. The buildings were actually so new that they did not become the official home of the Harvard Medical School until the following September, when the first class of students was admitted to what seemed very grand surroundings compared with the old cramped quarters on Boylston Street.

The first two years at Harvard had shown a pattern of college life which he would continue in his junior year. He was a studious young man with few extracurricular activities. Endowed with a short, slender physique, he could not achieve success in varsity sports. Without a natural musical talent, he did not attempt choral or instrumental groups. He chose not to participate in student journalism. Not belonging to the upper social stratum, he did not join a select "final" club and cultivate friendships within its limited membership. Further, he was gradually losing enthusiasm for his close association with the Baptist Church and indeed had no interest in any other religious group, to the distress of his father. Gifted with an excellent mind, he chose to apply it to scholastic pursuits.

On beginning the junior year at Harvard he wrestled with a decision as to his career. He had expressed some interest in becoming a teacher, perhaps in history, but this was not apparently sufficiently attractive, and for some reason—perhaps because it involved nature, which he always enjoyed, and because it represented science which he was also learning to like yet a science very different from the medicine his father practiced—he decided to go into forestry. This choice seems to have been an impulsive one and was influenced by discussions he had with Dr. William B. Bolles, a senior surgeon at the Boston City Hospital. On September 25, 1906 he wrote: "Conference with Prof. Fisher in Cambridge—finally decided to take up Forestry as a profession; Fisher is head of it at Harvard." Within three weeks he was regretting his impulsiveness. On October 15, 1906 he was feeling poorly from a head cold and wrestling with his decision, the next day he cut his classes and had a conference with Assistant Dean Wells, and as a result changed into a premedical program which included three courses in chemistry, one of which was taught by the famous Professor L. J. Henderson. This proved a decisive turning-point in his life.

Thereafter he worked hard at his course work and did so with a new zest and enthusiasm. A zoology class on the dogfish viscera was "beautiful" as was an injection of the blood vessels of Necturus. His morale and his grades both improved, and his junior year marks were two A's, two A−'s, and one B. In February 1907 he saw his first professional theatrical production ("The Squaw Man") and later that month listened to President Theodore Roosevelt deliver a stirring speech which must have ended even more stirringly as the President led the students in the

Harvard Cheer. Booker T. Washington addressed the students in March of 1907 as did William Jennings Bryan whose subject was "Faith." Paul White's Harvard College education was to end in June 1907 (although he actually graduated A.B. cum laude June 24, 1908) as he had decided to enter the Harvard Medical School after only three years of college, an option existing then as now. Eighteen years later, he would write a bit sadly that "This saved a year but also deprived me of close affiliation with my college class." He did, however, take a one-month early summer chemistry course at the Massachusetts Institute of Technology by way of additional preparation. The summer was otherwise occupied by his month at Camp Becket and by an excursion to the White Mountains where he climbed to the summit of Mt. Washington typically getting to the top first in his group. He was now five feet eight inches in height and weighed only 120 lb stripped.

Registration at the Harvard Medical School occurred in September 1907, and in the ensuing nine months he was to study anatomy, histology, physiology and chemistry.* Once again he was living at home as the Medical School had no living accommodations. The year seems to have passed uneventfully except that he was studying very hard, but it was clear that he had found himself and was in the right niche. "To bed late as usual—must reform" he wrote on February 20, 1908 and again

---

* During the years in which Paul White attended the Harvard Medical School, the required course work took four years with the basic sciences (anatomy, physiology, histology and embryology, chemistry, bacteriology, pathology, and pharmacology) occupying most of the first two years. Medicine, surgery, pediatrics, and obstetrics and gynecology were presented in the second and third years. The fourth year was devoted to electives. The schedule was dominated by lectures and the clinical training was conducted by a combination of these and outpatient clinics. The number of hospitals which Paul White mentioned visiting for teaching exercise was large. These included the Boston City Hospital, the Boston Dispensary, Boston Lying-in Hospital, Boston State Insane Hospital, Carney Hospital, Children's Hospital, Infants Hospital, Long Island Hospital, Massachusetts Charitable Eye and Ear Infirmary, Massachusetts General Hospital, McLean Hospital, Municipal Tuberculosis Sanitarium, and the Samaritan Hospital. Paul White was taught by an eminent faculty which included Walter Bradford Cannon in physiology, Henry A. Christian in medicine, William T. Councilman and Frank Burr Mallory in pathology, James Jackson Putnam in neurology, Maurice H. Richardson in surgery, Thomas Morgan Rotch in pediatrics, and Theobald Smith in comparative pathology. He does not appear to have developed a close association with any of his instructors, although he did have life-long friendships with many of his classmates.

on February 27, 1908. A high point of the year occurred on March 10, 1908 when he and a classmate assisted the great physiologist, Walter Bradford Cannon, in a demonstration of decerebrate rigidity in the cat.

That year he also reluctantly accepted the Chairmanship of the Membership Committee of the Page Class at the Dudley Street Baptist Church (now merged with the Ruggles Street Baptist Church) but turned down an offer of its presidency. However, he was elected its Vice President in 1909. The Page Class had been founded in 1888 under Charles L. Page and was described in the Twentieth Anniversary Booklet of 1908 as "Seeking to discover and aid men to fulfill the obligation of manhood, it presents an attractive opportunity to study together their Maker's Book; to upbuild the body politic; to cheer each other and others up life's incline; to strengthen and purify the physical and mental nature to best conserve well-being of two worlds." From time to time he would address the class on a scientific subject. Paul White was also elected President of the Young People's Society of Christian Endeavor on February 16, 1910, but this was to be his last close attachment to the Dudley Street Baptist Church. Thereafter medicine occupied more and more of his time, there was correspondingly less for the church, and it was clear that his heart was not in church activities and that he had accepted these elected positions only out of a sense of duty. He continued to be physically very active whenever his schedule permitted, walking 18 miles from Boston to Dedham, Dover and Westwood on April 24, and that summer he went to Camp Becket for a month again, this being the last time.

The second year at the Harvard Medical School started on a happy note. As one of the best students (with an A average), he was chosen as a prosector to assist in anatomy demonstrations under Professor Thomas Dwight. He was also excited by starting to attend clinics in January 1909 at the Boston City Hospital. On May 20, 1909 he wrote in his diary that he had heard the very eminent Dr. William Osler, Regius Professor of Medicine at Oxford, speak at the Medical School. This event which should have been an exceptional one, to be savored and long remembered, seems not to have made much of an impact. That this great physician, so profoundly admired on both sides of the Atlantic, a singularly gifted scientist, writer and speaker, should have failed to make more of an impression may have meant that the speaker was fatigued and not at his best or that the listener was—or both. Fifty-nine years later, in responding to an inquiry from a preparatory school student, Paul White observed that Osler once "visited when I was a medical student at the Out Patient Department of the Massachusetts General Hospital and gave a brief talk, but he was dog-tired and almost went to sleep." One suspects that with the passage of time Paul White had moved the site of the talk from the Medical School to the Massachusetts General and that indeed the occasion was not up to expectations for a good reason.

Paul White spent nearly two months of the summer of 1909 as a camp doctor at Camp Wellesley in West Ossipee, New Hampshire, returning in time to sign on for two weeks of service in the North End of Boston for the Boston Lying-In Hospital. At the end of his fortnight there, he had delivered twelve babies. It was characteristic of his thoughtfulness that on the next December 24 he returned to the North End to give presents to the children of one of his obstetrical patients. The third year of medical school saw him elected to the Boylston Medical Society in the fall and to Alpha Omega Alpha (with three other classmates) in the spring, evidence of recognition of his excellent mind. On May 6, 1910, he read a paper on "Physiology of Digestion in Infancy" before the Boylston Medical Society, his first presentation of a scientific subject before a scientific audience.

There was one tragic happening in the White family at this time and this was the death of his younger sister Dorothy on May 1, 1910 at the age of 10½ years. She had developed rheumatic fever as a young child, thereafter was delicate, and probably had a series of recurrences, both active endocarditis and pericarditis being present six weeks before her death. Paul, her elder brother, seems to have been very good to her, and for many years on many occasions and especially on weekends would read to her or play games with her or take her out walking. Doubtless this illness and its sad ending were factors in his later interest in rheumatic fever as a disease. A month after Dorothy's death, on June 4, 1910 his older sister Miriam was married in a small wedding to Andrew F. Faden.

The summer of 1910 was again occupied with time spent as a camp doctor at Camp Wellesley, time also spent in growing a mustache, which thereafter became a permanent fixture. In September he worked 12-hour days at the Haymarket Square Relief Station of the Boston City Hospital caring for emergencies. The load of work was heavy and he saw 141 cases on September 9 including lacerations, fractures, and poisonings. His final year at Medical School was devoted to a series of one-month electives which, in Paul White's case, included pediatrics, obstetrics, theory and practice of physic, pathology, surgery, clinical medicine, neurology and bacteriology. However, the most exciting event during this fourth year was the news that he had won a coveted 16-month internship appointment to the West Medical Service of the Massachusetts General Hospital (the "MGH") to begin March 1912. This was tremendous news and he was thus confronted with the pleasant dilemma of how to spend his time between graduation in 1911 and starting his internship eight months later. He applied to the Children's Department at the Massachusetts General Hospital, and fortunately its Chief, Dr. Fritz B. Talbot, liked him and awarded him a six-month appointment as the third intern ever appointed to that new service. Paul White graduated in June from the Harvard Medical School, M.D. cum laude, second in his class. The first in the class was James Howard Means, later to be the Chief of Medicine at the Massachusetts General and thus for many years Paul White's department chairman. His father celebrated the ending of this phase of his son's formal education by taking him to Bermuda for nine days.

CHAPTER TWO

A Devoted Slave and Other Roles

Paul White's first eight years after graduation from medical school were a preparation for a life-long career in a specialty—the study and treatment of heart disease, called cardiology. That the interval was so long did not however mean eight years of learning to be a heart specialist. The actual training phase was limited to 22 months in pediatrics and internal medicine at the MGH, plus nine months in cardiology in England. This in turn was followed over the next five years by six other phases including two more forays in Europe, affected in part by the exigencies of World War I but also significantly by Paul White's proclivity for seeking out new and interesting experiences. Unlike most of the physician trainees of today, he seemed to show little sign of impatience and anxiety to be launched promptly into a career. Indeed, his varied pattern of life from 1911 to 1919 was indicative of a style that was to characterize the next 60 years. It was as if his agile mind found the confines of being a doctor in Boston too limiting, and he periodically would seek out a world with more adventure and broader horizons, even though Boston and environs were always to remain the base for his family and his professional home and the working center of his research, practice, and teaching.

The first phase began when he started as a house officer on the Children's Service at the MGH on July 1, 1911. The hospital was located in the west end of Boston on the Charles River, and the original building, designed by Charles Bulfinch and opened in 1821, was still the center of all activities. There were four medical wards on the east end of the structure and four surgical wards on the west end. Each ward was located in a large, high-ceilinged, square room with, in the middle, a double brick fireplace and chimney. Approximately 28 beds were arranged around the periphery of the room, with a nurse's desk in the center adjacent to the chimney. In the summer, the wards would move out-of-doors into tents set up on the lawn in front of the hospital as this was an era that believed in the health-giving qualities of sunlight and fresh air—even though it might be somewhat dirty city air. The patients were all adults, except for the few children admitted from 1910 on to the new pediatric service which was located on the third floor in the center of the building. There were no private patients until 1917, a reflection of the 19th century reputation of hospitals as housing mainly the indigent members of the community who, if not already dying, would doubtless end up that way shortly.

The young medical house officers served for a total of 16 months, progressing in four-month periods through the positions of Sub-Pup (or extern), Pup, Junior, and Senior, with increasing responsibility at each level but without salary. The Sub-Pup was to work in the outpatient clinics in the mornings and help in the wards in the afternoon. The Pup performed all the laboratory work himself, including blood counts, urinalyses, stool examinations, and all cultures. The Junior and Senior House Officers were responsible, under a senior attending physician, for the work-ups and care of the patients. In contrast to the medical service, the new small pediatric service only had one house officer assigned to it and that was for only six months. Theoretically, each house officer had every other afternoon and evening free, but the load of work was such that these "off" hours frequently had to be spent on the wards. On medicine, Paul White's fellow house staff members included James Howard Means, destined to be the Chief of Medicine at the MGH, and George R. Minot, who went on to win the Nobel Prize for his historic research in discovering the treatment of pernicious anemia with liver.

The Sub-Pup and Pup were not provided with living accommodations in the hospital, but the Juniors and Seniors lived over the Accident Room on the second and third floors in what was named the Flat which contained a sitting room (furnished importantly with an icebox) and several small bedrooms. There was a single bathroom on the third floor with four washbasins and three large tubs. Dr. Francis M. Rackemann who has described the life vividly in his biography of George Minot wrote:

> In the morning, the water in all the tubs was left running so that they were always full. The end tubs had hot water; the middle one had cold. On getting

up, most men would lie in the hot tub for a minute or so and then would jump directly into the cold tub, usually with a yell, and with the water splashing all over.

Dr. Rackemann also has written:

There was no telephone on the wards, but the Flat had a sort of local house phone, with a set of bell buttons at the bottom of the stairs. By ringing the appropriate bell, the nurse could reach any one of us in the middle of the night. In the daytime or evening, when she wanted a doctor, she pushed the big button, which rang a much louder bell. Whenever this bell rang, all noise stopped instantly, and then the nurse would call plaintively, "Dr. Minot," or "Dr. Wilson." If he were there, the "callee" went downstairs to the "caller," but if the "callee" was not in the Flat, one of us started counting softly, "One, Two, Three" and at the "Go," everyone joined in a roaring "NO!"

The young doctors were subject to the rigid discipline of the hospital director, Dr. Frederic A. Washburn, who considered it unseemly for them to go about with their hands in their pockets—hence, their trousers were made without side pockets.

One July 12, 1911, Paul White wrote a letter to his brother Warren about his first twelve days on the Children's Service where he was the only house officer.

Hello, Wally. Got your letter, also your postal—but too busy to write till today. It was hard getting started here in my new service since I am Senior, Junior, Pup and Extern all at one and the same time. I had to get on to myriads of new tricks, but now I am fairly on my way. It is great fun and I am having a wonderful time. The heat early last week bothered us all, of course, and made my start a little more strenuous still, not counting a fine coryza which all my nurses and I suffered.

My service is going to be very good and extremely instructive. Every morning except Sundays and holidays I run the outpatient for children. At noon or 1:00 o'clock I make my daily ward visit with the visiting physician (on Sundays and holidays @ 10:00 a.m. The rest of the time early in a.m.—before outpatient—and in afternoon and evening). I run the ward—examine patients, prescribe treatment, do the clinical lab. work (bloods, urines, stools, cultures, etc.), write up records and do a little surgery (such as lancing ear-drums—have done six so far), doing lumbar punctures (did my third this a.m.—pretty fair for one week), infuse patients, arrange seepage, tap chests, etc., etc.

We have all sorts of cases—hearts, kidneys, lungs, feeding, ears, nervous diseases, joint diseases, mouth diseases, gastro-intestinal infections (esp. in the summer now), heat prostrations, etc., etc. Also blood diseases. Ages range from two or three weeks to 12 years.

School was fairly interesting, but this is great. Medicine certainly is a thing that has a live interest.

The staff of house-officers is very good—decent, wholesome, jolly fellows and we have good times together.

The nurses are also excellent. They are certainly of a high grade socially and I have a fine cordial bunch in my ward.

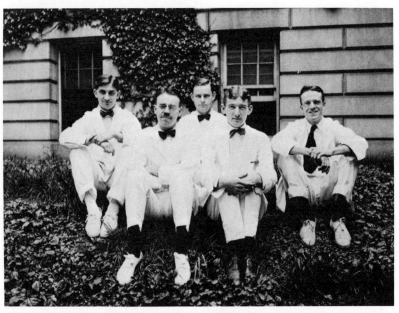

House officers of the Massachusetts General Hospital, 1916.
Front row, left to right: Paul Dudley White, Elliott C. Cutler.
Back row, left to right: John J. Morton, H. H. Crabtree, Orville F. Rogers, Jr.

That all was not work was indicated in another letter to his brother dated July 30, 1911 in which he wrote:

We get together in "the Flat" and have a good time—keep an ice chest with drinks, have cookies, etc. about, have a pianola with many pieces, etc., etc. The other night, I was initiated into the "Owls" which is a sort of fraternity of the whole bunch, very informal. Initiation consisted chiefly in being suddenly awakened at night by being "rotated" by the five seniors—i.e. the bed in which I slept turned upside-down and very neatly too at 2:30 a.m. and then beating it upstairs to a very fine party (almost a full course dinner).

The six months spent on pediatrics were thus exciting and excellent training. At their end on December 30, 1911, he noted in his diary that while he had been a house officer in the Children's Service, he had admitted 152 cases. Not remarkable then, but appalling if it were today, was the further statistic of 26 deaths—a mortality of 17%. His Chief, Dr. Fritz B. Talbot, expressed his appreciation of his loyal service by presenting him with a silver cigarette case appropriately engraved. Quite bowled over by this exhilarating introduction to the clinical world, Paul White accepted the offer of young Dr. Richard M. Smith to become his assistant in the practice of pediatrics in Boston when he finished the 16 months of his regular MGH appointment in medicine. With the Children's Service behind him, he indulged in two months' vacation, mainly spent in New Hampshire skating and hiking and tobogganing.

Paul White returned to the MGH to begin as house officer on the West Medical Service on March 14, 1912. He passed through the stages of Sub-Pup, Junior and Senior and concluded his appointment on July 31, 1913, having had two particularly eventful episodes. The first was collaboration while Pup with Dr. Roger I. Lee, a young staff member of the hospital, in a research project to develop a method for measuring the clotting time of blood. The results of this joint effort, "A Clinical Study of the Coagulation Time of Blood," were published in 1913 in the *American Journal of Medical Sciences*. The method described soon became known as the Lee-White Coagulation Time and was used throughout the world for the next 50 or more years. Indeed Dr. Maxwell M. Wintrobe, in the sixth edition of his *Clinical Hematology* published in 1967, wrote: "Although many different procedures have been proposed, the method of Lee and White, devised in 1913, remains the accepted technique." This was Paul White's first publication, albeit a joint publication. It came in an era when methodologic research publications were not common (most were clinical reports) and particularly were not common from young doctors in their first year of hospital appointment. It proposed a technique which proved reasonably reproducible and reliable, inexpensive, not unduly time-consuming, and useful. Indeed this modest scientific paper has the distinction of being a landmark publication. In later years, it was usually forgotten that the White of Lee-White was Paul White, the famous heart specialist.

The second event was recorded in his diary on February 6, 1913 with the following entry: "Have been offered a remarkable opportunity by Drs. Edsall and W. H. Smith to be an expert on *hearts*. To go abroad in Fall with expenses paid, to study in London with Lewis for six or nine months, then back to MGH next year to run the new electrocardiogram [sic] for two years and then—." There was no evidence that Paul White in his medical school and hospital training had become especially enamored of the subject of heart disease. Further, he had already agreed to stay in Boston and practice pediatrics. His only investigation had been in the field of blood clotting. However, the lure of an offer for study in a foreign country under a leading scientist in an exciting new area (his diary entry indicated that he did not know that the correct word for the equipment he was to use was electrocardiograph and not electrocardiogram) and with expenses paid was too enticing.

The genius behind this attractive offer was Dr. David L. Edsall, Jackson Professor of Clinical Medicine at the Harvard Medical School and Chief of the East Medical Service at the MGH. Edsall, who was a graduate of Princeton and of the University of Pennsylvania Medical School, had acquired an enviable reputation as an outstanding investigator and teacher in a number of areas, including metabolism and infectious disease. He was also a most astute bed-side clinician and was rapidly becoming a medical statesman with progressive ideas for improvements in medical education. Although a professor of therapeutics and pharmacology and then of medicine at the University of Pennsylvania, he had become unhappy with the conservative element in that medical community and left in 1911 to become Chairman of the Department of Medicine at Washington University in St. Louis. It soon became apparent that he had jumped from the frying-pan into the fire, for the reactionary physicians in St. Louis were even more obstructionist than their Philadelphia counterparts. Edsall therefore had accepted in 1912 an invitation to come to the Harvard Medical School to succeed Dr. Frederick Shattuck as Professor of Medicine and also to be a service chief at the MGH. It was greatly to the credit of both the School and the Hospital that they reached outside Boston in making the appointment, as there were powerful local forces believing that Boston was indeed the hub of the medical universe and the repository of all medical brain-power. Then and later, when he became Dean of the Medical School, he was recognized as an extraordinary, far-sighted leader, to become one of the greatest forces for constructive change in the long history of Harvard University and United States medicine.

It was Edsall's belief that the U.S. medical schools and teaching hospitals urgently needed to acquire greater competence in physiological processes in health and disease in order to better understand and treat human illnesses. With this specific aim in mind, he promptly undertook, as the new leader at the MGH, to see to it that some of its brightest young men went away for post-graduate research training in physiology, to return later to Boston to apply and expand on their newly acquired knowledge. Thus he sent J. Howard Means and Cecil Drinker to Denmark to work on respiratory exchange under August Krogh, and George R. Minot to Johns Hopkins to work with Drs. William S. Thayer and W. H. Howell on problems of blood. On a grant of $1,000 as a Frederick Sheldon Traveling Scholar, Paul White was to go to London to study with Thomas Lewis and James Mackenzie in cardiology and especially in the new and exciting field of recording the electrical activity of the heart—electrocardiography. This was especially timely, as a patient of Dr. William H. Smith, Mr. Francis Skinner, had donated money to the hospital for purchase of its first electrocardiograph. There was no electrocardiograph in Boston as yet, although ones were beginning to be used in several locations, including the Pennsylvania Hospital in Philadelphia, and in New York at the Presbyterian Hospital, the Hospital of Rockefeller Institute for Medical Research, and the New York Postgraduate Hospital.

Paul White accepted Edsall's invitation gladly, but first he had to extricate himself from his agreement to work with Dr. Richard M. Smith in pediatrics. Fortunately Smith was understanding and generous and imposed no barrier to the plan for study in Europe. On the last day of Paul White's house officer appointment in medicine, Dr. Richard C. Cabot kindly gave him a letter of introduction to Osler—now Sir William

Osler, the Regius Professor of Medicine at Oxford, to be used once he
was settled in England:

Dear Sir William
Paul White is a recent Mass. General Hospital graduate with a bent for studying circulation.
    He is in pursuit of wisdom *via* Lewis, Mackenzie, & Co. but needs also a
draught of true Oslerian *Aequanimitas*.
    Affectionately,
    Richard C. Cabot, July 31.

The next phase in the 1911–1919 period began when Paul White sailed
for Europe in August 1913 in the company of his classmate J. Howard
Means and Means' mother. They stopped briefly in London where White
paid a courtesy call on Dr. Lewis. In a talk Paul White gave at the University College Hospital in 1955, he described this first meeting with
Lewis:

When I went to the University College Hospital Medical School to see him, I
was ushered into the basement and there met his "diener" who said that Dr.
Lewis was about to leave for luncheon but would doubtless see me for a moment, whereupon I entered the laboratory where he was engaged in physiological studies on the heart of a dog, at the time under anesthesia on the table.
Dr. Lewis himself, about to leave for luncheon was dressed, as was the custom
of the day, in morning coat, a silk hat on his head, his left hand gloved and
holding the other glove, and his right hand massaging the heart of the dog
which had momentarily ceased to maintain an adequate beat. He turned briefly
to me, acknowledged my presence by a nod, and asked me to come back a few
weeks later in the fall.

Paul White and Howard Means and the latter's mother then went to
Holland, visiting Amsterdam and Vollendam briefly and arriving in
Groningen on September 1 to attend the ninth International Physiological Congress which was in session from September 2 through 6. The
presence of many great scientists was an exhilarating experience and Paul
White much later wrote: "My own most vivid memory of the Congress
was that of the demonstration repeated by Prof. A. D. Waller of London
of the initial human electrocardiogram by primitive capillary electrome-
ter, which he had just shown at an earlier congress of the same sort in
1887, when I was one year old." Following the Congress, the trio went

on to visit both the medical and tourist sights in Berlin, Vienna and Bavaria. Paul White then went on alone to Italy and Switzerland. He arrived in London in mid-October to start work primarily with Dr. Thomas Lewis but to spend some time also with Dr. James Mackenzie.

Dr. James Mackenzie (later Sir James Mackenzie), then age 60, was the international eminence on clinical observations and research on the heart. He was from the parish of Scone near the city of Perth in Scotland and received his medical training in Edinburgh. In 1879, he joined two physicians in Burnley in Lancashire, England in general practice. Here he had the opportunity to watch and document the natural history of disease as seen in patients whom he followed year after year. Becoming challenged by the apparently insoluble and ill-understood heart problems of some of these patients he showed extraordinary ingenuity and scientific curiosity in recording on a piece of smoked paper tracings of the pulses in the neck veins, and in the arteries of the neck and the wrist, as well as of the heart beat on the chest wall. Later, with the help of a watchmaker, he developed an ink-writing recording instrument called a polygraph. He carefully pored over the thousands of records he made correlating the findings with the clinical states of the patients. Finally in 1902, after 23 years of practice and observation, he published a book on *The Study of the Pulse* which brought the Burnley physician international recognition, a recognition which had been largely withheld in his own country where it was considered that little valid science could come from a general practitioner in an unsophisticated community such as Burnley. In 1907, he moved to London where he opened a counsulting practice on Harley Street and the following year published a large volume, *Diseases of the Heart,* which further established his growing fame. He was keenly interested in and supportive of the investigations in electrocardiography of young Thomas Lewis, though he considered this to be a field in which he was not qualified to take an active part. Deeply aware of the crucial importance of carefully listening to and examining and following the patient, he was skeptical of what seemed to him to be the trend toward excessive preoccupation with technology, including x-rays of the chest and the new electrocardiograms.

Thomas Lewis (later Sir Thomas Lewis), although only 31 years of age, was rapidly becoming an acknowledged world leader in basic cardiological research. He was born in Cardiff, Wales where he received his initial university education. He entered University College Hospital, London in 1902 for his clinical training and was awarded an M.D. in 1907. Beginning in 1910, he devoted most of his time to research as he did not find the routine of practice at all congenial. Especially in the early years of his research, he was a pioneer in investigating the nature of normal and abnormal impulse formation in the heart as well as of conduction and rhythm disturbances, studies which were undertaken in the basement of University College Hospital in a room intended for charwomen's implements. An extremely hard worker and not an easy personality to get to know and like, he attracted many students from outside the British Isles by his scientific brilliance. Of him, Sir Harold Himsworth wrote: "Lewis had great gifts—men have been gifted before, but few have used their gifts to such advantage."

Sir Alan Drury's description of the Lewis laboratory paints a grim picture, but a picture not unusual in an era in which most medical research while mentioned in respectful tones was provided with inadequate facilities and precious little money.

> The laboratory was an unattractive half basement and low ceilinged room with an inner dark room for the galvanometer and experimental animals. It was dark, crowded with equipment and uninviting. Into it came patients for electrocardiography, dogs for experiments, trays with coffee and buns for lunch. It was hot and dusty in summer and cold in winter. True a large fire burnt brightly in the winter but anyone who found time to warm his backside at it was not beloved by Lewis. It was no good to try and look out of the window for relaxation, for it was glazed with opaque glass. The scientific peaks were our only scenery, and it was our job to try and find the pathways to the top.

Paul White wrote to his father on October 22, 1913 from London about his start in the laboratory. His letter suggests that he had already acquired a British style of writing.

> Am now at it although I am not worked so hard as I should like to be. Lewis returned a few days ago and meets us every day. I find, however, that he is rather an elusive chap, that is just now at any rate; if I want to learn much I

see that I must make him make me work. He is agreeable enough, you know, but seems naturally rather retiring and absent-minded. Yesterday I took my first electrocardiographic tracings, they are not so difficult to obtain; the difficulty comes rather, I suppose, in the interpretation of them after they have been acquired. Yesterday also I bought the new edition of Mackenzie on the *Heart*.

On October 29, he called on Mackenzie for the first time and found him extremely cordial. Mackenzie invited him to spend the afternoons with him or his assistants at the London Hospital, a possibility which had been encouraged by Lewis, with whom he would spend the mornings. Paul White did indeed start with this schedule, but it was soon apparent that Lewis and not Mackenzie was the real magnet for him. Writing on November 9 to his father, he sounded as if he and three other visiting students were learning how to relate to their young mentor:

In regard to Lewis, I am now quite enthusiastic about him and I don't think unwisely so. He's "coming fast" and before many years if my guess is correct will be the world's greatest cardiologist. Even at present I think he probably is, but he hasn't become widely known yet. Mackenzie still is regarded as the foremost heart-man but his day is done. From what I have seen of the two men, I think there is no comparison. Mackenzie's fundamental idea is right but it is for others to carry it out—in fact now he rests heavily on Lewis for all his new facts about the heart and for application of older principles.
. . . Lewis is a real Welshman—hence he is quite eccentric, very taciturn and difficult to understand at first. He frightens lots of men away at first undoubtedly—few ever stay with him more than two, three or four weeks, which makes him all the more cynical. But we—the four of us—being in earnest are hanging on like leeches and he is now just beginning to open up well. I think he sees now that we mean business. He certainly has changed quite a bit which delights us. We have passed the most elementary stage and actually begin to show him that we have some intelligence.

This was the beginning of a highly successful and productive and intensive nine-month indoctrination, both into the world of research as well as into the specialty of cardiology. It was greatly to the credit of Edsall that he had suggested this training in the laboratory of a young newcomer. Paul White could not have found as favorable auspices to launch his career anywhere else in Europe or in the United States, even though, as he wrote, he was "a devoted slave of the master." It was to

Paul White's credit that he did not bridle at the initial, slow, relatively inhospitable reception, but stuck to it and showed Lewis that he was an intelligent assistant, worth encouraging. He showed himself that he could profit from this London experience. Edsall would indeed have been pleased if he could have read Paul White's letter to his mother written on December 21 in which he said: ". . . I am realizing that to get the most out of clinical cases one must see and help in considerable experimental work where fundamental principles are brought out and worked upon. My ideas have quite undergone a revolution in this respect—I've always paid more attention to results without first having grounded myself on elements."

His hours of work soon came to be exclusively with Lewis. He admired Lewis for his intellect and Lewis in turn came to rely upon him more and more, in part, as Paul White wrote, because Paul White was the better of the two at arithmetic. He gave up his informal role as an observer with Mackenzie as he found Lewis so much more advanced in cardiology.

The work with Lewis was done in the dark basement laboratory and was of several kinds, much of it shared with a Canadian, Dr. Jonathan C. Meakins, who would later become Physician-in-Chief at the Royal Victoria Hospital in Montreal and Dean of the Faculty of Medicine at McGill. One task was taking electrocardiograms on patients and laboratory animals using a large machine with a string galvanometer with the actual tracings being recorded on glass plates.* At times, pulse tracings of the type introduced by Mackenzie were also taken. Another task occupying many hours was helping his teacher in painstaking analysis of the findings in the electrocardiograms. Yet another was the injection and dissection of hearts from various species—fish, cat, dog, pig, sheep, ox, monkey, and human—to observe the pathways conducting the electrical impulses.

---

* The electrocardiograph was introduced by Einthoven in 1903, making use of the fact that a magnet and a conductor of electric current will interact. Einthoven employed a string galvanometer in which a straight conducting "string" (a platinum or silver-coated glass or quartz thread) lay between two poles of a magnet and moved in relation to changes in the electrical field detected on the surface of the body, changes which resulted from the beating of the heart. A record of these sequential changes was called an electrocardiogram.

That the laboratory was sometimes also used for non-scientific purposes was indicated in a letter sent to Paul White in December 1914 by
the laboratory helper after Paul White's return to Boston:

> Hope you excuse me for taking the liberty in writing to you, I have often
> thought about you especially about this time last year when we us to stay to
> work untill the early hours of the morning, and have football practice in the
> laboratory none of that now & very little work I wish you were here now it
> seems a dead & alive hole ever since you left I have no one to talk to.

Only occasionally would he see patients with Lewis, leading him to
write at the end of his stay in London: "I've forgotten what a patient
looks like . . ." However, Paul White did have opportunities to visit
hospitals and laboratories in greater London. He attended what must
have been an exciting meeting of the Physiological Society in March, a
meeting heavy with scientific giants, including Cushny, A. V. Hill, Bay-
liss, Starling, Barcroft, Waller, Keith, Flack, and Lewis. He also spent
some time arranging for the purchase and shipment to the Massachusetts
General Hospital of a Cambridge electrocardiograph with a string galvanometer with silvered glass fiber plus camera, projection lantern, rotary
time-marker, control board and glass slides, priced $1,427.37.

Paul White did not become a laboratory recluse. Like any American
visitor, he saw the sights in the greater London area, particularly on the
weekends. Not surprisingly when he visited the now famous Futurist and
Post-Impressionist Exhibition of paintings on Bond Street, he found it
amusing and grotesque and noted that one visit to such a gallery should
last a lifetime. He went to the theater and enjoyed Bernard Shaw's "The
Doctor's Dilemma," and also saw Sir Herbert Tree in Belasco's "The
Darling of the Gods." Sunday, February 15 saw a combination of England
versus Ireland in rugby in the afternoon, attended also by King George
V and Prime Minister Asquith, and "Tristan and Isolde" in the evening
at Covent Garden, attended by Queen Mother Alexandra. He reported
becoming quite addicted to afternoon tea and even started to smoke—a
habit which proved very short-lived. The Suffragettes were getting public
attention through a variety of noisy and disruptive tactics, and the doctor
from Boston who witnessed some of these scenes was unsympathetic

with their violent approach, writing home that the long series of recent outrages was atrocious. At the end of March, he watched the Oxford-Cambridge boat race, which Cambridge won, and afterward saw in London swarms of Oxford and Cambridge students everywhere all in dress suits and silk hats, some on top of taxis and some wrestling with the bobbies. There seem to have been no attractive young English ladies who caught his eye, and he wrote to his mother: "Are there any strikingly beautiful wealthy girls you've seen about lately (probably none in Dudley Street) who you think would be apt to pine for an old, baldheaded, dried-up specialist?"

Paul White was to take away from this London apprenticeship several lessons which had an indelible impact. One was that results in science come in large part from hard work. Lewis was an extremely hard worker, he set an example by his industry which was coupled with his success, and Paul White clearly felt challenged and rewarded to find he could keep up with him. He acknowledged: "I thought I used to work hard at the MGH but a winter with Lewis has shown me how a man can work." Paul White's life in medicine was to be at the Lewis pace. A second lesson was that although he learned a great deal about the physiology of the heart, he found that a life of laboratory research was not for him; however, he wanted to be in a position to share somehow in the excitement of the pursuit of this new knowledge. Writing on May 17 he concluded: ". . . I realize that I shall not do much of any experimental work probably not only because I think I should prefer the clinical side but also because of my relative unfitness. Nor do I expect to become a Mackenzie. Nevertheless, the examples of these Englishmen and what Germans I've seen make me want to contribute something in the way of research (perhaps clinical) in the future." Both Mackenzie and Lewis were gifted with minds having the rare, precious ingredient of originality, an attribute usually evident early in a scientific career. Paul White's talents did include the ability to look at problems involving medical science in new ways, an ability eminently helpful throughout his career. However, contributions to basic new knowledge would not be his forte; rather it would be his role to combine the intelligent synthesis of clinical observations with an unusually wide experience, a well-developed common sense, and an attractive and energetic personality. A third lesson was that the study of the anatomy and pathology of non-human hearts was important and rewarding. Lewis had arranged with the London Zoo to obtain the hearts of all animals dying there. Paul White would return to the United States to undertake repeatedly the study of the hearts of various species, including those of animals dying at the Franklin Park Zoo in Boston.

Paul White left London for good on June 16 having as one of his last acts ordered a new suit of clothes at a tailor on Chancery Lane for £4. Instead of returning promptly to Boston after the ten-month absence to see his family, install the new electrocardiograph, and begin his career, he chose characteristically to spend two weeks in travel. This was not to be a leisurely vacation—a quiet well-deserved respite from his laboratory labors. As he wrote on June 14, 1914: "I've planned a merry and very busy schedule, but as I have the wanderlust again and am anxious once more to 'hit the trail' my energies will quite suffice." "Hit the trail" was a phrase prophetic of things to come. He visited Oxford but chose not to use there his introduction from Richard Cabot to William Osler. One wonders if the exciting experience of working with the youthful Thomas Lewis had not made encounters with distinguished but aging personalities like James Mackenzie and William Osler seem less rewarding. He went on to visit Wales and Scotland and sailed for Boston from Liverpool on June 30.

The third phase in the 1911–1919 period began when Paul White returned to the MGH on August 1, 1914, age 28, still unmarried, and the beneficiary through his own efforts and those of Edsall and Lewis of an exceptional training. Here was an opportunity to get back into patient care as well as to make use of his special knowledge regarding the heart—special because he was the only physician in Boston versed in electrocardiography. He was appointed to be a house physician to the Medical Service, a position first created in 1913 and later, in 1922, renamed resident. The house physicians were between the attending staff and the regular house officers in age and experience, would provide advice and instruction to the house officers and students, and would also assist with very sick patients in the hospital as well as with outpatients. Dr. Walter W. Palmer, who was the first one appointed, held the post from 1913–1915, and Paul White, who was the next to be selected, served in that capacity from 1914–1917. Palmer went on to be appointed Director of the Medical Service at the Presbyterian Hospital in New York in 1921 as well as Bard Professor of Medicine at the College of Physicians and Surgeons of Columbia.

Soon after Paul White's return, Drs. Edsall and Cabot sent a notice to the MGH staff that "In view of Dr. Paul D. White's recent work with Thomas Lewis on electrocardiography, we thought it would be best to ask Dr. White to enlighten the depths of our ignorance on that subject and he will talk to us in the House Physicians' room at the Hospital on Wednesday, September 30 at 12:00." He was also asked to demonstrate the new equipment on Ether Day at the MGH in October—a demonstration which was possible because of the good fortune of the safe arrival of the apparatus after a voyage across the Atlantic under newly hazardous war-time conditions. Space, as always, had proved to be in short supply at the MGH; so the equipment had to be given an undignified home in the basement, under the Skin Ward and next to the bathroom used by the patients who had syphilis.

Thanks to ample case material on the wards and in the clinic, Paul White began putting together articles for publication and was able to write his brother Warren on July 29, 1915 that six were in preparation and another one had already been published. "The field I'm in is fertile," he wrote, "for some of the ground has as yet hardly been touched. Never can I regret having gone into it. The clinical side alone is inexhaustible. . . ." Referring to abnormalities of pulse and heart rhythm he had found in his patients, he commented that he had already seen 99 cases of alternation and 101 cases of auricular fibrillation—more of the former than anyone on record except Mackenzie. His name came to be known outside of the Boston area, and during the summer of 1915, he was asked to give lectures in Virginia and Kentucky, events which were followed by other similar invitations. In the spring of 1916, he was authorized to establish for the first time a Cardiac Clinic in a basement room of the Bulfinch Building of the Hospital on Saturday mornings in order to promote more effective investigation and treatment of cardiac cases. He also received a Harvard appointment as a Teaching Fellow in medicine. He began to receive letters from practitioners from around the country who wished to come to Boston to study under him, requests which were to continue and grow over the next 35 years. Thus was set in place a solid base of clinical opportunities and experience, clinical research and reports, and professional education, all under the auspices of a great hospital and medical school. The ingredients for a successful career as a heart specialist were at hand. Lacking, but in prospect, would be financial security from a private practice or, less likely at that time, from a small academic salary.

Becoming a heart specialist (cardiologist) was actually a novelty in 1916. There had always been eminent physicians who, through their practice, investigations and writings, had become recognized as more knowledgeable than the great mass of doctors in matters pertaining to the heart. Such a one early in the 20th century was Professor Karel Frederik Wenckebach, chief of the first medical clinic in Vienna, and another was Sir William Osler, Regius Professor of Medicine at Oxford; yet another was Paul White's former teacher Sir James Mackenzie of Burnley and London. However, partly because the traditional basis of teaching had emphasized the wisdom of a broad knowledge of human illnesses, partly because the fund of knowledge about heart disease and its treatment was scant, and partly because few physicians could expect to earn a living from a practice restricted to heart patients, such doctors preferred not to be known as heart specialists. They set a standard for the others. Physicians even in the larger cities liked to consider themselves qualified to handle essentially all medical problems that were not obstetrical or surgical; and with considerable justification, they viewed specialization as unduly limiting the scope of their understanding of human disease. Dr. James B. Herrick of Chicago, one of the early giants in the field, stoutly resisted the label of heart specialist ("this term against which I long fought"), desiring only to be known as an internist, one whose practice is limited to internal medicine of which heart disease was a part. Moreover, in 1916, heart disease was not the number one cause of death as it was to become in the middle of the century. For example, in New York City in that year, there were 53,108 deaths recorded of which 31,660 were attributed to infections and nephritis, a third as many (10,687) to heart ailments, 5,060 to violence, and 4,701 to cancer. It was not surprising that organized certification of professional competence in cardiology actually did not take place until 1941.

Paul White could have returned to the MGH to become a top internist but with a special interest and qualification in heart problems including electrocardiography. However, he deliberately chose to proceed down the new path of specialization, limiting his professional work to diseases of the heart, and was the first in Boston and one of the first in the United States to do so. He wrote how Dr. Richard C. Cabot, who was a leader in medicine at the MGH and the Harvard Medical School advised him strongly against specialization in heart disease. This was all the more significant since Cabot was very experienced and was to publish in 1926 a 781-page book entitled *Facts on The Heart*.

That Paul White's favorable start in becoming a specialist in the problems of heart disease was interrupted was due to the existence of the Great War in Europe and the Middle East combined with his readiness once again to "hit the trail," as he had written in 1914. He had obtained a commission as first lieutenant in the Medical Reserve Corps of the U.S. Army early in 1916, and shortly thereafter, he with 21 others became members of an MGH-based hospital unit which was on a stand-by basis. Meanwhile the British forces were being hard-pressed in the war, and United States physicians and surgeons were sought to volunteer for tours of duty in British military hospitals in Great Britain or on the continent. Paul White chose to be such a volunteer and was notified on July 25, 1916 that his application to serve with a Harvard-sponsored unit for six months had been accepted and he would sail from New York on August 17. Elements in his decision to serve may have included his fondness for new experiences, the general war fervor, and a particular sympathy for the British cause as a result of his year in England. The venture clearly was not an unusual opportunity to learn more about heart disease. Items of personal equipment recommended for the expedition included six negligee shirts, twelve collars, one steamer rug, one woolen wrapper, and one pair of bedroom slippers, all suggesting a proper Bostonian's idea of wartime needs. Pay would range from $3.00 to $5.00 a day.

The next phase in the 1911–1919 interval thus started when the Harvard unit departed from New York two days late on the blacked-out *S.S. Lapland* with a group of 11 doctors, mostly from the MGH, plus 15 nurses. They docked in Liverpool eight days later and entrained to London. While there, Paul White went out to Hampstead Heath to the Hampstead Military Hospital, a research hospital for the study of certain heart cases believed to result from military service. The condition had been given various labels including that of "soldier's heart," and the investigation was under the direction of Paul White's old London teachers headed by Lewis and Mackenzie assisted by some of his former fellow students, including Meakins. Later, Paul White himself became intensely interested in this problem which was characterized by chest pains, shortness of breath, sighing respirations and fatigue but without any clear evidence of structural heart damage.

On September 3 while still in London, Paul White's diary noted that there was the greatest excitement with "a sight never to be forgotten." He and his hotel roommate, Dr. George Denny, were awakened at 2:08 a.m. (PDW typically gave the time precisely) by an uproar outside the window, and they watched a large zeppelin float overhead outlined by search lights with shells bursting near it in the sky. It disappeared toward the north, but at 2:25 a.m. "a sudden brilliant flare appeared in the sky to the North, died down after a few seconds and then increased rapidly to an incredible brilliancy. In a few seconds more, only a dim glow remained in the sky and in a minute from the beginning of the flare, it was all over. The zeppelin was dead. People leaned out of the windows, stood on the Strand and in the Court Yard and clapped and cheered for a long time." This was the first dirigible ever to be a war-time casualty, having been shot down by a British airplane.

A week later they were in France at the British expeditionary force's General Hospital No. 22 in Camiers, six miles south of Boulogne and only two miles from the Channel, where they remained for three months. Paul White was made medical officer of a 48-bed medical ward and was also named Sanitary Officer. His first admissions included two cases of shell shock, one acute nephritis, one epilepsy, one bronchitis, one tuberculosis, one myalgia, and two fevers of unknown origin. Heart cases were to be scarce indeed. The load of work was very uneven and in the afternoons, he was often able to take seven- to ten-mile walks or bicycle rides of up to 40 miles. After only three months of active hospital duty, he and George Denny travelled to Paris where they heard "Aphrodite" at the Opera Comique, found the Louvre was almost closed, and attended the Folies Bergeres. They crossed the Channel and sailed from Liverpool for home on December 15. Thus ended a relatively brief contribution to the British wartime medical needs, in truth a limited contribution but one which also signalled a very personal support for the Allied cause by these as yet officially neutral Americans.

He returned to a United States more and more distracted by the events in Europe to resume his role at the MGH, but only for a brief period. On April 2, 1917, President Wilson appeared before Congress and requested that a State of War be declared to exist between the United States and the German government, a request promptly approved by the House of Representatives and the Senate. Almost a month later, on May 1, Paul White spoke on "The Electrocardiogram in Cardiac Hypertrophy" at the Hotel Traymore in Atlantic City before a meeting of the American Society of Clinical Investigation. And on May 24, he found himself on temporary active military duty examining personnel applying for enlistment in the MGH Base Hospital No. 6. He was indeed the first member of the unit to go on full active service on July 2, 1917. The hospital was headed by Major Frederic A. Washburn, the Director of the MGH, with Dr. Richard C. Cabot as Chief of the Medical Service and Dr. Lincoln Davis as Chief of the Surgical Service. The initial complement was to consist of 28 officers, 64 nurses, 153 enlisted men, one chaplain, one dietitian, and six secretaries. Several of the group were to go on after the war to very distinguished careers including W. Jason Mixter, who became an important neurosurgeon at the MGH; Frederick C. Irving, later professor of obstetrics at the Harvard Medical School; James Howard Means, who would become chief of medicine at the MGH; Carl A. L. Binger, who became prominent in psychiatry and psychosomatic medicine at the New York Hospital and at Cornell Medical School; Joseph C. Aub, subsequently a noted investigator and physician-in-chief of the Collis P. Huntington Memorial Hospital; and the chaplain, Henry Knox

Sherrill, destined to be Presiding Bishop of the Episcopal Church and President of the National Council of Churches of Christ of America.

It was early in the summer of 1917 shortly prior to going overseas that Paul White received an unusual letter from his father, combining praise and criticism, joy and sadness, clearly composed with great care and thoughtfulness:

Dear Paul,

Just a steamer letter to say to you a few things quietly and privately that couldn't find time & place very well else. One is, though I'm very sorry to have you go again into the work in France to do routine and drudgery which seems as tho *any* body could do, yet I'm proud to feel that there is no shirking and if that was all you can do at first, your special work may wait as many another's special work has to wait. . . . Be reasonably careful *do:* eat regularly and sleep more than Warren does if you want to have any reserve strength for experiences.

It takes one of the White family as a rule half a lifetime to get into his own physically . . . you need two or three years more to be at your best I believe.

Now one other thing I do worry about is your apparent *neglect* of *spiritual* things. I suppose it may be disagreeable to be reminded that no part of your nature can be ignored or disregarded without a real loss to the whole man. No man living can *afford* to go without worship as you have & not kill every spark of Christian *fellowship* with His Heavenly Father. No work in this world is so important that it can safely be allowed to *displace* Him in any way without a real insult to His tender love for you. I can not understand you in all this and it really grieves me more than I can express! Are you truly honest about this? However much your particular views of God and Christ & His Church may have changed I can not view your *indifference* without real alarm for your future! I fear you do not regularly pray unless you should see threatening disaster and I wonder if you would then. In no sanctimonious fashion do I write this, for *I know* if you think you are superior to these eternal beings you have made the *gravest mistake of your life!!* We do not outgrow the old Bible or religious efforts and desires unless we're *blind* spiritually or have departed from Christian ways and have become ashamed.

All this is such a sweetness & joy to my own life & I love you and am so proud of your intellectual attainments that I can not abide your living on so indifferent spiritually! You have my constant prayers & anxious solicitude for I know you are missing *the big thing* in this life afterall & in spite of other successes. For my sake give these things a little more time in your life & all life will be so *much sweeter & happier!* Faithfully lovingly,
Your Pater.

This moving appeal does not seem to have persuaded Paul White to return to a greater involvement in religion. Yet, the exemplary lives of his parents, their deep concern for his spiritual well-being, and his intense early exposure to Christian teaching and morality clearly influenced his behavior throughout a life which was to be a credit to his Baptist inheritance even though he largely separated himself from the orthodox church. Four months later while overseas, he was to copy in his diary a quotation from the wartime writings of H. G. Wells. He noted that the quotation represented his own faith as well as that of Wells who had written:

> In the last few years I have developed a religious belief that has become now to me as real as any commonplace effect. I think that mankind is still, as it were, collectively dreaming and hardly more awakened to reality than a very young child. It has these dreams that we express by the flags of nationalities, by strange loyalties, and by irrational creeds and ceremonies, and its dreams at times become such nightmares as this war. But the time draws near when mankind will awake and the dreams will fade away and then there will be no nationality in all the world but humanity, and no king, no emperor nor leader but the one God of mankind. This is my faith.

Base Hospital No. 6, which was a part of the first U.S. expeditionary force of 25,000 men, arrived in Bordeaux on July 28, 1917 via Liverpool, Southampton and Le Havre. Typically, one of Paul White's first purchases on arriving in France was a French bicycle, which was promptly put to good use as he rode about the countryside while waiting to begin medical duties. On August 17, the group was settled in a former school located in the village of Talence just south of Bordeaux which had been serving as a 1000-bed French military hospital. Thus began yet another and sixth phase of the 1911–1919 period. After several brief assignments, Paul White was placed in charge of all medical supplies and the pharmacy, a dull administrative role which he was to fill for four months, when he hungrily began to take over ward medical officer duties. The early admissions to the hospital were largely soldiers with infections. There was much severe pneumonia in December 1917 and January 1918 which was especially prevalent among the black troops from the south in whom the mortality was as high as fifty percent. In February he was at last placed in charge of a heart ward which included patients with rheumatic fever, but these cases were to be only a part of his area of responsibility. Begin-

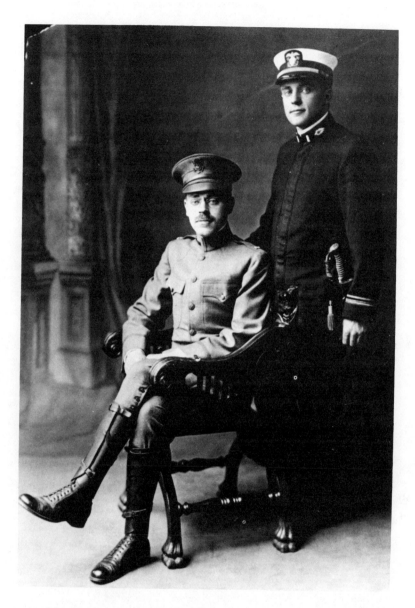

Dr. Paul Dudley White, seated, and brother, Dr. J. Warren White, standing, in uniform at the end of World War I.

ning in the spring of 1918, gas casualties started to be admitted in numbers, and he was appointed chairman of a committee to study the problem
and undertake lung-function testing. A constant and heavy stream of
wounded and gassed soldiers flowed in during the summer and fall of
1918 as the American forces went into action, and by the time of the
armistice, the original 1000-bed hospital had grown to nearly 4500 beds.
Paul White, whose initial obligations had been very modest, shared in
handling this tremendous load and in October, he was responsible for
wards holding nearly 500 patients. Thereafter, with the welcome coming
of peace, the hospital census shrank rapidly and the medical staff became
relatively idle again. The Base Hospital was finally closed on January 14,
1919. It had been frustrating for him to remain attached to the same unit
throughout this whole period as most of his colleagues in the original
MGH group were transferred out to other, more interesting or at least
different assignments as the war proceeded.

The 17-month period was not all just army hospital routine. He made
trips to Paris in November and again in June, the latter at a time when
the city was being shelled. He also while on a brief leave in March had
an exhilarating trip along the French Riviera with Chaplain Henry K.
Sherrill and his medical colleague, Henry Marble. When the wife of the
American consul appeared at the hospital on May 21 about to deliver a
baby, "an extraordinary thing happened" as he wrote in his diary. No
obstetrician was available, the surgeons "refused to conduct the party,"
and Paul White accomplished a successful delivery of a 7½-pound baby
boy of which he later became godfather. This was the first delivery he
had done since 1911 in medical school. At the end of November, he also
had a fortnight of travel about France, visiting what had been the front
battle lines east of Paris including the Moselle Valley.

That the many months of conscientious ward work, often unexciting,
very little of which was cardiological, were appreciated by some was indicated by an item which appeared in the December 24, 1920 issue of the
Boston Globe in a letter to the editor. If Paul White's father read it, he
should have been pleased. Corporal Calvin Davis of Rochester, New

Hampshire, responding to complaints about the way some of the soldiers had been treated in the military hospitals wrote to the newspaper:

> . . . I am an over-seas fellow and was a patient in base hospital no. 6 composed of the unit from Mass. Gen. Hosp. in Boston. Now, let me tell you, there was no lack of care, and tender care at that, in that large ark of a hospital. It was a splendid bunch who took care of us fellows, and one especially, a Capt. Paul White of the staff, was a regular pal to us sick ones, and he never was too tired or rushed for a friendly word or a change of dressing, which counts so much when you are trussed up like a fowl. He was a prince and a fine doctor, and right on his job and gentle; say, his hands never made you wince or yell out. . . .

With peace at hand, it would have been expected for him to have left the U.S. Army as soon as he could escape, to return to his family, his home, his hospital and medical school colleagues, and his professional work. He had completed what he and so many others had been required to do and more, for not only was he the first to be called up in his unit, but he had also gone out of his way to volunteer several months of his time in 1916 for the British Expeditionary Force. He would have seemed to have more than adequately served his nation, the allied cause, and suffering mankind. But he was not to see Boston for another half-year. Once more, he would "hit the trail."

Early in January 1919, Paul White had a conversation one evening with Francis W. Peabody, a major in the Army medical corps, who had been a fellow member of the Harvard Medical School faculty and was a rising star at the Peter Bent Brigham Hospital. In two years he would be appointed Director of the new Thorndike Memorial Laboratory at the Boston City Hospital. Peabody told Paul White that the Red Cross was making up medical missions to undertake relief work in the Balkans where there were serious health problems due to the breakdown of civil administration and public health in the aftermath of the war. Peabody himself was not to be actively involved, as he was on his way back to Boston to resume his teaching. Immediately, Paul White was attracted—"It would interest me considerably to join such a mission in any capacity, preferably medical." Thereafter, negotiations between Paul White and the Red Cross proceeded rapidly. On January 31, 1919, he was demobilized from the army at St. Aignan; and on February 3, 1919 in Paris, he signed a five-month contract with the American Red Cross as head of a unit of five medical officers to work in Eastern Macedonia. Going with him would be four of his army medical colleagues, Drs. Robert H. Crawford, John S. Hodgson, Dewitt S. Clark, and Carl A. L. Binger. After the usual administrative and travel delays, he arrived in Athens with most of his group on February 28, having had his ferryboat trip from the tip of Italy across the Ionian Sea to Greece in the company of numerous rats and fleas. This was the prophetic introduction to the final phase of the 1911–1919 period.

What did Paul White contribute and get from this Balkan experience which lasted from February until the end of July 1919? His contribution was essentially one in public health, at first in Northern Greece in Carvalla and Drama. A major epidemic of typhus was already waning there when the team arrived, but Paul White and his colleagues had to make daily inspections to identify typhus cases, see that the family of a case was deloused, have the house fumigated, and review the delousing centers. Further, they had to make sure that all citizens in the area received a delousing every week, regardless of whether or not there were any cases in the family. During the course of their work, one member of their team, John Hodgson, contracted typhus but fortunately made a good recovery. After several months of this activity, the epidemic had ended and Paul White spent yet another four weeks inspecting hospitals in Thessaly and the Peloponnesus.

What he got from this mission to Greece aside from being awarded the Greek Silver Cross Order of the Redeemer were very mixed impressions. He learned first-hand about typhus and typhus epidemics and helped in their control, he saw how catastrophic wartime and post-wartime conditions can be on civilian health, and he learned about Greek military and civilian hospitals. Much of the mountainous and coastal scenery was magnificent, and since he visited both northern and southern Greece stopping at many small towns, he witnessed a range of local architecture, customs, food, and cultural traits. He also saw in 1919 Greece a veritable melting pot of ethnic groups. In Salonica, on the way to Carvalla, there were civilians and soldiers from France, England, Australia, Canada, Italy, Serbia, Albania, Turkey, Austria, Bulgaria and Indonesia. On the road to Drama, he passed Greek cavalry, teams of oxen, caravans of camels and horses carrying bales of tobacco, and Macedonian peasants riding on mules or walking. In addition, during the month of July before returning to Paris, he left Greece and visited Constantinople as well as Constanza, Galatz, and Bucharest in Rumania. There was much that was strange and new and colorful to impress one as well as much that was dirty and squalid.

Another and very different impression involved the incompetence found in the Red Cross staff and administration. Whereas Paul White had praise for many of the Greek military and medical leaders with whom he worked, he was very disillusioned by what he witnessed in the echelons of the Red Cross. He soon found that the American leadership of the Greek Red Cross commission was absurdly inefficient and at swords' points with other Red Cross commissions. It was discouraging when the New York lawyer, who had been placed in charge of the operations in Macedonia and who was one of the few cooperative and able Red Cross administrators, resigned in disgust. On April 14, 1919, Paul White wrote regarding the Red Cross staff: "Most of them are nice enough fellows but are doing work that trained businessmen should handle. As in the army, there is a great misapplication of personnel and much of the American money is being squandered in the process of doing some good. I suppose in the end it is worthwhile, but one hates to see so much waste of time and money. Our own present work in this grand international joy ride is open to the same criticism, but we are helpless under the present administrative regime." Toward the end of his tour when he had been ordered to distribute hospital supplies, he looked forward to the time when "I can start homewards to some more worthwhile work than this sketchy Red Cross distribution—often to places that don't need or want the stuff. It's a pity there hasn't been a better administration to manage things—especially in Athens. There have been too many unintelligent amateurs in the game disposing of millions of dollars of good American money."

Finally, his tour of duty was completed. After visits to Turkey and Rumania, he took the Simplon Express from Bucharest to Paris, arriving there on July 29, 1919. He reported to the Red Cross Headquarters for passage home and once more was exposed to the pitiful muddle obvious there and declined offers of other assignments. He sailed from Brest on August 7 on the *New Amsterdam* and was back in Boston on August 19, more than two years after he had departed.

CHAPTER THREE

Getting in Stride

"My advice to medical students contemplating a career is to select some field for concentration of endeavor after they have finished an internship and possibly another year of laboratory or clinical experience. It does not matter in the least which field is the choice. I believe that in our profession every field of activity is of great interest, and a certain amount of time spent in any one quickly results in absorption in that work that has been chosen. For the greatest accomplishment there should not be too much dispersion of interests or changing from one to another. It is the perpetual digging away at one thing that makes a man master in the field he selects. Years of hard work are necessary and it is the willingness to stick at such work that counts much more than any amount of so-called brilliance or political pull."

Such was Paul White's advice to aspirants to a career in medicine, written in 1925 to Dr. Cecil K. Drinker who had requested a brief account of his professional life. It was a clear statement of his views as he settled into medicine and reflected exactly his own career. Because he enjoyed what he was doing and because he was successful, he urged others to emulate him—and many did. The age of specialization was at hand.

Also in the letter was a summary of his post-war activities:

After returning to America in 1919, I spent an additional year as West Medical Research Resident at the Massachusetts General Hospital.

In 1920 I began outside residence, continuing to spend, however, the bulk of my time in cardiovascular research. This I have carried on in the five years that have elapsed since 1920. During the same interval I have been practicing medicine, most of my patients being sent to me in consultation in order to study the condition of their hearts. I have seen nearly all of them at my office and laboratory at the Massachusetts General Hospital. At the present time my chief interests are two, first, clinical research, and second, the practice of medicine. A small portion of my time I devote to teaching and administrative work of one kind or another, but neither of these last mentioned fields attracts me as do the other activities which I place first. I admit, however, that I have gained a great deal of benefit in the past from my teaching, both of undergraduates and graduates in the Harvard Medical School, and a little of this I desire to continue always. Also I have enjoyed experiencing various positions such as Secretary and Chairman of the Section of Pharmacology and Therapeutics of the American Medical Association. . . .

Each year I have had a small group of medical men, mostly recent graduates, who have been associated with me in my clinical research and this association has been stimulating and delightful.

Here was Paul White's ranking of the priorities in his world of 1925— first came his research which unlike that of Thomas Lewis was closely related to patients and was therefore clinical and not basic in nature, and second came the practice which was a prerequisite for the first. Finally, and seemingly a low third, came teaching and various administrative and medical society roles. Later, as his experience in training young men and women from Harvard and from all over the world broadened, he came to value increasingly his teaching role and to give to it a significant portion of his time. All of this was wrapped up with the admonitions that one must specialize and must work hard.

That the clinical research was active and was foremost in absorbing Paul White's energy and interest was obvious from his output of scientific articles. In the seven-year interval 1913–1920, he was author or co-author of 26 publications, which was surprising in view of the interruptions imposed by World War I. During the seven-year period 1920–1927, the number had risen to 80 and these were not abstracts but full papers. Further, they were not, as was commonly the case with others, multiple slightly different elaborations of the same limited scientific theme; on the contrary they covered a wide range of different cardiological subjects.

The clinical research and practice were of course both dependent on his position at the Massachusetts General Hospital. Whereas a medical school appointment was essential for becoming a staff member of the Hospital, and being a faculty member at Harvard added a certain lustre to Paul White's name and gave him access to students, it was the Hospital and not the School which was functionally the important element.

The MGH had long been distinguished by its age—old for the United States, by the frequent reminder that it was at the MGH that there had been a notable premier public demonstration of the use of ether as an anesthetic agent in 1846, by the calibre of its staff and its scientific publications, and by its affiliation with the Harvard Medical School. Entering into the twentieth century blessed with the vision of leaders like Edsall whose horizons were not constricted by Bostonian smugness, it not only maintained but enhanced its reputation for excellence. It was to be through the strong personalities and the scientific achievements of men like James H. Means, Chester M. Jones, Fuller Albright, Walter Bauer, Stanley Cobb, Joe Vincent Meigs, and Edward D. Churchill, that this was accomplished. Paul White was destined to be a member of this elite group and to make his own important contributions, but he first had to get his foot well over the door sill.

That he was welcomed back to the hospital with warmth when he returned in 1919 was not surprising. On September 19, 1919, he was once again, by action of the trustees, appointed a House Physician (i.e., resident) at the munificent salary of $500 a year, and he was informed that a new obligation would be to answer emergency calls and supervise the laboratory work at the Phillips House, the new private patient pavilion which had been opened in 1917. A special consideration granted by Dr. Edsall and by the trustees of the Hospital was "the privilege of seeing two private patients daily at the Massachusetts General Hospital. It is understood that Dr. Edsall will furnish you the use of his suite for this purpose." Paul White resumed responsibility for the electrocardiograph laboratory in the basement which was becoming increasingly busy with more than 1400 electrocardiograms being taken in 1921.

Soon he was seeing private patients downstairs in the spartan office and basement laboratory of the Bulfinch Building rather than in Dr. Edsall's office. Mrs. Natalie Kreisle, who saw him as a patient there in 1924 when she was seven years old, recalls the very simple waiting room with its small cellar windows and straight chairs. The electrocardiogram was taken with the patient seated in a closet holding a wet sea sponge soaked in salt solution in each hand and with the left foot placed on a third sponge from which went wires to the large electrocardiograph machine. There was also a fluoroscope to permit Paul White to view and measure the heart by x-ray using an orthodiagraph, which gave a rough estimate of heart shape and size. His office in which he examined patients had a bookcase in which were bottles containing hearts showing various abnormalities which somehow and remarkably did not seem ghoulish to her or other patients, doubtless because he would take the time to explain them to his patients so that they acquired some of his own enthusiasm and fascination for what they saw. In 1925 the office and laboratory were moved up to the ground floor of the building to more adequate and convenient, but still exceedingly simple quarters which had housed the apothecary shop. He was to have his headquarters there for the next quarter century. It is said that the change was stimulated by the untimely death of one of his prominent patients who succumbed while traversing the long walk from the front door of the hospital along the corridors and then downstairs to the far corner of the basement.

Perhaps the first notable private patient seen by Paul White was John C. Coolidge, age 80 years, of Plymouth, Vermont, who came to the office at the MGH on May 1, 1925 at the request of his son, President Calvin Coolidge. Dr. James M. Faulkner described him as "a tall, weather beaten, old man with rugged features grasping a straw suitcase in one huge hand." Mr. Coolidge was clearly uncomfortable at being so far from home, refused to let the accompanying secret servicemen carry his suitcase for him, and when the visit with Paul White had been concluded, seemed reluctant to leave. It turned out that he had brought with him a urine specimen in a Horlick's Malted Milk bottle—which had been entrusted to Dr. Howard Sprague to analyze—and he would not return home until Dr. Sprague had returned the bottle to him.

His position as House Officer had ended in 1920 when Paul White was appointed to the new position of Chief of the Medical Out-Patient Department, a post he was to hold for five years. If ever there was a position in which insoluble problems abounded, this was it. The OPD, as it was called, received a constant stream of new and old patients, mainly with marginal or no incomes, who would arrive early in the morning and wait for long hours seated on hard benches until seen by a young doctor in training or perhaps by a senior attending physician with or without students. The chronic difficulty was that the supply of patients was almost unlimited whereas the reservoir of doctors, while on paper reasonably adequate, in fact was never enough. Both the senior and junior physicians tended to give priority to other demands and particularly to the sick patients in the hospital beds, begrudgingly giving whatever time was left over to the clinic.

Paul White took the clinic job seriously. He went around the country visiting similar clinics in New York, Baltimore, Chicago, Rochester (Minnesota), Minneapolis, St. Louis and Cleveland. A committee was appointed, of which he was chairman, to query the staff and make recommendations for change. The usual drearily repetitious staff comment was "we need about half as many as patients and twice as many visiting men." Finally in 1922, measures to limit the number of new cases and provide better medical staff service were adopted. These met with general approval but it appears that any improvements achieved were quickly eroded, both because the pressure for care from numerous ailing, indigent patients continued and because the habits of the attending and house staff doctors proved quite permanent.

Meanwhile, clinics only for heart cases were well established, but that also meant that they too demanded a great deal of time. Paul White had begun a cardiac outpatient clinic in 1916, based on a cardiac class for children and adults which had been started by Drs. Richard Eustis and Joseph H. Pratt in 1913. A separate cardiac clinic for children, chiefly those having or having had rheumatic fever, was also held, and White attended both of these as well as acting as their Director. Through his influence, he recruited physicians in practice to work in the clinics and he also arranged to have the young doctors training in cardiology under him spend time there on a regular basis. The extent of his personal commitment to these low income outpatients may be judged by his comment written in 1930 that his experience to date with the clinical observation of heart disease was based on seeing 4000 private patients and 8000 clinic patients. As the result of his hard work and in recognition of his stature as a heart specialist, Paul White was elevated in 1925 to the level of Associate Physician at the MGH and three years later in 1928 reached the top level of Physician.

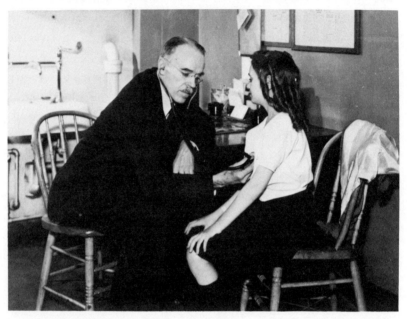

Dr. Paul White examining a patient in the old outpatient clinic of the Massachusetts General Hospital about 1930.

His climb up the academic ladder at the Harvard Medical School was nowhere near as rapid as it was at the hospital, and indeed to most outsiders, it seemed disgracefully slow. He was made an Instructor in Medicine in 1921 but it was not until 1933 that he became an Assistant Professor of Medicine. He was made a Lecturer in Medicine in 1936 and finally in 1946 was promoted to the rank of Clinical Professor of Medicine. He never did become a Professor without the descriptive term "clinical," a rank far more august than that of Clinical Professor, even though by 1946 he had been internationally recognized as a top authority in his field for at least 15 years.

The reasons for the lethargic pace of his promotions starting in 1921 would seem to be several. His research throughout was clinical, that is very much patient-related, as contrasted to basic more laboratory-oriented investigation which was more highly prized. Clinical research traditionally was given low marks by promotion committees unless it was unusually imaginative and exciting. Further, especially in those days, he would have been given minimal or no credit for his teaching and practitioner roles. Also, he disliked committee work and hence avoided it, and since this distaste was joined with quite frequent absences from Boston, he was less and less available to take his turn with hospital and medical school administrative and committee assignments. This last may have been a factor in the mind of the person who became his chief—Dr. James Howard Means, who had been his colleague from medical school, house staff, European travel and wartime days. It was indeed the duty of Means more than anyone else to recommend and push his promotion at the Harvard Medical School if he felt it to be deserved and it appears that he was not in a hurry to do so. However, Paul White did very well for many years without the professorial title and there is no evidence that he craved it or exerted pressure to obtain it any earlier. He was not a political person. It was, in a sense, amusing that he at last became Clinical Professor at the Medical School in 1946 just before he received an honorary degree in Prague from Charles University; and then only four years later in 1950 Harvard University gave him its highest recognition of all, an honorary Doctor of Science degree. At that time, Means wrote him a generous letter which included "This is a very distinguished tribute to you, and extraordinarily well deserved. It is also an honor to the MGH of which you are one of the most distinguished sons."

By the spring of 1922 Paul White was ready for a good vacation and glad to have a change from what was rapidly becoming a very busy professional life with clinic and private patients, supervision of the out-patient program in medicine, writing and lecturing. On May 19, 1922 he paid the Boston Buick Company $995 for a new automobile. However, his vacation plans did not involve use of the car as a month later he and Dr. Joseph C. Aub left for Europe on the *Empress of France*. Joseph Aub had been an intern at the MGH in 1915, became a House Physician the following year, and like Paul White was unmarried and ready for a respite from hospital duties. The two were very good friends then and remained so for the rest of their lives. Their voyage on the *Empress of France* was uneventful except for one incident which subsequently received a full exposure in "Our Hearts Were Young and Gay" by Cornelia Otis Skinner and Emily Kimbrough published in 1942, as well as in a condensed version which appeared later in the *Reader's Digest*.

Emily Kimbrough and Cornelia Otis Skinner, the latter the daughter of the famous actor Otis Skinner, were also on that boat and the former recalled the episode very clearly in conversation in 1983:

> Cornelia Skinner and I had set out for Europe, and with considerable difficulty we persuaded our parents to let us go alone. They were to meet us at Southampton. That was as much independence as we were allowed. . . . We took the Empress of France and shortly after leaving Quebec we were invited to have tea with the Captain, and Paul and Joe Aub were there. That's when we met them. They were older than we—enough to make them terribly interesting to us. We felt very grown up and awfully sophisticated and they were sort of men of the world. We had a very, very good time on the ship. Then just before we were to dock at Southampton, Cornelia became mysteriously ill. She had a wretched sore throat and felt quite awful.
>
> Something prompted me *not* to report to the ship's doctor. I don't know why but I thought about our two friends so I asked Paul and Joe if they would come and take a look at Cornelia. She was frightfully embarrassed about it. At any rate, they came in and they looked her over and then they asked me to come out into the corridor with them. When I got out there, Paul said "There's no question about it, she's got measles!"
>
> Measles! Good heavens, what to do? Because I knew right away that anything that was contagious should be reported. I also felt that we would be quarantined. There were Mr. and Mrs. Skinner waiting for us in Southampton and the ship was going on to dock in Bremen and we would be incarcerated and not released until we reached Bremen. It was not to be thought of! The situation was hideous. Joe had some definite commitments. He was going to Paris and he could not leave the ship at Southampton. Paul said: "I am taking a terrible risk. If I should take responsibility for this, and only because Mr. and Mrs. Skinner are going to be there at Southampton, I could leave the ship with both of you and with Mr. and Mrs. Skinner and I could stay for perhaps 24 hours to make sure how she is and I would not report this to the ship's doctor. I want you to understand that I've got to work this out myself because I'm

really violating everything that is practically sacred to a physician. I could be jeopardizing my whole career."

By this time we had told Cornelia. It frightened both of us that between us we were going to be the ruin of him and his life would be ended. However, he wrestled with himself, and he decided that he would make the sacrifice. So he did not report it to the ship's doctor and when we docked, we got Cornelia up on her feet, and with the true sense of the theater, she had applied makeup and was overlaid with a white kind of enamel to cover the spots which had come out as Paul predicted they would and had come out profusely. She was really one of the most macabre looking sights. She was terribly ill by that time and running a very high temperature.

We sat her down in a chair in the lounge telling her not to move while we went through all the passport business, etc. While she was there we learned afterwards, a little child came over and stood staring at her with a solemnity that only a child has and finally asked in a tone of awe "Do you tell fortunes?" Mr. and Mrs. Skinner were waiting on the dock and I leaned over the rail and waved and then they waved back and called "Where is Cornelia?" "Oh she's coming, she's here," I said. As soon as I could, I went down the gangplank and I said: "You must not say a word, be absolutely quiet, Cornelia has measles." Mr. Otis Skinner in that voice which had reached the back row of the top gallery echoed, "MEASLES!" It reverberated throughout Southampton. Well we silenced him and no one was the wiser, but the ship's doctor was very suspicious. He suddenly turned up at the hotel and sent up his card and asked to call. He hoped that the young ladies had docked satisfactorily and felt no ill effects from the voyage. They assured him that no, no, we were fine, splendid and told him we'd gone off on an excursion of some sort. The wretched man left and from then on all was clear sailing. Paul moved on within the next 24–36 hours.

The European jaunt was essentially a pleasure trip including visits to London, the Rhineland, Munich, Oberammergau (where Paul White and Joe Aub saw the Passion Play), Vienna, Northern Italy, France including a visit to the buildings used in 1917–19 by Base Hospital No.6, and Berlin. This phase ended with a 2¼ hour flight in a DeHaviland airplane across the English Channel from Brussels to England. Paul White had a brief reunion with Sir Thomas Lewis in London, and with the Mackenzies in St. Andrews in Scotland, where he also bought a set of golf clubs. He finally embarked from England on August 12, 1922 after eight weeks of very pleasant sight-seeing and essentially no medical work. This was to be his last major vacation without a wife.

In the summer of 1923, Paul White journeyed to Northampton, Massachusetts to talk about heart disease at Smith College before a class of future social workers. One of the students listening to him was Ina Helen Reid who had been born and brought up in West Roxbury, five miles from the Herbert Warren White family. Ina Reid was the daughter of Winfield Scott Reid, a Boston businessman who had come from Nova Scotia, and Hannah Alexander, who had been born in Eastport, Maine. Ina Reid had been educated at Miss Hewin's School in West Roxbury, then attended the Girls' Latin School, and entered Smith College from which she graduated in 1923. She had the goal of entering social work and so started after graduation at the Smith College Training School for Social Work. She was impressed by Paul White's lecture and met him briefly at that time.

The following winter of 1924 when she was required to have a session of practical work, she was assigned to the MGH and was given the topic of chorea (also known as St. Vitus' dance), which was a manifestation of rheumatic fever. This was a time in which Paul White and two of his young trainees, James M. Faulkner and Harold Segall, were engaged in a study of rheumatic fever in families which involved making a large number of home visits. Indeed over 1000 people were actually examined and it was natural that Ina Reid, with her interest in social work, fitted into the project very neatly. Harold Segall had hoped that this very attractive young lady would be working with him but it soon became apparent that she was spending most of her time with Paul White who clearly outranked him. That White got to know her only after the first of the year is clear from his daily reminder cards which referred for the first time on January 7 and January 8, 1924 to the Smith student as "Miss Reed." The end results were very happy and were two: first, a scientific paper by Faulkner and White on "The Incidence of Rheumatic Fever, Chorea and Rheumatic Heart Disease With Especial Reference to the Occurrence in Families" which was presented at a meeting of the American Medical Association in June 1924 and subsequently published in the *Journal of the American Medical Association;* and second the engagement of Paul White and his social work trainee who thereby forfeited her prospects of a career. They were married June 28, 1924 by the Rev. Henry K. Sherrill, Paul Dudley White being 38 years of age and Ina Helen Reid being 22. They departed for a European vacation which Ina White recalls as being somewhat less than idyllic due to seasickness on the way over and "terrible hay fever and Paul was always taking pictures in hay fields; and no matter where we were, my eyes were streaming all the time. Poor Paul didn't have a very good introduction to me. . . ."

Paul White had waited a long time to choose a wife and when he did make his choice, he certainly chose with consummate skill and taste. Ina White was to charm all who knew her by her personal loveliness, her warmth of manner and genuine interest in people, her willingness to adapt graciously to many varied situations, and her high intelligence. As Paul White had written when his mother had died, being the wife of a physician is not easy. This was to be true in his own marriage. Being Mrs. Paul White provided a loving partnership in what was to be an extraordinarily interesting, active, successful and varied life. But because of her husband's enormous energy and life style which included long hours and long days and much reading and study and a great amount of travel, she was to find that his career consumed most of his time. Not well organized like her husband and not surprisingly lacking his extraordinary energy, she yet had a very busy productive life with him and on her own, with a broad range of interests. For many years she was active at the MGH as a member and at one time Chairman of the Committee for the Home Care of Children with Heart Disease. When the marriage unhappily failed to provide a family, Paul and Ina White adopted an infant girl, Penelope Dudley White in June 1936, and an infant boy, Alexander Warren White in December 1939. Here too, Paul White's obligations were such that his wife was to assume a very large responsibility for rearing the children. She was indeed a remarkable wife, a devoted mother, and a very rare person. For Paul White, there was simple truth in the Proverb "Whoso findeth a wife, findeth a good thing."

On returning from their European wedding trip, the Paul Whites had begun their married life at 110 Charles Street in Boston in an apartment consisting of a first floor and basement with a small city backyard. The location was wonderfully convenient for the hospital, the rent was low, there was a certain charm living there among the old buildings at the foot of Beacon Hill, and the cockroaches thrived. A stray cat adopted the Whites (Ina White was always very partial to animals) and moved in as a boarder despite the landlady's edict that the tenants could have no pets. In the course of time, the cat had the usual litter of kittens. One day when the landlady came to call, the mother cat acknowledged the occasion by carrying the kittens into the room one by one for admiring inspection. The landlady evidently had a warm heart for she said nothing despite this violation of the local ground-rule, and the Whites were allowed to stay. Ina White recalls that it was in this apartment that her father-in-law, Dr. H. Warren White, came for dinner one night and was rewarded at the end of the meal with an apple pie which the new bride had baked as the *pièce de résistance*. This culinary triumph was not received with the enthusiasm it seemed to deserve because Ina had no cheese to go with it—an omission which was clearly pointed out at the time by her father-in-law and which she never forgot. Subsequently, the Paul Whites lived briefly on Linnaean Street in Cambridge and then in a rented house on Hawes Street in Brookline.

The first home that they owned was a good-sized house which they built in 1933 at 300 Woodland Road in Chestnut Hill, at a cost of $40,000. The building lot was large, Paul White's mother was now a widow, and therefore a small house was also built for her on the place fronting on Laurel Road. There she settled and lived for several years before moving to an apartment nearer the city. She was not the only additional member of the family to live on that property. Paul White's older sister Miriam Faden died in 1932, and her husband was hard pressed with the problems of the Depression and with four children to support and raise. It was therefore decided that their second daughter, Dorothy, should live at 300 Woodland Road during the week and go to the nearby Beaver Country Day School. This arrangement persisted for the nine-year period 1934–1943. For several years, Paul White also helped with the educational expenses of the other children.

Yet another addition to 300 Woodland Road came later as a result of World War II and the wartime conditions in Britain. As the aerial bombing of Britain accelerated and with no immediate relief in sight, Paul White wrote to his old chief, Sir Thomas Lewis, suggesting to him and Lady Lewis that their daughter Philippa, known as "Pippa," then aged

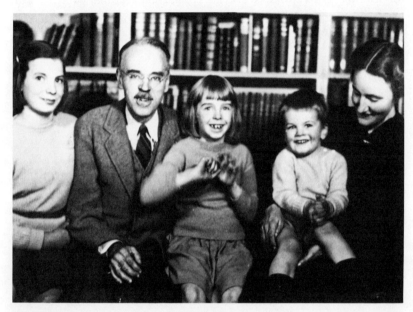

The White family in wartime, about 1942.
Left to right: Philippa Lewis, daughter of Sir Thomas and Lady Lewis; Dr. Paul White; Penelope Dudley White; Alexander Warren White; Mrs. Ina Reid White.

nine, come to the United States to live with the Paul Whites until conditions improved. The Lewises were glad to accept this invitation, and Pippa arrived and stayed for the next four years. The household was therefore a busy one, with the Whites' own two children Penny and Sandy, their niece Dorothy during the week, and Pippa. Penny was very fond of animals as was her mother (Paul White, while not a real animal lover, went along with this agreeably), so the family circle also included various dogs and cats, a pony, and later horses.

Shortly after their marriage, Paul and Ina White seeking an alternative to suburban living for the summers and week-ends also had purchased an old colonial house on Prospect Hill in the town of Harvard, located some 35 miles northwest of Boston. When this area became too popular with visitors and sightseers, they moved in 1936 to a second charming old place on Poor Farm Road also in Harvard and kept that house for the next 39 years. The family went to Harvard every summer and for brief visits at other times, and it was here that many of the gatherings of students and associates of Paul White took place. Isolated from the city and the hospital and office and in a country setting, with no telephone and for many years no electricity, it served as a refuge for Paul White from what was to become a frantic professional life.

CHAPTER FOUR

Writing and Research

Paul White had written in 1925 that he considered clinical research to be his chief interest. The number of his scientific publications and other writings rose steadily from a few in the War years to many during the 1920's and 1930's. His most significant studies were reported in this 25-year interval in which he was getting in stride professionally. Although the volume of his publications continued large after 1940, investigations reported prior to this were the ones which made the greatest impact on medical science. As is well known, medical researchers tend to be most productive of good work during the earlier years of their careers. Several of these most notable contributions by Paul White need to be cited.

Paul White had brought the exciting new electrocardiograph from England to the Massachusetts General Hospital in 1914, and it was natural that he would soon make use of it in clinical research. One early study begun in 1915 involved giving the commonly used heart drug digitalis, derived from the purple foxglove, to himself and a group of his young colleagues and following the electrocardiographic findings. As a consequence, on January 26, 1916, Paul White wrote a letter to Alfred E. Cohn* at the Hospital of the Rockefeller Institute of New York, in part as follows:

Dear Dr. Cohn, I have been studying the effect of digitalis leaf on the normal human electrocardiogram with especial reference to the P–R interval. During the past year and a half I have occasionally seen cases in the wards, usually toxic as from typhoid fever or definitely cardiac at the outset, who showed considerable prolongation of conduction time even to the stage of 2:1 and 3:2

* Alfred Cohn to whom the letter was written was a distinguished practitioner as well as investigator of cardiovascular phenomena at the Rockefeller Institute who two years earlier had published observations of the action of digitalis on patients in "an early stage of heart disease." Cohn, like White, had studied with Sir Thomas Lewis in London and he had brought the first electrocardiograph to North America.

block on small amounts of digitalis. To satisfy myself as to the effect on perfectly normal P–R intervals I fed myself and four others of the men here
digitalis leaf up to 2.0, 2.5, and 3.5 grams in a week to ten days. I took careful
records daily and have made fairly accurate measurements of the intervals in
about 75 plates, with other observations (especially on the amplitude of deflec-
tions) in about 75 more. The *T* deflection obeyed your rule of digitalis action
perfectly in all. I also tested the effect of exercise and atropine with and without
digitalis. All together the results are interesting and it seems to me worth
publishing. Do you think a paper on this work would be suitable for the Journal
of Experimental Medicine?

This was written while White was house physician (i.e., resident)
to the medical service at the MGH. He had already as a house officer
published one paper on blood clotting with Roger I. Lee (discussed in
Chapter Two) as well as several with Sir Thomas Lewis and others on his
own. This was to be his fourteenth publication—it did indeed appear in
the *Journal of Experimental Medicine* later in 1916 with 6 tables and 5
beautiful figures.

Digitalis was a drug used to strengthen the heart muscle and also reduce the heart rate when it was rapid and irregular. One of its effects was
to slow the passage of the electrical impulse through certain portions of
the heart and it was this that excited Paul White's interest. It was a tribute
to his persuasive abilities that he induced four of his fellow house physicians and officers to take the drug with him and to have several electrocardiograms taken—they were recorded on glass plates at that time—as
well as receive another drug (atropine) and study the effects of exercise.
The detailed study did show a significant effect on conduction beginning
5 to 6 days after the drug had been started and lasting up to two weeks
after it had been stopped. The effect on conduction was completely but
temporarily eliminated by giving the other drug, atropine. Not surprisingly, several of the young men became somewhat ill from the medicine,
with loss of appetite, nausea, and palpitation, referred to in the article as
"mild subjective sensations." Writing nearly 60 years later, Paul White
recalled "I can still taste it from memory . . . Some of the medical staff
prophesied that we had shortened our lives." This was the first of eight
papers Paul White wrote on the subject of digitalis, for many years

the most widely prescribed drug for heart disease and one still in common use.*

After his death, a memorial referring to this work was written for *The Pharmacologist* by Dr. J. Worth Estes, Professor of Pharmacology at Boston University. Dr. Estes had known Paul White since the summer of 1952 when, having just finished his freshman year at Harvard College, he obtained a summer job helping with the chores and the children at the Whites' place in Harvard. From this and subsequent contacts he came to know the White family well and was almost like their adopted son. Dr. Estes wrote:

> Dr. White's superbly detailed studies of the effects of digitalis on the electrocardiogram provided the ground-work for his later studies which permitted the

---

* It is impossible to describe all of Paul White's research and his publications. Some 758 scientific papers, books, discussions, and reviews are to be found in his bibliography, many of course the result of collaborative work with associates. In 1964 in two letters to Dr. Carleton B. Chapman, he identified 18 of his papers as being his most important efforts, as well as three of his books and his one historical chart published in 1947. The papers he listed were: Alternation of the Pulse: A Common Clinical Condition (1915), A Study of Atrioventricular Rhythm Following Auricular Flutter (1915), The Classification of Cardiac Diagnosis (with Merrill M. Myers) (1921), The Problem of Heart Disease in the Industrial Worker (1921), Observations on the Electrical Axis of the Heart (with C. Sidney Burwell) (1921), Bundle-Branch Block with Short P–R Interval in Healthy Young People Prone to Paroxysmal Tachycardia (with Louis Wolff and John Parkinson) (1930), Congenital Anomalies of the Coronary Arteries: Report of an Unusual Case Associated with Cardiac Hypertrophy (with Edward F. Bland and Joseph Garland) (1933), Weakness and Failure of the Left Ventricle Without Failure of the Right Ventricle. Clinical Recognition (1933), Acute Cor Pulmonale Resulting from Pulmonary Embolism: Its Clinical Recognition (with Sylvester McGinn) (1935), Chronic Constrictive Pericarditis (Pick's Disease). Treated by Pericardial Resection (1935), The Commonest Cause of Hypertrophy of the Right Ventricle—Left Ventricular Strain and Failure (with William Paul Thompson) (1936), The Speed of Healing of Myocardial Infarction (with G. Kenneth Mallory and Jorge Salcedo-Salgar) (1939), Heart Disease: A World Problem (1940), The Reversibility of Heart Disease (1944), Pulmonary Embolism in Medical Patients. A Comparison of Incidence, Diagnosis and Effect of Treatment in 273 Cases at the Massachusetts General Hospital in Two 5-Year Periods (1936 to 1940 and 1941 to 1945 inclusive) (with Jacques Carlotti, Irad B. Hardy, Jr., and Robert R. Linton) (1947), The Psyche and the Soma: The Spiritual and Physical Attributes of the Heart (1951), The Long Follow-up (1956), A Completed Twenty-Five-Year Follow-up Study of 200 Patients with Myocardial Infarction (with David W. Richards and Edward F. Bland) (1956). The writer has chosen to discuss only a few of these areas, selecting certain ones which illustrate both Paul White's range of interest and what were probably the most exciting contributions to scientific knowledge.

rapid abandonment of squill, apocynum, and convallaria as substitutes for digitalis. He emphasized the need to consider selectivity of action, bioavailability,
potency, efficacy, safety, and patient acceptability in the choice of appropriate
therapeutic agents. These investigations earned him membership in the American Society for Pharmacology and Experimental Therapeutics in 1921, and the
Chairmanship of the American Medical Association's Section on Pharmacology and Therapeutics in 1925. Later, his own clinical applications of the same
pharmacological principles enabled him to lead efforts towards the standardization of digitalis dosage forms.

*   *   *

Early in the Civil War, Dr. J. M. DaCosta, who had been appointed to
the Turner's Lane Army Hospital in Philadelphia, began to observe "a
peculiar form of functional disorder of the heart, to which I gave the name
of irritable heart." He looked up earlier military reports and found that
a similar condition had been described among the British troops during
the Crimean War and in the Indian campaigns. In 1871, he published a
paper describing as a typical case a soldier who, after recovering from an
intestinal infection, returned to full duty but "he got out of breath, could
not keep up with his comrades, was annoyed with dizziness and palpitation, and with pain in the chest; his accoutrements oppressed him, and
all this though he appeared well and healthy." The condition was a puz-
zle, there being a clear discrepancy between the symptoms and the lack
of physical evidence of any heart or other disease. In World War I, so
many of these cases were recognized that it became a serious problem to
the British troops, so serious that the Hampstead Military Hospital was
designated early in 1916 as the center for the study of these patients
under Sir Thomas Lewis. Paul White visited the Hospital briefly early in
the fall of 1916. Lewis published a short book on the subject of "The
Soldier's Heart and the Effort Syndrome" in 1919, describing essentially
the same symptoms as DaCosta and concluding that the condition was a
mixed bag. The largest group he believed had "constitutional weakness,
nervous or physical or both," but some were exhausted by war-time
conditions, some were recovering from or had infection, a few were convalescent from being gassed, and even fewer had incipient heart disease.

That same year, Dr. Alfred E. Cohn also wrote a comprehensive article on the subject and decided that "no matter what predisposing cause . . . the disorder is essentially a neurosis, depending on anxiety and fear. . . ."

Paul White began to write about this intriguing and elusive problem in 1920, and he continued to do so intermittently for 50 years, especially aided by Dr. Mandel E. Cohen. Paul White's short 1920 article in the *Journal of the American Medical Association* was an important one since for the first time it called attention to the frequency of the condition (variously named irritable heart, soldiers' heart, effort syndrome, and neurocirculatory asthenia) in civilian life. He wrote

> Since my return to civil life, I have noticed a group of cases, particularly in young women, which had been diagnosed as heart disease, sometimes for years, not infrequently as mitral stenosis which I feel were no more heart disease than were cases of effort syndrome encountered in soldiers during the war. In the Massachusetts General Hospital I have seen 12 such cases in the past six or eight weeks.

Later he and his associates described how this (which they preferred to label neurocirculatory asthenia or NCA) was indeed a common condition in civilian practice and how many patients were erroneously diagnosed as having coronary, valvular and other types of organic heart problems. They also found that it tended to occur in families and when present in one parent, approximately one-third of the children might be affected. Symptoms could occur without known provocation or at times with emotion or strenuous muscular effort. There might be an intolerance of crowds. Signs such as sighing respirations and a flushed face and neck were particularly common.

Various studies were undertaken, chiefly by Mandel Cohen, revealing how these patients were especially sensitive to pain, and showed unusual physiological and biochemical responses during and after muscular work. A twenty-year follow-up of 173 patients by E. O. Wheeler, E. W. Reed, Cohen and Paul White found that the majority continued to have some symptoms over this period and only about 10% had recovered completely.

This work served to call attention to NCA as a chronic, familial problem which was common in civilian life, and helped to delineate its characteristics. These contributions have endured. The origin of the condition remains obscure, but simple reassurance was found by Cohen and White to be the most helpful therapy.

* * *

A brief two-page report by Paul D. White and Merrill M. Myers appeared in the *Journal of the American Medical Association* in 1921, intitled "The Classification of Cardiac Diagnosis." Toward the end of his life, Paul White called this "probably the most important paper I ever wrote, for it was the basis of our current diagnostic plan and of my own book, *Heart Disease* written a few years later." In this short paper which came from ten years of hospital experience, Paul White did something very simple, so simple that its obvious message had escaped nearly all physicians. He pointed out that a diagnosis of heart disease was woefully incomplete and inadequate without inclusion of three important considerations: 1. the cause or origin of the condition—that is, the etiology; 2. the nature of any structural change, if any, in the heart; and 3. the functional state of the patient—especially the presence or absence of heart failure. By forcing the physician to think in these terms, it was his belief that there would be a better understanding of what was going on, studies and treatment could be more usefully directed, statistical data could be collected, the outlook for the patient more intelligently considered, and the possibility of actual prevention entertained.

While some of the ingredients of this classification had been emphasized in England by Sir James Mackenzie and Sir Thomas Lewis, and in the United States at the MGH by Richard Cabot, and at Bellevue Hospital in New York by John Wyckoff, they had failed to change the habits of most physicians largely because a lucid, easy to use, and rational classification had not been clearly spelled out. In many doctors' offices and hospitals, a single entry in the patient's chart under diagnosis such as "dilation of the heart" or "heart failure" had been thought to be enough without forcing the physician to reflect on why such processes were present and what could be best done about them. Under Paul White's influence all the patient records of the Boston hospitals and their clinics began gradually to use such a schema, and it spread to the practitioners in their offices, especially to any doctor who had any exposure to Paul White and the group around him. Most important of all, the Association for the Prevention and Relief of Heart Disease in New York, which was the predecessor of the New York Heart Association, published in the *Journal of the American Medical Association* in 1922 under the name of the same Dr. Alfred E. Cohn of Rockefeller University, a similar recommendation. This recommendation gave credit to Drs. White and Myers for their classification of diagnosis published a year earlier. Subsequently the classification endorsed by the New York Heart Association incorporating the ideas of White and Myers was adopted worldwide and with some revisions continues extraordinarily useful and influential to this day.

*   *   *

On March 20, 1928, Paul White saw in his office David H. Clement, an 18-year-old Yale College freshman who was on the freshman swimming team. The young man gave a story that for 4 years he had observed episodes of rapid beating of his heart, starting and stopping suddenly, and lasting about 15 minutes. The attacks were not usually related to exercise or emotion. The physical examination was entirely normal but the electrocardiogram was most unusual, showing at rest two apparent abnormalities in the conduction of the electrical impulse through the heart, in that the P–R interval was short and the QRS interval was prolonged. Both of these findings disappeared with exercise. Dr. Clement, now an emeritus professor of pediatrics at Yale, has written

> Dr. White had never seen an ECG like mine. (He recorded them on glass plates in his lab/office in the basement of the Bulfinch building.) He gave me injections of atropine and had me run up flights of stairs and recorded the influence of exercise. Finally he said "Yes, David, you can go on swimming for Yale."

This from a *Harvard* professor! He became my instant hero. A lesser physician might have grounded me indefinitely and I might have developed a cardiac neurosis. And now, as I swim my lengths some 56 years later, we all know how correct his decision was and my appreciation knows no bounds.

Paul White entered as the diagnosis of this unique case in his day book, the nonspecific words "Paroxysmal Tachycardia. Abnormal ECG."

On April 1, 1928 some eleven days later, a 35-year-old male gymnastics instructor with the remarkable initials S.O.S. came to the Cardiac Laboratory of the MGH having been referred to Paul White by Dr. Hyman Morrison of Boston. He was seen first by Dr. Louis Wolff, then a fellow in the department working under Paul White. The patient gave a history of ten years of frequent episodes of rapid irregular beating of his heart precipitated by excitement or effort and lasting about a half hour. The physical examination was normal. The electrocardiogram (taken the next day) was similar but not identical to that of the previous patient David Clement and also became briefly normal after exercise as well as after injection of the drug atropine. At a later date the electrocardiogram also showed a very irregular heart rhythm of the type called atrial fibrillation. Dr. Wolff discussed the case with Paul White, showing him the electrocardiogram, and suggesting that here was something distinctly unusual meriting further study, with which the latter totally agreed. Patient S.O.S. was examined several more times in subsequent months and further observations were made. Paul White apparently only later recalled the patient David Clement seen by him earlier with a quite similar story and findings. Dr. Wolff, thus encouraged, combed the scientific literature and could find no reports of this condition, but he did locate the records of two similar patients, males ages 16 and 21, who had been seen earlier at the Hospital.

Later that year, Paul White went to Europe taking with him the electrocardiograms on S.O.S. and the first draft of a manuscript on the subject. While in London he wrote on October 24, 1928 to Wolff:

I talked over with Sir Thomas [Lewis] the electrocardiograms of our case of Bundle Branch Block. He was much interested but had absolutely no explanation, especially for the short P–R interval. He thinks that this sort of a case along with a few others of different nature upset our present conception of things and that there are new discoveries to be made. I did not offer the paper for *Heart* because on reflection I believe it worthwhile to observe our man longer (another 6 months or so until we have him under our eyes for a year at least, with repetition of our tests at the end of that time) and because [Dr. John] Parkinson showed me the other day an electrocardiogram just taken by him showing wide QRS waves and short P–R intervals in a healthy boy of 18 or so. As yet, he has done no tests but I shall get him to repeat our studies on this lad and if they pan out, as ours did, ask him to join with us in the description of these two cases. More of that later, but after a bit I shall probably return our paper to you to hold until Spring, and then, with the new additions of the present status of our case and the accounts of Parkinson's case, send it in for publication, probably to the *American Heart Journal*.

The fact that Paul White mentioned only the one case seen by him and Wolff suggests strongly that the 18-year-old college student David Clement seen by Paul White alone on March 20 was not as yet recognized as having the same problem as patient S.O.S. seen by Wolff and Paul White on April 1. Paul White's office record on the latter case also has the words "first case of WPW syndrome" (which is what the condition was often called later) written on the front sheet in red ink in Paul White's own handwriting. Paul White also took to Vienna the electrocardiograms on their patient S.O.S., but the best minds there could only suggest that this was a bundle branch block and what was called an AV nodal rhythm.

Finally in August 1930 in the *American Heart Journal* a paper was published by Wolff, Parkinson and White entitled "Bundle-Branch Block with Short P–R Interval in Healthy Young People Prone to Paroxysmal Tachycardia" describing 11 patients in all, 4 from the MGH including S.O.S. and David Clement, and 7 from Parkinson at the London Hospital. This landmark article describing what was soon called the Wolff-Parkinson-White or WPW syndrome (and later the pre-excitation syndrome) established that such an entity existed, discussed the changes in the electrocardiograms with exercise and atropine, emphasized that the findings occurred in healthy young people, and concluded that "this mechanism is apparently not indicative of disease of the heart." That the authors were not convinced that this was the usual bundle-branch block is suggested by their cautious reference to "aberrant ventricular complexes of the type generally recognized as indicating bundle-branch block" but they did not provide an explanation of the phenomenon. However, they did comment that a congenital anomaly could be responsible. The importance of the publication was two-fold: by calling attention to a new entity, it encouraged investigation by others; and by stressing its occurrence in these 11 healthy young people without signs of organic heart disease, it helped to remove the label of a serious heart condition from many persons. Louis Wolff should have the credit for flagging patient S.O.S. as something unusual, and Paul White for agreeing and encouraging further study as well as for withholding publication until a reasonably sized series had been collected and observed. He also obtained the opinion and participation of Parkinson.

The unraveling of what was going on in such cases has taken 50 years, the leadership gradually being taken over by the electrophysiologist from the practicing doctor. It was in 1932 that Holzmann and Scherf suggested in the German literature that in these patients the electrical impulses going from the upper to the lower portions of the heart were travelling by a special by-pass tract present since birth, a shrewd and critically important concept also proposed a year later by Wolferth and Wood of Philadelphia. The subject has ever since been of intense interest to pathologists, physiologists and clinicians and more than a thousand reports on the condition and its nature have been published. As Sherf and Neufeld have written, it has "presented a kind of Rosetta stone" for electrocardiography. These publications have enormously enlarged our understanding of the unusual electrical events occurring in the hearts of these patients, and have shown that the process is far more varied and complex than was realized by the original authors or by Holzmann and Scherf and their immediate successors. Great credit must be given to the three collaborators for recognizing and describing the problem in the first place, a problem which has kept many investigators busy in the laboratory ever since.

*   *   *

A young girl, K.S. had been under the observation of the Medical Service in the Cardiac Clinic of the MGH since January 1925 at which time she was 15 years old. She was complaining of shortness of breath and fatigue, her neck veins were prominent and pulsating, her liver was distinctly enlarged, and there was fluid in the abdomen. It was considered by Paul White and others who saw her that her difficulties were due to disease of the normally thin capsule called the pericardium which surrounded the heart, which had for some reason become thickened and was constricting the movements and function of the heart muscle. Over the next three and a half years, she steadily became more ill. She was limited in activity and her legs began to swell. Up to 10 quarts of fluid had to be removed from her abdomen to provide relief.

Finally on July 18, 1928 on the advice of Paul White, Dr. Edward D. Churchill, a surgeon at the MGH and later its Chief of Surgery, who had received training in chest surgery from Ludolf Brauer and Ernst Sauerbruch in Germany, operated upon her. He removed a considerable portion of the offending pericardium in an operation considered at the time a daring feat. In those days, one just did not operate on the heart because of the presumed extraordinary risk. Dr. Churchill could see at the operating table that relief from the constriction produced an immediate and encouraging improvement in the contractions of the heart muscle. Following the procedure, the patient recovered dramatically, losing 20 pounds of water in three weeks. She subsequently resumed a completely normal life, married, had two children, and finally died of cancer at the age of 59.

The operation on this patient clearly had exciting and tremendously satisfying consequences and not just for the one patient. It was the first successful operation to remove a constricting pericardium done in the United States and indeed the English-speaking world, although several had been done in Germany dating back to 1920. It called attention to the importance of chronic disease of the pericardium and what might be done to provide relief. In subsequent years the same procedure was offered to many other similar patients in medical centers all over the United States and abroad. Paul White and Churchill took the leadership in describing this in the medical literature beginning with the publication of this first case in the *New England Journal of Medicine* in 1930. Ten other articles appeared from Paul White and his associates over the succeeding 30 years describing more fully the pathology and clinical features of other cases encountered and the long-term course after surgical relief. Paul White also chose this as the topic for his St. Cyres lecture at the National Hospital for Diseases of the Heart in London in 1935. Altogether July 18, 1928 was a highly significant morning in the operating room for the history of acquired heart disease.*

The publication in the medical literature of a single clinical case such as the above has generally been frowned upon as being inadequate for any general conclusions and as showing evidence of a disposition in an undue hurry for recognition and lacking the patience to collect a decent series with proper observations. The story of this patient with chronic constrictive pericarditis was a justified exception since it demonstrated what was for the United States a successful new approach. Paul White occasionally described other single cases in an article when he felt they were unique, and such another one was his description in 1929 with Dr. Howard Sprague of a noted musician, Henry F. Gilbert, who lived a very productive life to his 60th year despite a serious congenital heart problem, the tetralogy of Fallot. This publication provoked the following interesting letter from Dr. Harvey Cushing, the famous father of brain surgery, Chief of Surgery at the Peter Bent Brigham Hospital, and the author of a Pulitzer Prize biography of Sir William Osler:

March 12, 1929

Dear White: My compliments on your account of the case of Henry F. Gilbert. It is not only a tribute to an heroic fellow but to your clinico-pathological

---

* It is of interest that the first successful operation for a congenital heart condition also took place in Boston ten years later on August 26, 1938. At that time Dr. Robert E. Gross successfully ligated for the first time a patent ductus arteriosus in a 7½-year-old child. The procedure was done at the Children's Hospital in Boston and Dr. John P. Hubbard was the attending pediatrician. Because this too was a courageous and unprecedented event, the little girl was referred prior to surgery to Paul White who concurred in the recommendation to operate.

acumen. My father once made a wise remark which I am prone to quote to the effect that some of the best work in the world is done in the face of chronic invalidism, which is an aspect that does not often appear in case histories.

Your paper is the type of biographico-pathological case report such as used to be seen in the heyday of English medical literature but which has disappeared in these squeamish times when we refrain from mentioning the names of our departed patients and if we take photographs of them, only show them masked.

Much power to your elbow.

Sincerely yours,

Harvey Cushing

*　*　*

One of the sudden disasters which all too often ended the lives of both medical and surgical patients was the passage of blood clots from the veins to the lungs. For a long time, this relatively common and unexpected event was regarded as an enigma, a strange and terrible act of God, striking without warning, difficult to diagnose when it happened, and indeed often diagnosed only at autopsy. Textbooks provided little information, and those on heart disease by Reid, Crummer, Mackenzie, Vaquez and Cabot did not even discuss the condition, although Paul White included it in *Heart Disease* published in 1931. Henderson reported that 6% of post-operative deaths at the Mayo Clinic between 1917 and 1927 were due to this complication, and it was also seen even more frequently in patients with heart disease. Commonly, patients with this condition were incorrectly diagnosed as heart attacks or pneumonia.

In 1935, Paul White and his associate Sylvester McGinn wrote an article which appeared in the *Journal of the American Medical Association* describing nine patients with this condition. Electrocardiograms were available in seven of the nine, four of whom died.

A typical case was that of a 60-year-old man who underwent an uneventful operation for removal of his gallbladder and who on the eighth day after surgery suddenly became very short of breath and coughed frequently raising some blood; his blood pressure dropped, and the color of his skin became dusky. He improved for a time but abruptly collapsed and died on the 15th post-operative day. At autopsy, there was a large clot in the right lung and a few smaller ones on the left.

McGinn and Paul White introduced their presentation of the problem with a scholarly historical review of the pertinent literature going back to 1889. In all, there were 27 references to prior articles germane to the subject. There followed a discussion in which the authors pointed to the symptoms and clinical findings present in these cases, including in some a change in the heart tones with a prominence of the pulmonary component of the second heart sound related to acute strain on the right side of the heart from the presence of the lung clot. They also described for the first time changes in the electrocardiograms—new findings which, when present, helped to establish the diagnosis. These highly significant observations were soon confirmed by others and were particularly important since at that time, the tools available to help establish a diagnosis were few indeed. McGinn and Paul White's interest in this problem helped measurably to alert practitioners to the possibility of early and more accurate diagnosis, and later to prevention through the use of anti-clotting drugs. Over the next twelve years, he and his colleagues on the surgery, pathology and x-ray staffs of the MGH published a series of papers which pointed to the leg veins as the commonest source of the blood clots and discussed a vigorous approach to the whole issue. Their efforts contributed importantly to the progress made in illuminating and coping with this serious problem.

*   *   *

It has been said by a few that a defect in Paul White's role as an investigator was that he believed that almost everything he published was so significant. Those engrossed with more basic investigations were especially prone to regard with faint praise his patient-related studies and wondered why he did not produce really "important" work. It is true that he was not at all humble in talking about the projects which he and his colleagues and students developed and completed, but his attitude was more one of uninhibited, almost childlike enthusiasm for the work than of egotism, although the latter was a factor in his later years. It was this enthusiasm which he used to good advantage to obtain contributions from many patients to support a modest research fund at the MGH. Quite rarely, his enthusiasm was disproportionate to what in time was demonstrated to be the long-term scientific worth, as with the operation of sympathectomy for the relief of high blood pressure which he promoted vigorously for several years until he saw that the results were variable and often disappointing and that simpler and better measures were at hand.

It is also true that when some of Paul White's admirers later proposed that he receive the Nobel Prize, it was not because of his achievements in research but because of his role in furthering the quest for peace through scientific exchange. He did not make any brilliant scientific discoveries. However, his writings with Lee on blood clotting, and with Wolff and Parkinson on the Wolff-Parkinson-White syndrome, were pioneer original contributions to medicine; those on the effects of digitalis, on neurocirculatory asthenia, on the classification of cardiac diagnosis, on constrictive pericarditis, on pulmonary embolism and other topics were significant because he seized upon the early work of others on which he imposed his own personal experiences in a reasoned, effective, and memorable manner. His contributions to clinical research were numerous, well-written, and excellent in quality; they have stood up well through the passage of time. They did not provide new basic knowledge regarding electrical or biochemical or physiological processes because his talents did not lie in those directions, and he wisely chose not to pretend that they did. There were remarkably few errors in judgment in his work and no endorsements of what later was shown to be worthless or harmful, nor did he, like some well-known scientists, make a career of writing and rewriting the same material with only very minor changes from article to article. A comparison of his scientific productivity with that of his leading clinical contemporaries during his most productive period 1916–1940 is highly favorable to Paul White. It is also to be remembered that one of his most effective roles was that of assigning a scientific topic to the young men and women training under him so that through their efforts and his guidance, they could learn the techniques of research and of writing a scientific paper, and in time be rewarded by the pride of a joint authorship with their professor. His bibliography is a record of the fruits of this educational experience, one which each co-author now looks back upon with profound gratitude.

CHAPTER FIVE

Famous Patients and Others

Just as Paul White developed a solid base of scientific studies during the interval between the two World Wars, so too did he use this period to build a private practice which allowed him to counsel and treat many thousands of patients and which provided the income to support him and his family for his entire life. In this effort, he was supremely successful because the essential personal ingredients were all there.*

A patient with heart disease seeks, ideally, a doctor who will listen with respect and interest, is thorough and competent, kindly and warm in manner, who takes the time to explain the condition and treatment in understandable and encouraging terms, and whose fee is moderate. During the first two-thirds of this century, such a physician was not a mythical figure. He was Dr. Paul Dudley White. Yet his office at the MGH and later at 264 Beacon Street was modest to a degree. The rooms were small and crowded, the furniture simple and old, there was no soft music. Clearly no interior decorator had taken charge. The message was in the man, not the trappings.

"Listen to what the *patient* can tell you—it may be more important than anything else you do!" Louise Wheeler, who was in charge of the Cardiac Laboratory at the MGH, recalls that Paul White repeatedly emphasized this to his students and how it above all characterized his relation to his patients. In listening, he gave the patient a chance to describe the history of the illness and the symptoms and their effects in his or her own words. In listening, he also had an immensely valuable opportunity to observe the psychological makeup of the person. And by listening, he demonstrated his own genuine interest in and respect for that one patient. Just as Paul White's and Merrill Myers' classification of the diag-

* Paul White's private patient records numbered 14,486. His first private patient was seen November 21, 1914 and his last new patient on May 16, 1973.

nosis of heart disease discussed in Chapter Four was absurdly sensible and obvious, but it required someone like Paul White to introduce it as a concept; so too was listening to the patient a simple well-known technique which should not have required reaffirmation. Yet many individuals with heart disease came to see him because no one with a discerning mind had bothered to listen enough or indeed at all.

He would not only listen patiently and attentively. When it came time to tell the patient and often others in the family of his findings and conclusions, he would explain the diagnosis, studies, treatment and outlook in simple, uncomplicated terms. Then there would be generous opportunity for questions and answers. Paul White was a marvelous communicator, because he took the time to do it properly. He was able to give the time by working long hours and by limiting the size of his practice. Many patients were referred to his associates because his appointment book would be filled for months. But he realized that unless he listened, he was not doing his job well; and all his life, he encouraged his patients to talk and he paid attention to what they said. As he grew older, he began to talk to patients more and more, often about himself. Yet he never lost the arts of listening to the patient, of thoroughness, and of lucid explanation.

Dr. William Paul Thompson, one of his former residents, has told of a typical incident in which Paul White's style of practice was beautifully demonstrated.

He was the best practitioner of medicine I've ever known anywhere. He loved patients as human beings. He impressed me especially one time in 1953 after I had been in practice for several years. I had in the hospital an elderly man with a stroke who was going to die. Dr. White was coming out to Los Angeles to get an honorary Doctor of Science degree at the University of Southern California, and the patient's family heard that he was coming and arranged for him to see the patient as a consultant. So Dr. White asked me to meet him at the hospital after he received his honorary degree at a dinner that evening. Well, the dinner went on and on and on and finally he called me and said he was ready to leave the hotel where the meeting was held and would I meet him? I said, "Yes" and went down to the hospital about 11:30 at night and in came Dr. White in his tuxedo. I thought, "Well, here it is nearly midnight—nearly 3:00 a.m. in Dr. White's time—and I must be very brief and give him just a little sketch of this poor old gentleman who is obviously dying." But that didn't do for Dr. White. He had to talk with and examine the patient, go through every item on the chart, every item in the laboratory data, write them down in his own records, and then spend a great deal of time with the patient and the family discussing everything with them. Dr. White did all that not just for the patient and the family—he also did it for me. And he made an enormous impression on me.

Paul White's patients included many of the great names of the twentieth century. Most often seen in consultation, these included in government President Eisenhower, Vice President Barkley, the President and Prime Minister of Pakistan, the Presidents of Nicaragua and Colombia and the Philippines, the Prime Minister of Lebanon, a number of United States senators and representatives; in the world of business and finance, J. P. Morgan, Cornelius Vanderbilt, Andrew Carnegie, William Randolph Hearst, and Frederick Prince; in literature and the arts, Katherine Cornell, Kenneth Roberts, Fritz Reiner, Charles Munch, James Michener, and Pablo Casals; a large assortment of bishops; and a host of prominent physicians and other scientists. He was never a name-dropper and even his close associates often did not know of the eminence of the men and women who came to see him.

But most of Paul White's patients were ordinary people whose names would never appear in the newspaper or in *Who's Who*. George Shallcross, who served as general helper in the Cardiac Laboratory for 29 years, saw that Paul White "was as courteous to the lowest as to the highest on the social scale, there was no difference." Dr. Benedict Massell worked with him for years in the Rheumatic Fever Clinic at the MGH and observed: "He was very kind to people. Whether the people had money or not made no difference, he took care of them no matter what their means. . . ."

One of his former students, Dr. Royal Schaff, watched him "delivering the best care that he could for anybody and everybody, from the President of the United States to the poor little lady coming in from the clinic. Everybody was equally welcome. He treated them all as gentlefolk, not as kings and not as paupers, but with universal humanity which obviously sprang from the heart."

Dr. Massell saw an example of his concern for people when his wife-to-be, a schoolteacher, received a hand-written letter from Dr. Paul White, a person of whom she had never heard. He was writing to her, unaware that she was Massell's fiancée, regarding a young clinic patient whom he felt was being overprotected by his parents. Paul White was urging the boy to lead a normal life and wanted his teachers to know this and to help. He had taken the time to make sure that the school system received his message by writing it out in longhand. Often he would work long hours in the clinic seeing indigent cases and as a result would arrive late at his office to see his private patients.

One reason for his enormous success with patients was his ability to encourage and give hope. He was never one to appear solemn and grave or to impart his wisdom in sepulchral tones, even in the most dire circumstances. Mrs. Natalie Kreisle first saw him as a patient in 1924 when she was recovering from rheumatic fever, and she recalls that he had a wonderful personality—he was interested in her as a person—and would encourage her and encourage her parents that they were doing the right thing. Dr. Benedict Massell said similarly, "The patients all liked him, they thought he was wonderful because he gave them an optimistic outlook. He wasn't the type of person to tell a patient that he or she had a dangerous disease with such and such a prognosis, in contrast to other cardiologists at that time. He never said such things. He would encourage them to do whatever was reasonable." Dr. Massell recalled a young man with rheumatic heart disease who wanted to be a pitcher on a professional baseball team. Paul White saw him and encouraged him to go ahead with his plans and the young man did so with success. As Dr. Edward Bland, his long-time colleague, said, Paul White could make a patient feel that "this wasn't the end of the road. He would take the most dismal situation and look at the bright side, and the patient woud leave his office happy. He just had a knack of convincing the patient and you and himself that perhaps things weren't as bad as they appeared."

One special aspect of his relation with his patients was his flexibility. Because of his long experience and his good sense, he knew that some individuals with heart disease would do well and could safely be allowed latitude in their activities, activities which would usually be considered unwise and even dangerous. Dr. Florence Avitabile, who reviewed many of the records of his long-term patients, found that most of the time his conclusions and advice at the time of a patient's first visit proved correct over a span of many years and that he somehow had an instinct which allowed him to foresee the future with remarkable clarity.

Dr. Allan Friedlich remembers the case of an elderly Jewish lady who had a major heart attack for which she was hospitalized. She was terribly unhappy, not about her heart attack but because she was going to miss her grandson's Bar Mitzvah which was to occur two or three days later. Ordinarily it would be considered out of the question for a patient with a recent serious heart attack to leave the hospital that early and sit through such a service. However, she was a patient of Paul White, and after he heard her story, "he had the good sense and the humanity to realize that if she did not go, she would get so disturbed that she might get into more trouble and he said to my amazement, 'Well, if someone picked you up and you just sat there and did not dance and were brought back here right after the festivities, I think it would be all right'." And so it was.* On another occasion Paul White permitted an internationally prominent scientist who also had suffered a recent, major heart attack to attend an academic exercise because of its critical importance to the sci-

*Paul White had many Jewish patients as well as Jewish friends and close colleagues including Samuel A. Levine and Allan L. Friedlich. Prior to World War II, his attitude toward the Jews was flavored with some of the naive views of the white Anglo-Saxon Protestant group in which he was reared. As the Nazi threat grew, Paul White had a flurry of interest in how to combat anti-Semitism in the United States. On August 23, 1940, he wrote to his friend Justice Felix Frankfurter of the U.S. Supreme Court, referring to his friendship with many Jews and also indicating his belief that Jewish leaders should counsel their people on ways to alter their behavior so as to lessen anti-Semitism in the United States. In a meeting with Frankfurter and Dr. Alfred E. Cohn in New Milford, Connecticut on September 14, 1940 arranged to discuss this issue, Paul White spoke of three traits he considered common among his Jewish patients and liable to provoke antagonism: aggressiveness, bargaining, and neurotic tendencies. He also discussed this with department store executive Louis E. Kirstein in November of that year. These Jewish leaders seemed to have listened attentively but pointed to the prevalence of these traits among Gentiles. The matter ended there. During World War II, Paul White endeavored to find jobs for Jewish refugee physicians who had fled to America and he subsequently worked closely with many leading Jewish doctors and was supportive of their careers.

entist's peace of mind. The epoch-making decision that President Eisenhower might run for a second term after his heart attack also represented a flexibility considered by some prominent cardiologists to be foolhardy; yet his judgment regarding Eisenhower's heart was vindicated by the course of events.

Not all of Paul White's patients were easy to handle. It was not unusual for his associates helping with their care to become exasperated with the behavior of a demanding, petulant individual. A few were spoiled VIP's who wanted to show off, and a few had come to Dr. White because they had antagonized other physicians who were glad to get rid of them. Somehow Paul White never lost his temper and remained poised and tolerant despite major provocation. He realized that difficult personalities may become more difficult in the setting of illness with anxiety, fear, loneliness and pain. Dr. Gordon Myers remembers "One patient in the Phillips House was demanding in every possible way and complaining about nearly everything. One day we went by on rounds and she said: 'Among all the other things that are so terrible in this hospital is this chair by the bed. It is so uncomfortable that I can't stand to sit in it.' Dr. White inquired as to why it did not seem to be comfortable. Later he went to a furniture store in Boston, selected a chair, rented it, and had it sent to the patient to use by her bedside. This was to me almost incredible! But he did things like that for any number of patients who were terribly demanding. Most people would not have put up with it at all."

Many of his patients were seen in consultation with their own physicians. Paul White might see them in their hospital rooms at the MGH or at another hospital or occasionally at home. A good consultant must be authoritative, unhurried, skillful in handling the patient and his or her problem, and helpful and diplomatic with the regular attending physician. Paul White possessed all of these attributes. Dr. Ernest Craige, who trained with Dr. White and is Professor of Medicine at the University of North Carolina Medical School, has graphically described how his teacher functioned as a consultant.

> I will confine my comments to one facet of his practice which I found very instructive and which I sought to emulate. This had to do with his handling of

a consultation. A typical locale for this was in the Phillips House. The patient would have been doing poorly and that is what precipitated the request for Dr. White's opinion. I was always struck by his concern for each member of the professional team as well as the other employees—cleaning ladies, dietary, etc. He had some good words for the sullen and apathetic nurses who worked there and encouraged them to renewed efforts on behalf of the patient. He would then sit at the bedside giving the patient his undivided attention, perform his examination, look at the ECG, x-ray, etc. and then he would be prepared for the conference with the referring physician. Not infrequently the case had been mismanaged or at least drastic alterations in the program were urgently indicated. In his conversation with the referring physician, Dr. White would avoid any hint of censure for what had been done to that point. He adroitly guided the analysis of the case such that finally the referring physician would enunciate the correct course to be followed. At this point Dr. White would agree enthusiastically with the conclusions reached by this revelation. Then he and the referring doctor would join the patient and/or family and go over the situation. Dr. White would make a point of praising the referring physician for his contributions to the case, including his suggestions regarding the new course to be followed. In this manner, the stature of the latter would not be diminished. Dr. White had no need to enhance his own position by diminishing that of the referring physician. The referring doctor learned something from the consultation and was grateful for the experience and the manner in which it was handled. The patient and his family and the professional attendants all benefited from the encounter.

All of his life, Paul White related easily and warmly to other doctors, even those heart specialists who might be considered as arch competitors. It was a tribute both to Paul White at the MGH and Dr. Samuel A. Levine across the city of Boston at the Peter Bent Brigham Hospital that these two outstanding cardiologists in the same city and medical school and specialty at the same time had a comfortable and indeed affectionate relationship. Paul White would refer complicated diagnostic or therapeutic problems to "Sam" Levine for his advice, and Levine did the same with White. Paul White also invited and respected the opinions of even his youngest colleagues and residents at the MGH. He was secure enough to welcome their views and wise enough to acknowledge his own limitations. Furthermore, he almost never criticized others, a trait which sometimes annoyed his associates who found it hard to be so forebearing. This helped to explain why he had no enemies in the profession in Boston, in the United States, or in the world.

Dr. Richard C. Cabot was Clinical Professor of Medicine at the Harvard Medical School, an outstanding member of the staff of the MGH, a specialist in internal medicine with a particular interest in heart disease, and in the twilight of his life, a patient of Paul White. In addition to his Boston heritage and social and professional distinction, he could be eloquent and generous. A paragraph from a letter he sent to Paul White in 1938, in reference to an article White had written on "Doctors and Books," describes yet another side of Paul White and also reflects distinction on Cabot himself:

> As I read on page 11 of the average doctor "who writes illegibly, spells atrociously, and constructs barbaric sentences," I thought of the splendid contrast to all that which I have admired for so many years in your records, written before the War and in France and on consultation-slips in the MGH ward-records. I should like to write your biography so as to have the fun of quoting some of your daily records which no one will otherwise ever appreciate as much as I do. I wonder if even your wife knows what a wealth of splendid character is limned and pictured in your hand-written records? I have loved them for 30 years or more. The round, clear script that saved the reader from puzzle and labor, the short, clear sentences that record all that's essential and nothing more, are absolutely the best of all the thousands and thousands of pages of hand-written records that I read in gathering case material for my "Differential Diagnosis." I doubt if any man living has read so many hand-written records as I, or ever will, because now they're all typed. So it ought to mean something to you and to your wife, and some day to your little daughter too, that of all the records that I've read, yours are absolutely the best. In the MGH volumes, Thayer's, Harvey Cushing's, and Moffit's are splendid, but they are not up to yours. The greatest merit of all, perhaps, in yours is that you always *commit* yourself on the points that most men sidestep because they half-consciously fear that they may later be shown wrong. You always incur that danger because it is for the patient's benefit that you should do so. I could write a whole chapter on your records. Perhaps I will someday!

Not only was Paul White almost unique in the legibility and clarity and completeness of his notes, he was also decidedly unusual in his follow-up. When a physician referred a patient to him, that physician always promptly received a complete report. Further, he would keep an extraordinary interest in each patient, often writing in a few months or a year to get a report on any progress, and frequently, in his travels anywhere in the world meeting or getting word of patients he had seen in the past.

One aspect of his daily office schedule had its own special flavor. He early learned that if he left his office and went to lunch in the hospital cafeteria, he would be asked repeatedly for "curb-stone" consultations on patients, both while walking to and from the cafeteria and while trying to eat his lunch. He therefore devised the stratagem of slipping out the back door of his office at lunchtime, circumventing some of the hospital corridors by proceeding outside along the walk in front of the Bulfinch Building, and going one block to a small restaurant called Minnie's (run by the Minichiello family) at the corner of North Grove and Cambridge Streets. There he would pick up the morning newspaper from the counter, sit alone at a table and drink a milk-shake and eat a sandwich while scanning the news, and then leave paying for the lunch but never the newspaper which would be returned to the counter. Since members of the Minichiello family had become Paul White's patients, this routine was entirely acceptable to them. Rarely, a visitor or associate or student would be invited to eat with him in these very modest surroundings. After he moved his office from the MGH to 264 Beacon Street, he continued to go out for lunch at a corner drug store.

He was fortunate indeed to have had devoted and capable assistance from remarkable secretaries all his life. Agnes Donovan, who married Dr. Bernard Walsh, was his first full-time secretary beginning in 1927, and she was followed by her sister, Helen Donovan. From 1960 on, Dr. Florence Avitabile acted as "chief of staff" for him. These three particularly, with help from others, carried a tremendous load in the office and did it quietly and so well that Paul White probably did not appreciate his good fortune.

Paul White was always modest in his fees.* They were so modest that they upset some of his young assistants who tried to urge him to charge more. Dr. Edward Orgain, who later became Professor of Medicine at

---

* Examples of Paul White's charges are provided by his records for two days, twenty years apart, days which appear to have been quite typical. On December 6, 1943, he saw seven old patients in his office with two charges for $15.00, three for $25.00, one for $35.00, and one for $50.00 (a patient from Los Angeles). He also saw an old patient in the hospital and charged $25.00. On December 6, 1963, he saw five old patients in the office with two charges of only $10.00, two for $15.00, and one for $25.00; that same day, he also saw five patients in the hospital with one charge for $5.00, two for $10.00, and two for $15.00.

Duke, recalled how he and Dr. Ashton Graybiel as well as Agnes Donovan encouraged him to increase his charges, but to no avail. Orgain and Graybiel attempted to circumvent the established fee schedule, however; as when a prospective patient might call at off-hours, when the secretary was not there and inquiry was made as to the size of the fees, they would mention a figure considerably inflated above what Paul White was accustomed to charge. To very wealthy patients, Paul White might suggest that he send no bill, and instead a generous check should be given to a worthy medical cause. Once, in Paris, he saw a rich Greek ship owner and after the consultation was concluded announced that the fee was to be $5,000 made payable to a hospital in Athens which was sorely in need of funds. He got the check for the hospital and did not receive a cent himself. Relevant to the issue of fees was a letter Paul White received in August 1963 from a person unknown to him who wrote:

A story is being circulated about you which seems to me impossible. It is said that when you were in Washington at the time of Eisenhower's illness, you charged and received $5,000 for making one call on the daughter of a congressman of modest means. The story seems to me unlikely. Would you care to comment on it?

Paul White's reply was unusually spirited for him:

You ask about a bill that I might have sent to the daughter of some congressman. This is perfectly ridiculous. I never did any such thing. And I might add that when I saw the President himself, my fee was only $50 on each occasion—and there weren't very many occasions.

Such rumors and spurious anecdotes were not uncommon and continue to this day—the price of being before the public. Another story, for which there is excellent evidence, involved the widow of a President of the Philippines who came to Boston to see Paul White in consultation. In view of Dr. White's prestige, she is said to have brought with her $10,000 in cash, but became concerned that this amount might prove inadequate. Her fears were unjustified, as the bill was for $100.

The eminence of Paul White and his purported miraculous skill meant that there were many occasions when doctors and patients took advantage of him in order to get his opinion. This was most flagrant in the spring of 1948, when he was leading a medical mission of the Unitarian Service Committee to Greece. Not a day would go by without someone (usually a local host) imposing on him to see a special patient, which meant lengthening the already long workdays. One dividend came when after seeing the mother of the chief admiral in the Greek navy, Paul White, as usual when on a teaching mission, charged no fee. The admiral insisted that he must do something in return for this great favor. As a result, Paul White and his teaching team were loaned a Greek destroyer which allowed them to make an exciting visit to the monasteries on Mt. Athos. This was an unforgettable experience as they found that the monks were, in the words of Paul White, "living wholly in the past of 1,000 years ago (when the monasteries were founded) only not nearly so well. They are greatly depleted in numbers (from 5,500 to 2,000 now on the entire peninsula) and they are poor and ignorant. . . ." This rewarding payment for seeing one patient was offset by many fatiguing impositions throughout the five weeks in Greece. Paul White wrote two weeks after the start of the mission that "My greatest problem has been with private patients whom I have had to see under pressures of the university professors, the Embassy, AMAG [American Mission for Aid to Greece], the Greek cabinet and King, our own and the Greek army and navy—it's been a hard grind, but I haven't been able to avoid it." He wrote at the end of the mission: "We were all dead tired from a grueling last few days in Athens, grueling especially for some of us who were hopelessly beset by patients up to the last minute, interrupting meals and pursuing us everywhere without mercy and urged on by the professors themselves."

Once, while taking a local air flight in the Middle East, Paul White found that a would-be patient had bought a ticket on the same plane and next to his own seat in order to get his opinion. Paul White was impressed by his persistence and did the best he could in that noisy environment. Dr. Conger Williams recalled one rare occasion when Paul White got even with a man who was taking unfair advantage of him. This was in Mexico City where, on arriving for the usual late dinner, he found that his locally important host had invited as guests two friends whom he wished to have examined that very evening. Confronted with this un-expected and irritating request, Paul White thereupon announced that he would see them both but only before and not after dinner; and so he did, talking with them at length, examining them completely, and rendering his judgment in detail. The company had to wait, hungry and fretting, and did not sit down to dinner until nearly midnight. It was not until Paul White was in his eighties that this kind of pressure began to lessen.

Such was his world of practice, always in demand, with an interna-tional clientele, the rich and the poor, treated alike with a single standard, and handled with intelligence, experience, good sense and warmth.

This world of practice set a model for his colleagues, students, and patients. As the age of medical technology advanced and study of the patient with heart disease more and more involved special x-rays, detailed electrocardiograms including exercise tests, cardiac catheterization, echocardiograms, and cardiac scanning, Paul White's approach which did not emphasize these tools seemed and was old-fashioned. That his ap-proach continued to be valid was due partly to his own personal success with such a method; and partly because it was a reminder that what he learned from the history and physical examination and getting to know the patient was a necessary first-step to the proper use of the new tech-nology, and was often the only step necessary.

CHAPTER SIX

Text and Teaching

Paul White wrote to his mother from London in May of 1914 while still in the laboratory of Lewis that he was "a poor teacher." This self-appraisal may have influenced his comment made some 11 years later that his chief interests were clinical research and practice, with teaching and administration rated equally in third place. It is likely that this early rating of his interests and talent changed with time, for after his return to the Masssachusetts General Hospital in 1919 from his varied military obligations, he began to devote more and more time to teaching. It was not long before he had reached the saturation point in terms of hours available. The students found that he relished this role and did it extremely well; and this would hold true for the rest of his life. They in turn sought the opportunity to sit at his feet and he was besieged with applicants of all ages who wanted exposure to the White personality and the White method of instruction. This facet of his life became a major one, interrelating far more effectively than he initially realized with his clinical research and practice. An important medium for extending this influence as a teacher was his publications.

The largest writing task undertaken by Paul White was the preparation of his textbook on heart disease, published in 1931, which promptly became the standard for students all over the world. There were several books on heart disease available in the late 1920's when he began writing, but many such as those of William Duncan Reid, Frederick W. Bishop, and LeRoy Crummer were routine efforts without distinction. Sir James Mackenzie's large successful text on heart disease was first published in 1908 with a final fourth edition in 1925, the year of his death, but it already seemed to reflect the ideas of an earlier era. A large and inclusive volume for the heart had been written by Henri Vaquez of Paris and published in English translation in the United States in 1924, but some of its ideas were narrow and out-of-step with the times (angina pectoris was due to disease of the aorta, hypertension to disease of the adrenal medulla, etc.). Richard Cabot of the MGH had produced his "Facts on the Heart" in 1926, but this was an unusual and not appealing book as a large portion was occupied with the case histories of 1,906 patients seen at the hospital. Although Sir Thomas Lewis had written books about his special research areas, he did not publish a general volume on heart disease until 1933 and when it appeared, it was a brief effort.

Thus, there seemed to be a place for another text, written by a cardiologist with new ideas, exposure to research and practice, experience in teaching, and with many scientific articles to his credit. Further, Paul White had witnessed how his teachers Lewis and Mackenzie had written books and how much these had contributed to their reputation, not to mention their incomes. Mackenzie had attributed a sudden jump in his income to the appearance in 1908 of the first edition of his textbook. This was still an age in which one physician did not hesitate to write a textbook by himself, without the aid of collaborators, reflecting not so much the author's broad competence and perhaps self-confidence as the relative narrowness of the field and the lack of many advanced technological developments requiring special expertise.

In 1928, Paul White obtained from Harvard University a Moseley Traveling Fellowship in the amount of $2,500 to permit him to write his book away from Boston where he could have relative peace and quiet. He and his wife left New York for Plymouth, England on the S. S. American Shipper on September 20, 1928, and had a rough ten-day trip in which Ina White was quite miserable and remained cooped up in the stateroom the entire trip. After ten days of visiting in England and nearly a month in France, they left Paris for Vienna on the Orient Express on November 27 intending to settle down there for the winter. Paul White planned to begin writing the textbook in January. With him he took a trunk filled with 12,000 reference cards, 30 or 40 books in English, French and German, reprints, and "skates and a baseball bat and ball." The number of reference cards was powerful evidence of how widely and how much he read of the scientific literature.

Their stay in Vienna at Pension Schneider turned out to be relatively brief. At first, besides seeing the sights, Paul White attended rewarding pathology conferences with Professors Jakob Erdheim and Hermann Chiari, x-ray conferences with Hugo Roesler, took German lessons, and arranged for a course on the history of medicine given by Professor Max Neuburger. This last was to include Ina White and a group of Bostonians also in Vienna, Dr. Fuller Albright, Dr. and Mrs. Joseph Aub and Dr. Dwight O'Hara. Paul White also began to buy very cheaply some old medical books. However, this proved to be an exceptionally cold winter in Vienna, and fortunately an alternative attractive warm spot was available. The evening before the Whites had left Paris, they had tea with Dr. Alan Gregg, a Harvard Medical School graduate and a former intern at the MGH who was Medical Director in Europe for the Rockefeller Foundation. Two years earlier, the Greggs had spent a delightful winter and spring in a villa on the Island of Capri. At Gregg's strong recommendation, Paul White had investigated and found that Casa Surya, which the Greggs had occupied, was available. The rent for five rooms and bath was $80 a month, with two maids by the day for an additional $16 a month. The modest rent was an important feature as not only was his grant from Harvard small, but earnings from his practice had of course stopped for the moment; further, he had begun to send monthly checks to his sister to help in the support of her family, a subsidy which had to be continued for several years. The attractions—climate, geography, economy—were irresistible and at the end of January the Whites left Vienna for Casa Surya in Anacapri on the Island of Capri.

The change proved a complete success. Paul White wrote to his father on February 25:

This is the life of Riley! Never have we lived so leisurely or carefree an existence. No noise, no *autos* (only one or two on the whole island and they are down at Capri), no *telephone*, no patients, no medical meetings or doctors, no acquaintances except our amiable, old lady neighbor Miss DeSwart who doesn't bother us but helps whenever we ask her to.

His writing schedule involved two and a half hours in the morning, one hour in the afternoon, one hour in early evening and another hour at night. Ina White worked along with him helping in a variety of ways with the text and the references. In between, he and his wife enjoyed the sunny garden, the magnificent views of Vesuvius, Sorrento and the Bays of Naples and Salerno, the olive orchards and vineyards, and the many walks down to Capri itself. This proved to be an ideal environment for undisturbed productive writing, very different from Paul White's usual routine when faced with a publication deadline which meant long, late hours. He once told his associate Gordon S. Myers "Well, of course I have always found that the best time to write is between 1:00 and 4:00 or 5:00 in the morning. Hardly anyone ever bothers you and you can really do a lot of uninterrupted work." On another occasion, his colleague Howard Sprague shared a hotel room with him in Washington and woke at 4:00 a.m. to find Paul White busily writing—on the subject of the evils of overwork. When Louise Wheeler and Conger Williams collaborated with him in writing a textbook of electrocardiography, they would meet at night as the days were very full.

> We would sit down and Dr. White had marked ahead how far we would go that night. It was always beyond our endurance. We would be yawning. We would be hiding our yawns behind our hands or our papers, and he would plow straight ahead. We would work until midnight, 1:00 a.m., or later, and then have to go home.

The five-plus hours of work on the book each day in Capri were enough to allow him to make rapid progress without late nights. Indeed it is extraordinary that his output was so great. He obviously knew just what he wanted to say, wrote quickly, and all in his beautiful, clear script. His references were well organized. On February 25 he had finished nine chapters, by April 21 he had finished 22 chapters, and by May 26 the first draft of the entire book of 34 chapters had been completed. On June 3 he mailed the last portion of the manuscript back to his office where his excellent secretary, Agnes Donovan, was doing the typing. She found that transcription of the hand-written text was at times difficult because some of the sections were "written on transparent paper with additions and corrections which traveled up and around the sides of the paper." The entire book, which he titled *Heart Disease*, had been written in five months although revisions and proofreading were still to come. (The revisions were time-consuming as Paul White was a perfectionist and continued to make changes, and many of them, even in the final proof, to the consternation of the publisher.)

In keeping with the article which he and Myers had written in 1921, the published version was in four parts: first, the symptoms and signs; second, the incidence, causes and types of heart disease; third, the structural abnormalities; and fourth, disorders of function. There were 931 pages, nearly 200 of which were devoted to a massive bibliography including many historical references, and there were 9 tables and 119 illustrations. Evidence of his interest in medical history were lengthy quotations from some of the great figures in the past, including Withering and Laennec. The book was dedicated to the memory of his father, and Paul White said in the preface that he wrote it because of "the need of a clear, concise and comprehensive presentation of the diagnoses and treatment of heart disease in the light of our present knowledge."

The book was intended essentially for the student and practitioner, not for the investigator; it benefitted enormously from his ability to put down on paper in clear, lucid language his years of experience with patients as well as what he had absorbed from the literature. It promptly met with a very favorable reception and became a standard text used throughout the world. An example of the response it received was mentioned in a letter to Paul White from one of his medical school classmates, Ernest Gruening, who, while Governor of the Territory of Alaska, wrote that his own physician referred to *Heart Disease* as "our bible on the heart." The reviews the book received in the medical journals were generally very flattering. *The New England Journal of Medicine* commented that it was "The most important practical publication on the subject of heart disease that has appeared in this country during the past decade or two." The *British Medical Journal* reviewer wrote that "He has sifted an immense mass of important contributions to the subject in producing a treatise that must have a strong influence upon cardiological thought of today." Generally laudatory reviews appeared in many other journals. The most critical view came from the British journal *Lancet* which noted

"Its chief defect—namely a lack of perspective. There is too much detail, too little emphasis on some of the main points." The writer was evidently a member of the old school because he lamented the inadequate discussions of influenza, focal infections and gout.

Over the next twenty years, three more editions appeared, the last in 1951, and the book was translated into Spanish and Italian. One of his distinguished students, Dr. J. Willis Hurst, who later wrote with a number of collaborators a highly successful text on heart disease has described Paul White's book as "a turning point in cardiology", stressing its important organization of the clinical material, the happy reflection of his extensive patient experience, and the magnificent bibliography.

In time after World War II as the knowledge about the heart and circulation was vastly extended through new technological advances including cardiac catheterization and refined x-ray methods for visualizing the heart and arteries and veins, the book became considerably outdated. It became important for students and physicians to have a text which emphasized both the modern understanding of the physiological processes involved, and the wide range of methods employed to provide this information. Further, it became apparent that in the future it would be impossible for a single author to possess the competence to write such a book although Charles K. Friedberg did so with remarkable results for some years. However, *Heart Disease* by Paul Dudley White remains a classic, still very useful for reference and as a permanent record of the astute views of a great clinician.

As a lecturer, Paul White was sometimes superb and sometimes frankly dull. He enjoyed appearing before audiences of any size, would not be tense or nervous, always had made preparations for his talk including an outline or if the occasion was very important a written text, and made frequent use of slides. He liked to refer to patients he had known who demonstrated interesting aspects of his subject, or to an item of medical history; and he might make witty remarks which enlivened his presentation. His message was lucid and graceful. His voice was clear and his accent pure Bostonian. Short of stature and thin, balding, gray-haired and with rimless glasses, he lacked the impressive appearance and dynamic platform style of some of his surgical colleagues. Rather, he was articulate and authoritative and could be charming. Often, and indeed much of the time, his presentation came off well or even brilliantly and he was widely sought after as a speaker at medical meetings and at luncheons and dinners of various professional and lay groups. However, there were occasions when he seemed too dry and scholarly to appeal to his listeners. One of his largest and most appreciative audiences was in 1964 at the Coliseum in Portland, Oregon where he spoke before 12,000 people for the Oregon Heart Association. Yet, he never appeared bored or annoyed if the group he was asked to address turned out to be only a dozen people.

He was meticulous about appearing on time for lectures—although not always for other commitments—and was unhappy when he was forced to be late. Once when he missed his train to Montreal where he was to speak the next day, he got into his car and drove all night from Boston in order not to disappoint his audience. There was another episode when he had been in London and had accepted a commitment at the Medical School of the University of California in San Francisco to make a presentation to the outstanding graduating student. By flying from London to San Francisco over the North Pole, he found he would just have time to give the award and the lecture which went with it. The flight was unfortunately two hours late, however, and Paul White arrived to find the huge audience waiting patiently. Without any respite he proceeded to give an excellent talk with no sign of fatigue. He spent that night with his former student Dr. Francis Chamberlain who recalls how, before retiring, Paul White made the unusual request for a sedative as he felt worn out. When queried as to the type of sedative he wanted, Paul White replied "a walk up the hill with you and the dog."

Paul White was at his best in small groups or with a single student on the wards of the MGH and at the bedside of a patient. Here he was in his element. One of his associates, Dr. Edwin O. Wheeler stated what each of his former students and associates have said, ". . . on a one-to-one basis, or in a small group of individuals, he was a superb teacher. . . ."

There were several ingredients in this success. One was his knowledge and experience. He was an acute observer all his life and had a good memory for recalling events and situations and the work of others which could contribute to an understanding of the problem at hand. He was able to use this long and varied background judiciously and with common sense, arriving at conclusions in a quiet, logical and impressive manner. But he did not live solely in the past. Even though he was not primarily interested in laboratory medicine he was remarkably receptive to new ideas and new techniques, even in his 70's and 80's, especially if they related closely to the patient. He might refer to these in his teaching to the astonishment of many students who expected to be exposed only to

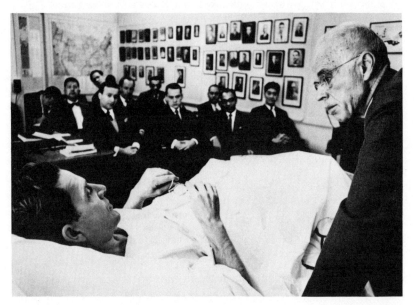

A teaching exercise in the Paul White conference room, basement of Bulfinch Building, Massachusetts General Hospital.

a series of aging clinical anecdotes. He always wanted to know more. Dr. Edgar Haber, who is now the Chief of Cardiology at the MGH in Paul White's old post, found that "When I talked about things which were really very far out of the range of his experience, he was immediately perceptive of their potential and extremely encouraging, feeling that it was time for this new direction to be undertaken. . . ."

Combined with this was his usual, almost boyish enthusiasm for his subject. One of his former students recalls how Paul White and a group consisting of the resident and two interns and four students would sit in the center of one of the old wards of the MGH discussing a patient. Paul White would so enjoy talking about the case, that he was oblivious to the absence of one of the students who, after having been attentive for a couple of hours, would quietly leave to get a glass of milk to relieve his ulcer pains. Dr. Benedict Massell, who worked with him in the Rheumatic Fever Clinic recalled: "He was extremely enthusiastic about everything. When we were going over patients together and there was a finding of interest, you would think it was the first time he had ever noticed it, although it was old hat to him; but he would be very enthusiastic about it and he imparted this to the students. I believe this was one of the things that made him a wonderful teacher."

Paul White's extraordinary ability to concentrate and ignore competing distractions was shown one night at home when with a group of associates, he was discussing clinical research problems and as was customary was leading the conversation. Distracting to the others but not to the host was a continuing playful chase of Penny's kitten about the room by the dachshund Jimmy, the little cat eluding Jimmy by getting on tables, the mantel piece, and book shelves. Finally, the kitten climbed up the side of Paul White's wing chair, stationed itself at the top overlooking his balding head, and extending one paw playfully patted the pate below. It was only then, when the others broke into laughter, that Paul White realized what had been going on, joined in the laughter himself, and then resumed his discussion having been interrupted for no more than 15 seconds.

This total happy preoccupation with a patient or a topic meant that he often forgot about time and might teach through the lunch hour. Gordon Myers has said that he became "So wrapped up in what he was doing and thinking that the fact that the time had come to catch a plane or to do something else didn't attract his attention." Paul White and Myers were discussing a patient in the lobby of the hospital late one afternoon when Paul White looked at his watch and exclaimed: "Oh my! My plane for Europe takes off in three minutes. Now what should I do?" Somehow, such minor crises were always resolved successfully, partly because of the tolerance of others and partly because in this area he seems to have led an unusually charmed life.

Much of his success as an instructor came through the example he set. The imprint of his style and his standards quickly became permanent in all of those who served as his residents or his associates. This imprint did not wash off. He was a master at sitting down with a patient and extracting a detailed history of the illness in a fashion which the patient thoroughly enjoyed. No one who saw him go through this exercise could help but be impressed by the tremendous importance of listening, and listening with the utmost courtesy and patience. Similarly, he was skillful in the physical examination, although this usually received less attention than what the patient said. He also set a standard by the record he kept of his observations with each patient, and his notes entered into the hospital charts were marvels of brevity, clarity and logic. When he found that he wished to change a word in a note he had written, he would not cross out the one to be changed but would take an ink eraser from his pocket, remove the ill-chosen word or phrase, and write in the new word or words. His handwriting was invariably legible, something which could not be said of most of his contemporaries. (The Chief of Gynecology at the MGH, Dr. Joe V. Meigs, once wrote a totally illegible consultation note in a ward patient's chart; the Chief of Medicine, Dr. James Howard Means, tried to decipher it and giving up wrote a note in the chart to Meigs asking him to write out the consultation report again; only to have Meigs return and find that he could not read the note Means had written.)

One limitation in his teaching for some was his lack of interest in the physiology (that is the study of function) of the processes he observed. He approved of what went on in the laboratory including research in cardiac physiology but he relied most on what he learned from the history and the examination of the patient and his teachings reflected this. Because he was widely read, and receptive to what was new, he was often informed, but not necessarily comfortable in applying basic new knowledge to the problem at hand. Such was of course not unusual among physicians who taught medicine, surgery and the various specialties during the nineteenth and the first third or more of the twentieth century.

Thereafter, as sophisticated methods for study of the heart and circulation were developed which were adapted for human subjects, the leaders in cardiology were exposed more and more to a new and exciting perspective. Paul White was an observer but not a participant in this perspective.

Yet, in the late 1940s he did indeed support and obtain funds for a new laboratory for cardiac catheterization at the MGH. At the same time, he encouraged the Chief of Surgery, Dr. Edward D. Churchill, to assign a young member of the surgical staff, Dr. J. Gordon Scannell, to work in this laboratory in addition to gaining experience in the rapidly developing field of heart surgery. He advised one of his students, Richard Cosby, to study in Cleveland with the very eminent physiologist Carl Wiggers, and was decidedly helpful to Dr. Lewis Dexter whose catheterization laboratory at the Peter Bent Brigham Hospital antedated that at the MGH. Dr. Dexter has told how early in his training he had been offered a position to work under Dr. White, but after some soul searching decided to study instead at the Boston City Hospital for a career in research under the exciting Dr. Soma Weiss who was an outstanding clinical investigator and teacher. Paul White "Never expressed any resentment that I didn't come to work with him. He seemed awfully pleased that I had a good job with somebody else that he admired." Later Paul White was very supportive of Dexter's own research work across town at the Peter Bent Brigham Hospital and indicated that "Anything he could do to push me ahead, he would do." In retrospect, it is a regretful item of Harvard Medical history that although the outstanding physiologist Walter B. Cannon was Professor of Physiology at the Harvard Medical School from 1906 to 1942 and therefore very accessible to Paul White and vice versa, and although they knew each other well socially, there is no record of any joint projects discussed, planned or completed. The pair, Cannon the physiologist and White the clinician, might have made an interesting complementary scientific team.

The opportunities for Paul White to teach were many, but because of his multiple interests and obligations, there had to be some limit. Since his teaching paid him nothing, and he received no salary from the Medical

School or hospital, his practice had to be maintained as his main base of support. Yet, throughout his active years at the MGH, he took his turn teaching on the medical wards, meeting a team of a medical resident, two interns and several medical students five mornings a week for eight weeks a year. In addition, beginning in the 1920's he started to accept for a month or more each year a few medical students as well as a few physicians who had already graduated from medical school and wanted an exposure to cardiology and to Paul White. This soon became very popular, especially for young doctors from Central and South America, and in time a formal one-year course for ten or so graduates was organized under the auspices of the Medical School. One 1944 testimonial to this experience was that of a young Brazilian doctor who wrote to the Institute of Inter American Affairs which had made the arrangements for his postgraduate study: "But I want to express my big gratitude and admiration to Dr. Paul D. White, the most skillful cardiologist I ever saw. Dr. White has discovered the way to associate in his own personality three individuals that I used to meet separately: the researchman, the clinician, and the professor, although I bet that teaching is his favorite hobby. I will never forget his magnificent lessons. . . ." There were also briefer review courses, especially in the summers, which attracted practitioners who could only afford to be away for a relatively short period.

Over the years, the alumni of these courses became scattered all over the world. Thus was built up a highly effective network of devoted, grateful former students and when Paul White travelled, they were eager to greet their former teacher, act as host, and arrange for lectures and tours as well as impose upon him for consultations with private patients. To have been a former student of Dr. Paul Dudley White, even if only for a short time, carried enormous prestige, particularly in Central and South America, Asia and Africa. Beginning in 1944 under the aegis of the American College of Physicians, an intensive one-week course in cardiology for physicians began to be presented each autumn at the hospital under the direction of Paul White. This proved very successful and indeed in its first year was oversubscribed by 150.

Needless to say, except for the annual eight weeks of ward teaching,

Paul White relied heavily upon his associates to share in the teaching load. As he became more and more committed to the activities of the National Heart Institute, the International Society of Cardiology and the International Cardiology Foundation, his colleagues assumed the largest share of this burden and his clinic and hospital teaching declined dramatically. His instruction orbit was not, of course, restricted to Boston, and starting early in his career he was invited to lecture before medical groups all over the United States. It was not long before his audience became international.

A special opportunity was provided each year from 1920 on to the lucky individual who served for twelve months as Cardiac Resident at the hospital under the supervision of Paul White and then usually stayed for another year with the title of fellow as an assistant to him in his practice

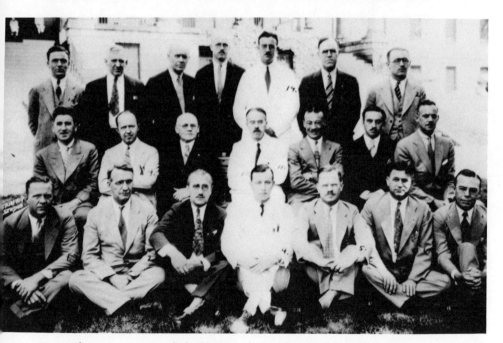

Postgraduate Course in cardiology, Massachusetts General Hospital, August, 1929.
Dr. Edward F. Bland, in white, front row center; Dr. Paul D. White, in white, middle row center; and Dr. Howard B. Sprague, in white, top row center.

and teaching. Dr. Howard B. Sprague, who was the resident in 1924, was the first of several who stayed on at the MGH at the conclusion of training as a permanent member of the cardiology group. From the former residents and fellows who trained under Paul White came four presidents of the American Heart Association, several full professors including department chairmen, and a long list of distinguished practicing cardiologists located from Seattle and Montreal in the north to Los Angeles and St. Petersburg in the south. These residents and fellows more than any others became aware of certain remarkable features of their leader. It was these qualities which helped explain why at the conclusion of their training, none of Paul White's young men ever went away disenchanted, or antagonistic.

For example, he never lost his temper and upbraided anyone. When displeased, it was apparent but it was very low key. Often this was indicated by absolute silence. Dr. Gordon Myers has commented: "I can remember a number of times when, having said something unwise, Dr. White would make a comment which sounded quite innocent at the time. It was only later on that I realized that the rug had been pulled gently out from under my feet. As an example, I recall after a rather pompous statement on my part about the diagnosis of a congenital heart disease patient, he said 'Isn't that interesting. Are you sure?' It was obvious that I was very sure at the time, but later on thinking about his remark, I became much less so."

He was generous with his young fellows and associates. He solicited their opinions, and respected them. He would often tell a patient that a procedure or drug which had worked out well was a suggestion of the resident or fellow. In writing a scientific paper with Paul White, the junior collaborator was almost always the one to be listed first in the roster of authors. Dr. Ashton Graybiel who was one of his early residents and who became a leader in naval aviation medicine collaborated with Paul White in writing a successful textbook on electrocardiography. Ashton Graybiel has written

> One did not need to be directly associated with Dr. White to deduce that he
> was a man of integrity, but such association revealed that he was a person of

great integrity. This is illustrated by an event which occurred just prior to the first appearance of *Electrocardiography in Practice*. The publishers strongly urged that the seniority of authorship be reversed [the authors were to be listed as Graybiel and White], pointing out the salutary influence on sales. If there had been a question in Dr. White's mind regarding seniority, which I doubt, this demarché quickly settled it. His instant decision cemented one inter-personal relation for good. That he was ambitious is evident, but it never led him into temptation.

He was tireless in trying to help people, particularly young people, to obtain favorable training positions or scholarships or practice opportunities. And he would make a major effort for anyone whom he had trained or held in respect. A review of his correspondence in this regard is an extraordinary experience, as he was constantly imposed upon by good, indifferent and bad people including many who had taken one of his courses for only a week who found that he would always answer their letters, usually give them the benefit of any doubt, and as often as possible would try to help. A letter from Paul White, even if noncommittal, was regarded by many as the ultimate recommendation for getting a research post, obtaining an industrial medical position, being appointed to an influential office in Washington, securing entree into Russia to do medical research, being awarded an honor, receiving state licensure in medicine, obtaining a research grant, getting a travel grant, and so on. He clearly found it hard to ignore an appeal or to say no.

An example of his generous spirit in helping young scientists was evident toward the end of his life in his role in the legal proceedings between Dr. Jeremiah Stamler and the Un-American Affairs Committee of the United States House of Representatives. Jeremiah Stamler was a young physician who had chosen a life of medical research and teaching and was attached to the Chicago Board of Health as Head of its Division of Adult Health and Aging. He had gotten to know Paul White through membership in the Research Committee of the International Society of Cardiology—indeed Paul White and Ancel Keys had placed him on the Committee and both had fostered his career. Like many young scientists, he was liberal in his political views. One day in the Spring of 1965, Stamler stepped off the elevator in the Health Department Building in

Chicago and was handed a subpoena to appear on May 25 before the House Committee on Un-American Activities which was conducting a hearing in Chicago on Communist influences in Chicago. The Committee, chaired by Representative Edwin E. Willis of Louisiana, was known for its flamboyant and intimidating interrogation of witnesses designed more to glorify the Committee members in the media than to ascertain the truth regarding alleged Communist activity.

Stamler obtained legal advice and sought a private hearing in Executive Session before the Committee as well as the right to question witnesses who might testify against him. Both of these requests were denied and he thereupon declined to testify. He (and Mrs. Yolanda Hall who had also received a subpoena) resolved to fight the Committee, believing that it had no right to force citizens to answer questions regarding their political views, especially without the opportunity to confront and interrogate any accusers.

Legal proceedings of this kind were clearly going to be protracted and expensive and so a Jeremiah Stamler Legal Aid Fund was set up. Paul White agreed to be its Chairman, a masterly selection since if anyone did not look or sound like a Communist it was he. Actually, Paul White's political views were quite liberal and it was in character for him to give his support to the Fund. In a letter Paul White wrote to *The New England Journal of Medicine* on April 27, 1966, he said: "The details of the techniques of the House Un-American Activities Committee are seriously and justifiably questioned in the suit brought against the Committee, because it is quite evident that they are both antiquated and undemocratic."

Stamler and his associates then began a major effort to raise money, chiefly but not entirely from scientists. Paul White repeatedly signed letters appealing for financial and moral support, wrote to various Congressmen and others of influence explaining the nature of the suit, and at the age of 83 in May 1970 flew to Chicago to speak at an art auction which raised $31,000 for the cause. The legal proceedings dragged on for eight years with the expenses mounting to $500,000, most of which was covered by the Fund. Finally, shortly after Paul White's death in October

1973, the United States Supreme Court decided in favor of Stamler and Hall, testimony to an effective and courageous stand against an abuse of Congressional privilege.

Unlike many of his peers who took advantage of their junior assistants who did the "scut" work for little pay, he was eminently fair in his financial dealings with his young associates. He did not exploit them. As Dr. Conger Williams has said: "We felt he was very fair. We were well paid by the standards of those days for being his fellows and taking care of his hospital patients. There was no feeling of resentment about that. I think he was very scrupulous about financial matters."

He was considerate in other ways too, such as when he was invited to come to Chicago on the occasion of the retirement of one of his former residents from the post of chief of medicine. The invitation came from the young members of the house staff in the Chicago hospital who said they could not afford an honorarium or first-class ticket, but would be able to pay for a round trip coach fare. Despite his age of 85 years, he accepted the invitation and flew to and from Boston in a coach seat in order not to disappoint his protege and the young doctors who had invited him. When one of his residents finished his training, he and if married, his wife, would be invited to dinner with the Whites and he would receive a valuable old medical book from Paul White's library.

Paul and Ina White also did their best to make the many students attached to the Cardiac Laboratory at the MGH and their wives feel at home. There would be regular visits to the White's farm in Harvard, Massachusetts to which the secretaries and technicians would also be invited. There would be a picnic, baseball or touch football, excellent food and drink, and sometimes a talk by Paul White about one of his books describing an interesting event in the history of cardiology. Agnes Donovan Walsh who was his first secretary wrote about one of these occasions:

> I recall that while we were playing baseball, Dr. White stole third, ran into a big Texan there and broke a rib, and then proceeded to steal home where I was at bat. He slid into me, feet first, knocking me down. He stayed down, and it was discovered that he had broken a bone in his leg. During his few days of

hospitalization thereafter, his patients came to his bedside, some in wheel-chairs, and he talked with them, leaning out from his bed to listen to the heart sounds. Soon he was running through the underground passages from the Phillips House [where he was a patient] to the Cardiac Lab on the iron which had been imbedded in the cast.

On another occasion, an admiral in the Navy Medical Corps who was taking one of Paul White's courses came out to a picnic, handsomely adorned in his white and gold uniform. There was a small pond on the place and the White's son Sandy invited the admiral to go out with him on a little rowboat that he had built. The naval officer did so somewhat apprehensively, and the picnic became a resounding success when the boat sank into the mud, leaving Sandy and the now wet and dirty admiral to struggle to the bank to the ill-concealed delight of the onlookers.

Personal relations between Paul White and his associates and students were characterized by a high degree of mutual respect. For most of the group around him, it was not an informal, relaxed, intimate relationship. Nearly all of them, including those who were full members of his cardiology department at the hospital called him "Dr. White" and not "Paul." Dr. Howard Sprague was one of the few who called him by his first name. There was warmth and there was affection and he was a decidedly friendly person, but also there was a limit, a barrier, imposed perhaps by a combination of differing generations and a New England family background which allowed intimacy to go only so far. As one former resident has said: "I felt as though I was very close to him, but I felt that his mission in life appeared to be stronger than his desire to relax and participate in what was going on at the moment." Paul White was not one to encourage his students and associates to discuss their personal, family and social problems with him, although sometimes this occurred, nor did he allude to his own problems with them. He was not a confidant. However, when aware that a problem existed in the life of a student or resident, he would be genuinely concerned and make a real effort to be helpful.

Dr. Gardner Middlebrook has described one episode in which what Paul White taught was very different from the usual clinical instruction.

It was December 1944, in the midst of World War II, and Paul White was that month assigned as the regular teacher for the indigent and low income patients on the West Medical Service at the MGH and Middlebrook was one of the interns there. On Christmas morning, Dr. Middlebrook was quietly making his ward rounds with the nurse, seeing each of the patients and reviewing the charts, when the door opened. In came Paul White, much to their surprise, as usually on a holiday the teacher, being a senior person, was not to be seen unless there was a major problem. Under one arm he had a bouquet of roses and he proceeded to give a Christmas greeting and several of the roses to the nurse and then walked slowly around the ward, saying a reassuring and friendly word to every patient and giving each a rose. The tour of the ward completed, he turned to Middlebrook and graciously gave him the book which was under his other arm, which was a copy of the latest edition of his textbook, suitably inscribed. He then left to return to his family. To the intern, to the nurse, to the patients, this was a Christmas in which they had seen a great physician and teacher who was also a great man.

CHAPTER SEVEN

Organization Man

The leading physicians of the first four decades of the twentieth century mainly occupied their time with seeing patients and, if located in academic centers, with teaching students without pay and perhaps, in a few instances, engaging in research. The era of the growth of professional scientific organizations, of research committees, and of voluntary health associations began around World War II. Thereafter, prominent doctors by choice or sense of duty or both began to devote more and more hours to medical society, health association, and other group scientific business. While they might grumble about these new demands on their time, most enjoyed the experience including the professional camaraderie. Paul White's life and his participation in these activities was typical of this evolution. His involvement in the United States with heart associations started in the 1920's and reached a peak in 1941–43. This was followed in 1948 by leadership in the new National Heart Institute, and this was succeeded in turn by involvement in international organizations. With his research, practice and teaching well established in the 1920's and 1930's, he was ready to put his energies into these new areas. In so doing, the successes he was to achieve were more a reflection of his personality and professional stature than of his organizational and administrative ability. He molded the image of the "organization man" to fit his own talents and leaned upon others to accomplish the tasks he neither did well nor enjoyed.

Voluntary health associations such as the American Heart Association started as scientific bodies with a coming together of physicians and others interested in a particular field for a discussion of scientific data, the presentation of the results of investigations, consideration of significant problems, and the promotion of a spirit of fellowship. With time, they became diverse in membership and broadened their programs to encompass varied community services and solicited financial support from the public. The first of these, the National Tuberculosis Association, which started in Pennsylvania in 1892, became a national movement in 1904. The American Society for the Control of Cancer was founded in 1913, and the American Social Hygiene Association was formed in 1914 as a merging of national and local services to control and prevent syphilis and gonorrhea.

The impetus to found a heart association came from an increasing awareness of the magnitude of the problems of heart disease. In New York City in the five-year period 1911–1915, deaths attributable to diseases of the cardiovascular system for the first time exceeded the numbers of deaths from pulmonary tuberculosis, hitherto number one in the mortality statistics. This reversal of the sequence in the vital statistics tables was a reflection in part of the decline in numbers of deaths from tuberculosis and other infectious diseases; and in part a consequence of the increasing age of the population, whereby more men and women acquired and died from heart disease. As Dr. Haven Emerson wrote in 1957: "We had saved the infant, the youth, the young manhood and womanhood to live into the seventh decade of life and die of causes which selectively attack the aged of the population and which are not in the present state of medical science preventable to any high degree. What appeared to be a sudden and ominous shift in mortality had its gradual origins over a half-century and was in fact an encouraging and calculable result of long-sustained public health efforts."

Leadership in developing a heart association came from New York City where Dr. Lewis A. Conner presided on July 14, 1915 at the New York Academy of Medicine at a meeting of physicians to consider the formation of a Society for the Prevention and Relief of Heart Disease. The group proposed to move forward, a constitution was written, articles of incorporation completed, and on December 15, 1915, Dr. Conner was formally elected President of the Association for Prevention and Relief of Heart Disease of New York City. Its aims included the dissemination of knowledge regarding prevention, research into methods of early detection and prevention, and organization of better facilities for care including convalescent care. Its program, as adopted in January 1916, was designed in part "to encourage the setting up of branch (or like) associations elsewhere." Financing was greatly helped by contributions from the Burke Foundation, but the budget was a small one averaging less than $4000 a year.

Similar activity got under way in Boston and in Philadelphia five years later. At 8:00 o'clock on the evening of February 3, 1921, there was a meeting in Boston at 202 Commonwealth Avenue, the home of Dr. William H. Robey, Jr. Present were nine doctors interested in the field of cardiology representing the Boston City Hospital, the Boston Dispensary, the children's and adult departments of the Massachusetts General Hospital, and the Peter Bent Brigham Hospital; the group included Drs. Samuel A. Levine, Joseph H. Pratt, and Paul White as well as the heads of social work at the Boston City Hospital and the Massachusetts General Hospital, Miss Gertrude Farmer and Miss Ida M. Cannon. The minutes, written by Paul White, stated that the "Meeting opened by outline of needs of association and cooperation of the cardiac clinics in Boston, more or less according to the experience of the New York Association of Cardiac Clinics" [i.e., the Association for Prevention and Relief of Heart Disease in New York City]. Topics for consideration and future action included diagnostic classifications, pooling of research interests, the issues of heart disease in industry and in the schools, and the "study and practice" of prevention. The final note in the minutes recorded that "Through the hospitality of Dr. Robey, a supper was served after the meeting."

A second meeting on April 15, 1921, also at the home of Dr. Robey, resulted in adoption of the name Boston Association of Cardiac Clinics, the election of Dr. Robey as Chairman and Paul White as Secretary, selection of an Executive Committee, and a report by Paul White that Dr. Robert H. Halsey, an officer of the New York City Association, would come to Boston to address the group at its next meeting. Dr. Halsey did so on May 20, 1921 at the Surgical Amphitheater of the Boston City Hospital before more than 100 persons. This was followed on Wednesday afternoon, June 15, 1921, by a meeting at the "Cardiographic Laboratory" of the MGH presided over by Paul White at which the group agreed to protest the proposed abandonment of the Social Service Department at the Children's Hospital. Dr. W. D. Reid of the Boston Dispensary and Paul White also reported on a conference at the New York Academy of Medicine on June 13, 1921 called to consider use of a common clinical record for the cardiac clinics in New York, Boston, and Philadelphia. Thus was a heart association launched in the Boston area.

At the first meeting of the new Association the next fall on October 14, 1921, a schedule of clinical meetings on alternate months at the major teaching hospitals was adopted, and these meetings constituted the principal program of the Association. This established a singularly happy format which was to last for more than 25 years, a routine which brought the doctors in the Boston area interested in heart disease together regularly. Each of the major teaching hospitals, by playing host once a year, had an opportunity to have staff members—especially the younger ones and trainees—prepare and present research material to an expert local audience. The best of these reports would be presented later at national meetings, and many would appear in print. Indeed, in the early years of the Association, the papers were regularly published by the *Boston Medical and Surgical Journal* (which was to become later the *New England Journal of Medicine*).

It is significant that in New York City, Boston, Philadelphia and also in Chicago, which organized its own association in April 1922, these young local associations from the outset included lay members on their boards of directors. To be sure, they constituted only a modest, usually affluent minority, but by their presence, they indicated the desirability of establishing a broad base of support in the community. Also significant in terms of the breadth of their interest were both the inclusion of social workers in the membership, and the frequent discussions and concerns regarding the cardiac clinics for the indigent, the health of the schoolchildren, the problems of heart disease in the workplace, and the need for prevention. It was not envisioned by the physician leaders that they would launch large fund-raising campaigns as the National Foundation for Infantile Paralysis was to do later, and indeed their reluctance to embark on a major fund-raising effort sharply limited the scope of their programs.

Writing to a prospective member of the Board of Governors of the Association on November 17, 1922, Paul White emphasized that now was the time to act: "We feel that Boston and New England should keep abreast of the times in this new field of work. . . . The problem is a big one but I do not think that it is to be regarded as a visionary one. When one sees, as we all do, the tremendous crippling of the young people of the community by heart disease [and here he was referring to the impact of rheumatic fever], it is obvious that something needs to be done. I am sure that eventually something will be done, and it seems to me that the present is a favorable time to make a start."

The succeeding years saw the slow growth of the Association which proved to be a healthy and successful, albeit limited undertaking. It was agreed on February 16, 1922 that the services of a paid secretary should be secured, but it was not until May 1923 that Paul White was requested to interview a lady and offer her $1,000 "or less" for part-time work. A Miss Ruth Symonds was finally hired who was to work out of her office at the Harvard Medical School, as no other office space was available. The following year, Paul White wrote to Miss Katherine Ham of the Social Service Department at the Allegheny General Hospital in Pittsburgh offering her the job of full-time executive secretary of the Association at a salary of $2,000 a year, but the offer was declined. Speakers from out-of-town were invited to address the group—Dr. William St. Lawrence of St. Luke's Hospital, New York City, in January 1922; Dr. Louis I. Dublin of the Metropolitan Life Insurance Company of New York in May 1922; Prof. K. F. Wenckebach of Vienna in May 1923; and Dr. Louis Gross of New York in December 1925.

At the meeting of December 21, 1922, it was resolved to change the name from the Boston Association of Cardiac Clinics to the Boston Association for the Prevention and Relief of Heart Disease and to seek incorporation; and as a result, there was a public hearing at the Massa-

chusetts State House before the Commissioner of Corporations on March
23, 1923. The session appears to have been uneventful, Paul White only
noting in the minutes in his own handwriting "Discussion in favor by
obese M.D.'s widow." A distinguished Board of Governors was selected
which included Dr. Richard Cabot, Miss Ida Cannon, Mr. C. E. Cotting,
Mr. Arthur S. Johnson, Dr. Roger I. Lee, Dr. Samuel A. Levine, Mrs.
Henry Lyman, Dr. Francis Peabody, Dr. Joseph H. Pratt, Mr. A. C.
Ratshesky, Mrs. Fritz B. Talbot, Dr. Conrad Wesselhoeft, and Miss Ma-
bel Wilson. It was considered wise to recruit additional well-to-do interested Bostonians who were not already over-committed—not an easy
task, as one of the physicians noted in writing apologetically to Paul
White that he was "sorry that I do not know of any rich people who I
think would do." On May 10, 1923, Paul White was elected Chairman
of the Board of Governors of the Association. He did not like the cum-
bersome name which had been adopted by the new corporation, writing
on October 17, 1924: "We hope to change the name of this organization
shortly to the Massachusetts Heart Association which should be quite an
improvement. . . ." A change, but to a yet different name, was finally
accomplished on December 18, 1924 when at a meeting of the Board of
Governors "The motion was made by Dr. White and passed that the
name of this Association be changed to the New England Heart
Association."

Paul White was elected President of the New England Heart Association on May 15, 1930 and was re-elected for a second one-year term on
June 3, 1931. That the Association had a frugal budget was attested to by
the treasurer's report at this latter meeting indicating expenditures of
$334.88 for the year, with receipts of $534.68, and a bank balance of
$2,024.87. Nothing was said by the treasurer at this time about the salary
of the paid secretary, and perhaps that was found to be a luxury which
could not be afforded. Finally, in November 1949, the New England
Heart Association legally changed its name again, this time to the Massachusetts Heart Association (the name suggested by Paul White 25 years
earlier) although under its aegis there continued to be a New England

Cardiovascular Society. Paul White demonstrated throughout his long life an extraordinary loyalty and interest in the Association. Repeatedly, he would, at its urging, speak before lay and professional or mixed groups. On numerous occasions, he assisted in fund-raising efforts through television and radio talks and public statements. He was indeed a founder who remained its true and faithful friend.

With the appearance of heart associations in New York, Boston, Philadelphia, Chicago, and elsewhere, there came an awareness of the desirability of some kind of national organization to which the local associations could relate. The New York group again took the lead and on April 24, 1922, sent invitations to about 100 physicians from the United States and Canada known to be interested in heart disease to attend a luncheon meeting at the Hotel Claridge in St. Louis on May 24, 1922 at the time of the annual meeting of the American Medical Association. Dr. Robert H. Halsey of New York acted as Chairman of the luncheon, which was attended by 46 physicians. At this luncheon, Dr. Haven Emerson, Professor of Public Health Administration at Columbia University, discussed the rationale for a national organization. He proposed that the "function of such a national group would be coordination of efforts, development of research, collection and distribution of information, public health and industrial education, to develop sound public opinion as to the true meaning and seriousness of the problem." Expressions of support then came from Dr. James B. Herrick of Chicago, the author of the classic 1912 description of coronary thrombosis; Dr. William S. Thayer, Professor of Medicine at Johns Hopkins in Baltimore; Dr. Joseph Sailer, Professor of Medicine at the University of Pennsylvania in Philadelphia; and Paul White. As a consequence, the chairman appointed a committee of five, composed of Drs. Lewis A. Conner, Chairman, James B. Herrick, Hugh McCulloch, Joseph Sailer and Paul D. White, to make specific recommendations.

Dr. Conner wrote a long letter to Paul White on January 3, 1923 suggesting that the new national association undertake chiefly educational work and not attempt to operate clinics or other facilities; he also mentioned that financial support would have to be mainly from foundations and a few large contributors, as membership dues and "ordinary contributions" would be "largely or wholly" expended locally. Paul White noted on the margin of the letter his preference for the name of the organization, the American Association for the Prevention and Relief of Heart Disease, and he formalized this in a letter to Dr. Conner dated February 27, 1923. This letter also suggested that "the type of organization best suited to the purpose would be one made up chiefly of coordinated associations now existing, taking in new local associations as they are formed in cities rather than states." Dr. Conner responded to Paul White on April 25, 1923 and advised following the organizational model of the American Society for the Control of Cancer but added: "The only serious difficulty that I can see is in determining the relation of the local Heart Association to the National Association. The Cancer Society provides for no such local organization." The Committee continued with its discussions, apparently at a measured pace, and finally the name of the new organization was decided upon—the American Heart Association, a certificate of incorporation in the State of New York was signed March 14, 1924, and on the evening of June 10, 1924 at the Drake Hotel on the Chicago lakefront, a board of directors, officers, and an executive committee were chosen. Unlike the Cancer Society, the American Heart Association (AHA) chose a federal type of organization, the national Association being composed of local units which were encouraged to continue with their own programs. Dr. Lewis A. Conner of New York became the first President, and Paul White was named as Treasurer.

Thus was ushered in a long 49-year relationship between the American Heart Association and Paul White, one which was beneficial to both, was characterized by warmth and mutual support, and even in later years was singularly lacking in the pettiness and rancor so apt to be seen as statesmen become elder and witness changes which they did not propose or understand. The American Heart Association provided opportunities for Paul White to meet and work with other leading United States physicians active in cardiology. These included especially Dr. H. M. Marvin of Yale, Dr. Arlie Barnes of the Mayo Clinic, Dr. Tinsley Harrison of the Vanderbilt, Southwestern, and University of Alabama Medical Schools, Dr.

Irvine Page of the Cleveland Clinic, Dr. Louis N. Katz of Michael Reese Hospital of Chicago and Dr. Irving Wright of the Cornell Medical School —to mention only a few.

Paul White served the Association in several ways. One of these was as an officer. He was, however, a people person who thrived not on official capacities but on relations with one patient or 1,000 people in an auditorium. He tended to avoid an administrative role unless he felt strongly that this was of especial importance and could be molded by him to emphasize the personal relations incident to the position. His long-term associate, Dr. Howard B. Sprague, was a natural organizer who thrived on making sense out of issues of structure and function, handing down parliamentary decisions, developing by-laws and budgets, and creating charts of committee relationships. Paul White seemed uninterested in these, did not do them well, and much preferred to see them taken over by others whom he trusted. That he did not seek out positions associated with authority and indeed often avoided them suggests that he would not have enjoyed and done well as a dean, chairman of a large department of medicine, or director of one of the National Institutes of Health. (He was Executive Director of the National Advisory Heart Council but never of an Institute.) Further, he found it difficult with his peripatetic lifestyle to hold an office which frequently required his physical presence.

His first official position with the AHA was as Treasurer, which was not very demanding because for years there was almost no money to account for. Thus in 1926, the organization had a bank balance of only $2,094.86. Local heart associations such as that in Boston paid annual dues of only $10, members of the Board of Directors were encouraged to make personal contributions, and the National Tuberculosis Association initially also made a small, annual contribution. Paul White was Treasurer from 1924 through 1932. He seemed to have kept the modest finances in order and perhaps left the office just in time. The Chairman of the Executive Committee, Dr. H. M. (Jack) Marvin was forced on December 20, 1934 to write to all the officers, directors and committee members as follows: "I am deeply embarrassed having to write to you about this matter, but no alternative is apparent to me at the moment. The financial outlook of this Association for the year 1935 is darker than at any time in the past six years. We will start the year with funds on hand sufficient for less than two months of normal activity, even though every possible expense has been reduced or eliminated." Dr. Marvin went on to request personal contributions, and in response, Paul White sent a check for $25. Paul White also served, in these early years, on the Board of Directors and on the Advisory Council, an entity abolished in 1936. In 1936, he was asked to be Chairman of the Program Committee, which was responsible for the annual scientific sessions, a demanding role which he fulfilled conscientiously for six years. Additionally, in 1937 he was a member of a committee to standardize the technique for electrocardiographic chest leads, and in 1938 was serving on a committee to standardize the recording of blood pressure. He became a member of the Executive Committee in 1939 and, in 1940, of the committee to review the arrangements for publication of the Association's scientific journal, the *American Heart Journal.*

He was elected President of the American Heart Association in February 1941 and was re-elected as President in 1942. He had undoubtedly been offered the presidency before but had turned it down due to lack of interest and many other obligations. Indeed, despite being a member of the Board of Directors all through the 1930's, it is apparent that he missed many of its meetings. In a letter to Dr. J. W. Wilce of Ohio State University, written on March 31, 1941, he wrote: "Thank you very much indeed for your letter of March 26, including your congratulations. As a matter of fact, I steered clear of the American Heart for some years, but now with the war emergency and on the job as Chairman of the Heart Committee of the National Research Council advising the Surgeons General, it seemed to me I could be of additional service by accepting the presidency of the American Heart Association in order to correlate the work toward the war effort in whatever direction may be needed." In February 1941, he was 54 years old and was not likely to see military service again. As he anticipated, many of the younger cardiologists in the country, including several in his own laboratory, were soon to go off to war. As a senior figure in the field and now involved with a responsible post in Washington, it was his turn to head the Association which he had helped to found 19 years earlier. The fact that his associate, Howard B. Sprague, was elected Secretary in 1941 nominally gave Paul White a person close to him geographically and familiar with his thinking who could help with many of the details on the job; but Howard Sprague in a few months was to depart for duty in the Navy.

The two-year period in which Dr. White was President of the AHA was a difficult one. With the existence of a state of war after December 7, 1941, it became increasingly awkward to have meetings, carry on committee work and have high-caliber presentations at the annual scientific sessions. Another new problem area surrounded the recent decision to create a subspecialty board to certify doctors as heart specialists, an undertaking in which the AHA was advising the American Board of Internal Medicine. This was a very sensitive issue, particularly for older, established physicians who wished to be certified as cardiologists, but did not want to take or were afraid to take the examination, and therefore sought inclusion under a "grandfather" clause which permitted certification without examination. Another chronic problem present since 1924 and to persist apparently permanently was that some local heart groups periodically made it known that they and their interests were inadequately recognized by the national Association and that something should be done about it, preferably at once. Each viewed its situation as unique and therefore deserving of special consideration. There was also the familiar petty but important problem of performance and morale of the small staff in the office. Fortunately these and most other details were handled with . extraordinary dedication by Jack Marvin who documented them in lengthy letters to Dr. White which the latter acknowledged with brevity and decisiveness.

Despite the pressures of the war, this was also a period in which questions were being asked as to the future role of the Association. Dr. Harold Rosenblum of San Francisco was appointed chairman of a committee to explore this problem, resulting in submission of a report to Paul White on September 24, 1942. The report advised an expanded program with four equal emphases—professional education of the physicians, promotion of cardiovascular research, promotion and standardization of community facilities for heart patients, and public education. It suggested that there be a National Heart Day to publicize the problem of heart disease, clarification of the status of local associations, cooperation with the U.S. Public Health Service and the Crippled Children's Bureau of the Federal Children's Bureau, emphasis on heart diseases in industry, and appointment of an Executive Secretary for public health work and cooperation with other associations. It also suggested modest measures to raise money from foundations, local associations, and individuals, but no major fund-raising drive. Paul White noted on the margin of this report: "I heartily approve. The chief problem is to raise money for our new Public Health Officer." His term of office came to an end without a solution to most of these considerations, especially the problem of the money. That these 24 months meant a lot of hard work without adequate finances, staff or volunteer help was apparent. (When Paul White took office, the membership was only 1575 and the bank balance was $2,285.69). That there were also occasional opportunities in New York for relaxation was indicated by one communication from Jack Marvin to Paul White mentioning "the theatre party after the meeting of the Board of Directors when Roy Scott took you, Bill Bunn, and me to see Gypsy Rose Lee in 'Star and Garter.' I emphasize particularly the great difficulty we had in keeping you from leaping onto the stage at some of the more exciting moments."

When after World War II the American Heart Association made the major decision to become a voluntary health association supported by funds raised widely from the public, Paul White took essentially no part in the process of redirection and reorganization. He was not entirely comfortable with the prospect of such a major change but wrote to Marvin on January 17, 1946, "Of course, we have in the past shrunk from all this publicity in keeping the Association very scientific and conservative, but obviously we have got to get away from that." Addressing the annual meeting of the American Heart Association in San Francisco in June 1946, he would say, ". . . a lot of publicity and money raising are often misleading—a few, simple, unhampered workers quietly toiling in laboratories and clinics may accomplish and have already accomplished in many fields in medicine more than a host of ignorant or ill-trained enthusiasts who have shouted of the need of doing something without knowing just what to do or how to do it." But, he would conclude that talk with an upbeat call to the audience to make "the American Heart Association second to none in the field of heart disease throughout the world. With its new program of progressive outlook and participation in public health as well as in scientific discussion, the American Heart Association seeks your aid and support."

A second area of involvement of Paul White in the American Heart Association was in his contributions along scientific lines. As discussed in Chapter Four, early in his professional career, he had acquired the ability to write scientific papers rapidly and well. This was a pattern very different from that of many physicians who might give effective lectures but found preparation of a manuscript so painful that the project would be indefinitely deferred. As his laboratory grew and he attracted more assistants and trainees, the opportunities to prepare jointly-authored scientific papers were numerous. Many of these publications were to appear in print in the official journal of the American Heart Association which from 1925 to 1950 was the *American Heart Journal.* In that 25-year span, Paul White alone or with his associates published 65 scientific papers in the *American Heart Journal.* After 1949 *Circulation* supplanted the *American Heart Journal* as the official major publication of the American Heart Association, and from 1950 until his death in 1973, Paul White and his group contributed seven more papers. Many of these reports were first presented at annual meetings of the Association. Paul White was also on the Editorial Board of the *American Heart Journal* from its inception in 1925 through 1964.

There were other scientific contributions which he made. He was author of a pamphlet on coronary disease published by the American Heart Association in 1943, he wrote two issues of *Modern Concepts of Cardiovascular Disease,* a small AHA leaflet having a very large circulation among physicians, and was responsible for at least two exhibits at the annual meetings of the Association. In his latter years, he showed a great interest in epidemiology and regularly attended and contributed to the scientific sessions of the AHA Council on Epidemiology of Cardiovascular Disease.

He was also Chairman of an AHA Committee on the Effect of Strain and Trauma on the Heart and Great Vessels. Paul White had been involved for many years in the broad area of work and its effects on the heart and circulation, including legal implications. Being an advocate of the benefits of physical exercise except for those individuals for whom it was clearly unwise, he found it difficult to accept the trend of decisions by compensation boards and jurists that the presence of heart disease in a worker was attributable to the physical and mental demands of employment. As a scientist, he found the evidence for such decisions unconvincing. As one concerned with encouraging employment, he also found it highly unfortunate that these decisions prejudiced employers against hiring both men and women with known heart disease, often only trivial and insignificant in amount, as well as older persons who might because of age be suspected of being candidates for future heart trouble. In 1946, he and Hubert Winston Smith, a professor of law, wrote a lengthy report on "Scientific Proof in Respect to Injuries of the Heart" which was published in the *North Carolina Law Review.*

In 1954, the AHA Committee on the Effect of Strain and Trauma on the Heart and Great Vessels, with Paul White its Chairman, began its deliberations which were to extend over 8 years. During this period, Paul White and the Committee persuaded Dean Harold F. McNiece of St. John's University School of Law in Brooklyn, New York, to embark on a research project financed by the National Heart Institute on the legal bases for awards in heart cases, which resulted in publication in 1961 of a comprehensive report entitled *Heart Disease and the Law.* The Committee, in its final important and controversial report in 1962, recommended that heart disease be removed from the provisions of the Workmen's Compensation Act because of the paucity of evidence that heart attacks are, except in rare instances, the result of employment—a view destined to be hotly disputed by labor unions and their attorneys. The report also called for an improved understanding between the medical and legal professions and supported a continuing study to define the relation of heart disease to physical and emotional stress.

A third area of involvement by Paul White in the AHA was in the broad field of public relations. Here he tried to educate the American public about heart disease and what to do to try to prevent it, as well as to urge widespread support for the Association. As the most prominent heart specialist in the country, he issued a statement in June 1959 supporting the need for an annual independent drive for funds by the American Heart Association as opposed to a simple united fund campaign encompassing all health and welfare needs which was endorsed by many. His reasoning was based upon his recognition of the large research and other needs in the heart field and the evidence that the Heart Association would raise substantially less money if its campaign was to lose its separate identity. He wrote that heart disease was "too serious a problem to hide in a segment of a United Fund." His forthright stand received considerable negative comment from editorial writers especially of medium-sized and small newspapers. Headings above editorials contained such language as "Dr. White Wrong in United Fund Views" (Sioux City, Iowa, *Journal Tribune*), "Dr. White Misses Point on Value of United Fund" (Charleston, West Virginia *Gazette-Mail*), and "Dr. White is Wrong" (North Adams, Massachusetts *Independent*). His view did, however, receive wide support elsewhere and the independent heart fund continued and prospered.

Especially after the publicity surrounding his role in President Eisenhower's heart attack, he was in enormous demand as a speaker, particularly by the American Heart Association and its affiliates during the month of February which, as Heart Month, represented the peak of the fund-raising effort. Few people realized the amount of time and effort he contributed to the Heart Association at a great sacrifice in terms of time and money. A heart association affiliate would cover his expenses, but any honorarium was bound to be very modest indeed. Heart associations did not pay well. Even when he spoke in Boston, it represented a very significant amount of time and effort.

In 1960 on February 1, he appeared on national television with Dave Garroway for the heart cause, on February 2 he went to the White House to help launch the national drive with Mrs. Eisenhower and President

Carlton Ernstene of the American Heart Association, on February 3 he attended and spoke at the annual dinner of the Massachusetts Heart Association, on February 7 he again spoke on national television on "Meet the Press" at the request of the AHA, on February 8 he went to another meeting of the Massachusetts Heart Association at the Museum of Science, on February 11 there was yet another interview on television, and

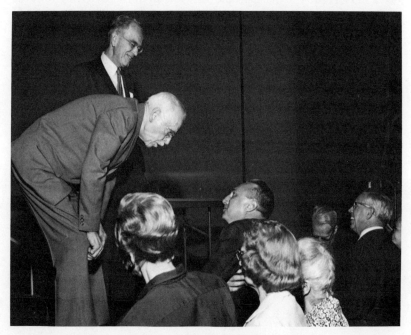

Dr. Irvine H. Page, standing, and Dr. Paul D. White, stooping over, answering questions at forum sponsored by Maricopa Heart Association and the Phoenix *Republic and Gazette*, Tempe, Arizona, April 17, 1968.

on February 17 there was still another fund-raising function at which he spoke. No other physician or lay person has ever done as much for the Association as Paul White, and it is very doubtful if any ever will.

He was honored by the American Heart Association with its Howard W. Blakeslee Award in 1956 for the way in which he had handled the media at the time of Eisenhower's illness, with its Gold Heart Award in 1964 because of his role as a founder of the AHA, and with its Distinguished Volunteer Service Award in 1969 (received from Mrs. Nixon at the White House). He received its James B. Herrick Award posthumously in 1973. At the time of receiving the Distinguished Volunteer Service Award from Mrs. Richard Nixon, Dr. Michael E. DeBakey, the eminent Houston surgeon, wrote him on April 8, 1969 a letter of congratulation which included, "I know of no one who has worked so tirelessly and fervently to make people conscious of the need to work towards eradicating heart disease." It is fitting that when the headquarters of the American Heart Association relocated from New York to Dallas, space was provided to include as a permanent exhibit the modest Boston office of Paul White including his old oak desk, chair, his pictures, and even his stethoscope.

CHAPTER EIGHT

The Promoter

The first half of the twentieth century saw a steady decline in numbers of deaths from infectious diseases in the United States, and a consequent lengthening of the life span. The medical profession and the public for the first time saw that men and women who had been dying from diphtheria, typhoid, tuberculosis and pneumonia lived into middle and old age to die from other diseases—chiefly heart disease and cancer. Concerned as to the causes and treatment of cancer—and the very name cancer was enough to create tremendous apprehension—a National Cancer Institute had been created by Congress in 1938 and it was expected that before long there would be pressure to create a similar institute for heart and blood vessel diseases. Compelling was the stark fact that there were more deaths from cardiovascular causes than from the next five causes of death combined including cancer. Further, organized groups such as the American Heart Association and energetic laymen and women and physicians were now at hand, restless and impatient to do something to promote research and service and education in this increasingly important area of chronic disease. Medical research in the past had been carried out by a few inspired leaders. They worked on small salaries, with limited laboratory space, with a handful of poorly paid assistants, little technical equipment, and shoestring budgets. However, it became apparent, especially after the experiences of World War II in handling problems such as malaria and rheumatic fever and trauma, that effective large-scale modern research programs required a change with investment of hundreds of thousands or perhaps millions of dollars—sums not then available from either public or private sources.

President Truman in a message to the Congress dated November 19, 1945, referred approvingly to the existence of the National Cancer Institute, and went on to make the cautious generalization that "We have not done enough in peace time for medical research and education . . ." The following October he appointed by Executive Order a President's Scientific Board to report on Science and Public Policy, chaired by John R. Steelman, a former professor of sociology and economics who had been in the Labor Department for some years and who was now assistant to the President. The Board was composed entirely of governmental officials including two physicians from the Veterans Administration. It received some suggestions from certain non-governmental sources among which were the Albert and Mary Lasker Foundation and the American Foundation for High Blood Pressure, but it evidently did not solicit comments from the American Heart Association. Among the findings reported on August 27, 1947 in the uninspired section on medical research was mention that "Diseases of the heart and arteries, other diseases associated with middle and old age, and acute respiratory diseases disable and kill large numbers of people, but little research is devoted to these conditions in the federal programs." The report noted that in the fiscal year 1947 the total national budget for research in medical and allied sciences was $110 million. The federal government's share was twenty eight million, half of it being spent by the public health service and one quarter each by the War and Navy Departments. The report recommended that the total national expenditures should be increased to $300 million—from both private and public sources, but mainly from the latter.

The Eightieth Congress of the United States showed very early in its deliberations that the time for a National Heart Institute and a federal program to support research in cardiovascular disease had come. Clearly the concept was politically attractive, and after some initial maneuvering it received wide bipartisan support. In its first session (1947), Senator Claude Pepper of Florida introduced into the Senate on February 26 a bill calling upon President Truman to arrange for a meeting of the world's experts "to discover new means of treating, caring [for] and preventing diseases of the heart and arteries." A companion bill was introduced into the House by Representative Arthur G. Klein, Democrat from New York City. The legislation was incorporated into the National Science Foundation Bill but came to naught as it was vetoed by the President. Much more important was House Bill #3762 introduced by Representative (later Senator) Jacob Javits of New York on June 9, which proposed the creation of a National Heart Disease Institute and a program for federal support of research in this area. This pioneering bill was not acted upon by the Congress, in part due to the press of other business and in part because this was Representative Javits' first year as a Congressman, and he was just getting to know his way around.

Meanwhile Senators H. Styles Bridges, Republican, of New Hampshire, and Claude Pepper, a Democrat, had conducted a hearing on April 24, 1947 as to the need for additional monies for heart research, and on July 19 Pepper spoke before the Senate Subcommittee on Supplemental Appropriations requesting an allocation of $2.9 million in the budget of the United States Public Health Service to meet this need. Supporting testimony was given by Dr. Rolla E. Dyer, Director of the National Institutes of Health, and by Dr. E. Cowles Andrus, Chairman of its Cardiovascular Study Section established in 1946. However, only $500,000 was finally approved.

Yet momentum had been established, and early in the second session of the Eightieth Congress on January 21, 1948, Representative Frank B. Keefe, of Wisconsin, introduced into the House a National Heart Act calling for creation of a National Heart Institute; and a similar bill (Senate Bill #2215) was introduced into the Senate on February 5 by Senators Bridges, Pepper, Ives of New York, and Murray of Montana, a bipartisan quartet. Subsequently, the Senate bill and the Senate hearings dominated the legislative activity.

On March 23, 1948, the text of a telegram received from 79 citizen "Sponsors of the National Heart Committee" was inserted into the Congressional Record by Senator Murray. This telegram called for an immediate hearing on pending legislation for a National Heart Institute and was signed by diverse public personages including actress Irene Dunne, radio stars Fibber McGee and Molly, motion picture producer Samuel Goldwyn, labor leader Walter Reuther, Reverend Harry Emerson Fosdick of New York's Riverside Church, radio commentator and author Lowell Thomas, Mrs. Franklin D. Roosevelt, Mary Lasker, and Drs. T. Duckett Jones and Paul D. White.

The most effective and both influential and affluent lay leader involved in all of this was the remarkable Mary Lasker, the third wife of Albert D. Lasker, a prominent Chicago advertising tycoon who had moved from Chicago to New York after his retirement from active business. Mary Lasker had an AB cum laude from Radcliffe College and during her first marriage had been active and well informed in the world of art. The Laskers had created the Albert and Mary Lasker Foundation mainly for the support of medical research, and Mary Lasker had gotten to know many of the top figures both in the world of medicine and in the area of politics. She was in a key position to exert pressure for her favorite causes. It appears that she, more than any other single person, should be credited with finally mobilizing and spear-heading the support necessary to create a federally financed center for the study and treatment of heart disease. She has described how, being convinced of the seriousness of the problem of heart attacks, she first went to Dr. Thomas Parran, then Surgeon General of the United States Public Health Service, to persuade him to recognize the problem and take some action. Parran was a renowned figure in the field of venereal disease, and he had received the Lasker Award of the American Public Health Service in 1947. Initially, he took a dim view of the suggestion coming from this energetic and informed lay person who clearly knew her way around the Washington scene, including the White House. A few days later, however, he notified her that he had decided that she was right and that he would support the idea of a national heart center. She was of tremendous assistance to Javits and other key members of Congress in seeing that the concept became a reality. Another influential lay figure also recognized by Javits as important in these negotiations was Mrs. Anna Rosenberg, prominent in New York and Washington in areas of industrial relations and personnel problems.

A physician intimately concerned with this activity was Dr. Thomas Duckett Jones. Duckett, as he was always called, was a member of a prominent Virginia medical family, had been educated at the University of Virginia, and in 1925 had spent a year as resident with Paul White.

This was followed by study in the laboratory of Sir Thomas Lewis in London. He developed a keen interest in rheumatic fever which was then the leading cause of death among children ages 5 to 19 years. The consequence of rheumatic fever, rheumatic heart disease, was well known as a frequent cause of death among adults. Beginning in 1929, Duckett began to work full-time on rheumatic fever at the House of the Good Samaritan in Boston as well as continuing active in the clinics of the Massachusetts General Hospital. In 1944 he proposed criteria for the diagnosis of acute rheumatic fever which were widely accepted and became known as the Jones Criteria. His concerns about rheumatic fever were broad and included psycho-social factors and community resources. A skilled and compassionate physician, his associates and students will always remember his anger when a block-head of a doctor visiting his rheumatic fever clinic asked him in front of the young girl who had just been examined "How long do you think this girl will live?"

He became the leading authority in the country on the subject of rheumatic fever and advised various governmental bodies and in particular the Children's Bureau on programs and national needs in this area. In 1947 at the age of 48, he accepted the position of Medical Director of the Helen Hay Whitney Foundation in New York. This move provided him with a more flexible schedule and increased opportunities to meet with and advise individuals and groups interested in seeing that heart disease received a larger share of national attention and public funds. As the expert consultant on rheumatic fever, he had developed useful contacts in Washington among members of Congress and others whose children and grandchildren he had seen as patients.

On April 8, 1948 the Subcommittee on Health of the Senate Labor and Public Welfare Committee, chaired by Senator Bridges heard testimony in favor of Senate Bill #2215 from a number of witnesses. These included Dr. Arlie Barnes, then President of the American Heart Association, Dr. Leonard A. Scheele, who had succeeded Parran as Surgeon General of the Public Health Service, and Duckett Jones. The full Senate passed the National Heart Act, which was the original Senate Bill #2215 with some amendments, on May 24, 1948, and the House did likewise on June 8,

1948. It became Public Law 655 after being signed by President Truman on June 16, 1948, representing the culmination of lobbying efforts by concerned lay citizens, scientists and political figures. It was of more than passing interest that Truman was away from Washington in Kansas at this time on a political tour as he was under heavy fire from Republicans who the next week in Philadelphia were to nominate Governor Thomas E. Dewey of New York as their own candidate for president with great expectations for success. The bill containing Public Law 655 was brought to Truman on the Presidential train for signature as a result of the influence of Mary Lasker who, concerned that the Bill might not be signed in time, went to her friend, Clark Clifford, Special Counsel to Truman, and made sure it was included in the mail being sent to the President from the White House. It was to this type of persistence and energy that Paul White would refer 16 years later when he spoke of "Mary Lasker, who with lay and medical friends and associates not only persuaded Congress to pass the National Heart Act but has ever since kept us on the job. . . ."

The National Heart Act, technically an amendment to the Public Health Service Act, established the National Heart Institute in the Public Health Service and within the National Institutes of Health. The intents were to encourage and support research in cardiovascular disease by grants to institutions and individuals and to create an information center on research, prevention, diagnosis and treatment. Funds could be granted for equipment and construction and for such patient care as was appropriate for research needs, and monies could be provided for training. A National Advisory Heart Council was to be established with the membership to include the Surgeons General of the Public Health Service, Army and Navy and the Chief Medical Officer of the Veterans Administration plus 12 others, six of whom should be authorities in the problems of heart disease. It was provided that leaders in education or public affairs could be included among the other six, thus importantly providing for lay representation. The Council was to review and approve the research proposals submitted to the National Heart Institute for funding as well as requests for funds for training, construction and equipment. All of this was subject to the technical approval of the Surgeon General who could not on his own approve a grant turned down by the Council. It was clear that the leadership and membership of the powerful Council were to be crucial in establishing the scientific standards and professional, lay, and political acceptance of the new Institute.

Paul White had been very much in the background to this point, attending to his own busy affairs including a visit with Pope Pius XII in Rome on May 28. On June 25, nine days after Truman had signed the National Heart Act, Duckett Jones came to see Paul White in his office at the Massachusetts General Hospital. He was there to persuade his former teacher to take an active role in the fledgling National Heart Institute and to do so forthwith. Paul White was unconvinced after the first meeting and Duckett Jones came to see him again on July 2 and found he was making headway. On July 6, Surgeon General Leonard A. Scheele phoned White to add to the urgency and on the following evening Paul White took the night train to Washington. There on July 8 he met with Scheele and later that day with Dr. Cassius J. Van Slyke who had been appointed the first Director of the National Heart Institute. Van Slyke was a graduate of the University of Minnesota Medical School and had been commissioned in the Regular Corps of the Public Health Service in 1932. He had no background in heart disease, indeed his chief area of experience had been that of venereal disease, and had been selected because of his administrative ability.

These meetings proved persuasive and in the short space of two weeks Paul White yielded to the arguments of Jones and Scheele and agreed to make a major change in his life. He would become the Executive Director of the National Advisory Heart Council and Chief Medical Advisor to the National Heart Institute. As he noted in his daily reminder on July 9, he would give up his position as Chief of the Cardiac Service at the Massachusetts General Hospital and would now work half time for the Institute receiving an annual grant to cover the time spent, office expenses and travel. He would continue to keep his office in Boston, having some continuing practice, follow-up his favorite research interests, and maintain an active international role. Two special items he listed were "no political control" and maintenance of cordial relations with private agencies including the American Heart Association and the medical schools.

Why was Paul White the man selected and why did he accept? He was chosen partly because he was greatly admired by Duckett Jones, partly because he was an experienced senior cardiologist who was known nationally and internationally, partly because his scientific views were widely respected and he was therefore not a controversial figure in the field, and partly because the Institute needed his prestige and authority at this time. Further, White was unusual in that as he had grown older he had kept his zest for innovations and new discoveries, unlike some of his colleagues for whom the tried and the proven were the cardinal guides justifying inaction. Although the Heart Act was now the law, there was as yet no provision for funds and a strong advocate was essential. Neither Scheele nor Van Slyke possessed any stature whatever as cardiologists.

For Paul White this came at a favorable moment. He was 62 years of age, was still full of energy and enthusiasm, was keenly interested in extending the horizon of knowledge of cardiovascular disease, liked the challenge of new ventures, and already had acquired some useful contacts in the Washington political scene and would shortly add others. Three of these political contacts were or would become patients, and they would prove invaluable in the years to come. One was Senator H. Styles Bridges of New Hampshire whom Paul White had known as a patient since 1944. He was a key figure in health legislation in the Senate. A second patient was Vice President Alben Barkley who first consulted Paul White about his health in the fall of 1950. His influence and support would be successfully solicited from time to time. A third and most important figure was Representative John Fogarty of Rhode Island, a former bricklayer and former President of the Bricklayers Union who became a patient in 1953. Fogarty was the extraordinarily skillful, well informed and dextrous advocate for the National Institutes of Health in the House of Representatives and was able to negotiate successfully key legislation for the National Heart Institute in its formative years.

The subsequent history of the National Heart Institute was to be a success story for Paul White, for the U.S. Public Health Service, for scientists concerned with heart and blood vessel disease and for the public. This was not, however, without considerable effort.

The first issue facing Paul White and Van Slyke was the composition of the National Advisory Heart Council which was to meet three times a year. A selection of six scientists and six lay persons was quickly made, the former including Duckett Jones, Tinsley Harrison, a distinguished teacher and clinician, Irvine H. Page, a senior investigator in high blood pressure, C. A. Elvehjem, a well known biochemist concerned with nutrition, B. O. Raulston, the Dean of the University of Southern California School of Medicine, and Paul White. The lay group was composed of one woman, Mary Lasker, and five men holding important positions in the business world and with records of an active interest in health, including James S. Adams, general partner of Lazard Freres & Company, and E. B. MacNaughton, Chairman of the Board of the First National Bank of Portland, Oregon. The Council had as its chairman C. J. Van Slyke who, as Director of the Institute, represented the Surgeon General of the Public Health Service.

Paul White's position as Executive Director of the Council was unique. Such a position did not exist in any of the other institutes and following his retirement from the job in 1957 after two four-year terms, the position was never filled again. He was an influential member of the Council, related more than any other member to Congress and to the staff, advised on the budget, and also served as chairman of the planning committee of the Council. When trips were made to visit medical schools and research laboratories which had applied for funds, he was often a member or a leader of the group. Paul White had what some looked upon as an idiosyncrasy, in that he insisted that each meeting of the Council start with a reading of what the members soon called the "Scriptures," which were the stated purposes of the National Heart Act and the responsibilities of the Council. As Dr. James Watt, Dr. Van Slyke's successor commented: "Paul felt that it was important to see to it that the Council never forgot that this was its job and that it had a high level of responsibility for it. I had the feeling that he was doing this as much for the benefit of the physician members of the Council as he was for the lay members." Lay members seemed to accept it with a degree of equanimity that was not always true of the more independent professional members.

By virtue of the respect with which Paul White was held and his friendly disposition and ease in working with others, he was able to assert his own views to a considerable extent. For one thing, he believed in granting funds to investigators in laboratories not merely because they had demonstrated scientific achievement or great promise, but because

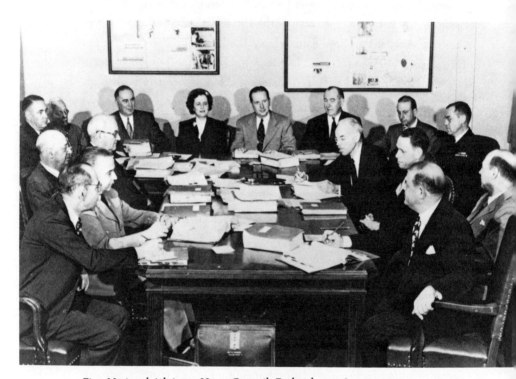

First National Advisory Heart Council, Bethesda, 1948–1949.

Seated at table, starting on left, clockwise: Dr. Tinsley R. Harrison; Col. James C. Taylor; Mr. Erwin Oreck; Mr. E. R. MacNaughton; Mrs. Mary Lasker; Surgeon General Leonard R. Scheele; Dr. Burrell O. Raulston; Dr. Paul D. White; Dr. Conrad A. Elvehjem; Mr. Maurice Goldblatt.

Seated back from the table, clockwise, starting on the left: Mr. Albert J. Wolf; Dr. C. J. Van Slyke, Director, National Heart Institute; Dr. Rolla E. Dyer, Director, National Institutes of Health; and on the right: Dr. H. M. Marvin; Cdr. R. C. Parker, Jr.; Dr. T. Duckett Jones.

they came from a region or institution needing encouragement and support. In so doing, he would not underwrite "bad" science, but he might favor what appeared to be only fair or marginal research if there was a chance of an eventual productive program in an area in which none presently existed. It would not have been difficult to limit grants to a few top investigators with proven records of accomplishment. It was more hazardous, but in Paul White's view more useful, for this new government-supported agency to spread the funds widely, helping the strong to keep strong but also assisting the weak in their search for strength. At times he was considered to have been gullible and susceptible to a persuasive personality or to a proposal without sufficient scientific merit, but such an occasional aberration would be expected to be balanced by the views of the other scientists.

A difficult issue was how to distribute funds between basic scientists working solely in the laboratory and those involved with patients or even with large population groups. Also how much would be granted to training, to equipment, to bricks and mortar? There was never any perfect formula to answer these questions. As Dr. James Watt commented, Paul White was by his presence an essential and stabilizing force in these controversial areas, particularly in the early years, and it was he "who kept Duckett from going off on some pretty big tangents on occasion. Duckett could not understand why we just could not go in all directions at once. . . ." Since Paul White was used to dealing with lay men and women through his experience in the American Heart Association, it was not difficult for him to relate easily to the non-scientists on the Council, to use their wisdom regarding broad social and scientific and financial issues, and thereby assure that they functioned as full members whose views and comments were encouraged and important.

Not everybody was enchanted with the presence of the Executive Director of the Council. There were those who considered the function of Paul White to be only that of reassuring the medical profession that this new federal intrusion into the health field would be limited in scope and not another wedge for governmental control of the whole health field. Further, on the one hand, Dr. Irvine H. Page, a member of the Council, was anxious to see a strong program for basic as well as clinical patient-related research and regarded Paul White's credentials in understanding and promoting the former with skepticism. Dr. James A. Shannon, Associate Director of the Institute in charge of research and later Director of the National Institutes of Health, had similar reservations. At the other extreme, Mary Lasker and Maurice Goldblatt, two of the lay members of the Council, particularly pushed for far more support for the application of research knowledge for the benefit of the patient and the community. They also considered that the Institute should have a much larger overall budget than it received in its early years.

The existence of the National Heart Institute meant a new item in the federal budget, and the Executive Director of the Council found very early that for the Council to have money for a meaningful program, he would have to lobby with the Congress and the administration, and lobby hard. This was an entirely new role for him but it was very familiar territory to Mary Lasker who thought that the doctors were far too timid in their approaches to the politicians. The budgetary process itself was complex. It involved a recommendation from the National Advisory Heart Council as to reasonable financial needs, agreement within the Institute staff and others in the administration including the Bureau of the Budget as to the next year's recommended budget, discussion of the budget before the concerned committees of the Senate and House, appropriate use of the lobbying efforts of interested individuals like Mary Lasker who would submit a citizens' budget, further consideration by the appropriations committees of the House and the Senate, passage by the full House and Senate, and finally, approval by the President. Generally, the budget proposed by the citizens' group was generous, that put forward by the administration relatively stingy, and the resolution by Congress somewhere in between.

Paul White first testified before Congress on February 15, 1949 when he appeared before the House Subcommittee on Appropriations, chaired by Representative John Fogarty. Here, as on other occasions, his testimony was that of a citizen expert, representing the budget proposed by the citizens' committee, and he was not speaking as a government employee. Thus he could criticize the administration's conservative fiscal posture toward the Institute. On this first occasion as well as in later years and influenced by Mary Lasker, it was his view that the administration's budget for the National Heart Institute was too modest. He emphasized that "only when the cause of a disease has been found, can adequate measures be developed against it;" and "research, like a series of stepping-stones, can lead to the eventual goal of the control of the diseases of the heart and circulation which have afflicted man since medical history began. But enough of the stones must be provided to permit progress." The next day, he sent a telegram to Senator J. Howard McGrath reiterating for the Senate the same appeal he had made to the House committee and saying: "It is a thrilling experience to have a share in this coordinated attack [on heart disease] and I am sure that we can look to you for leadership in the support of this program when it comes before the Senate."

Paul White, being a practitioner, liked to refer to individual patients and the lessons learned from them in his comments both to the press and to the Congressional committees. At times, he even brought patients to the hearings to tell their stories. These patient histories were often more effective than any amount of rhetoric about the general subject of heart disease. Representative Frank B. Keefe of Wisconsin on February 28, 1949 addressed the House of Representatives on the subject of Paul White, his persuasive testimony, and a newspaper article in which he had cited some of his patients. Representative Keefe had the article, which was written with reporter John E. Pfeiffer, reprinted in the *Congressional Record*, the first portion of which described an instructive patient:

Silly ideas about heart disease have worried thousands of persons. Men and women who were too frightened to visit their doctors have endured years of needless anguish—even died before their time.

Take the case of Joe Brown, a New England chicken farmer. At 3 o'clock one morning he turned off the alarm clock and dragged himself out of bed. He groped his way to the incubators and started turning the eggs over to make sure they'd be heated evenly on all sides. Then he noticed a pressing, slowly mounting pain in his chest, just behind the breastbone. The attack lasted half a minute or so, but Joe finished his chore and went back to bed.

An hour or two later the eggs had to be shifted again and Joe got up fearing a second spell. When nothing happened he heaved a sigh of relief and forgot about the incident. But a few weeks later he had another pain in the same place and a fortnight or so after that still another.

Finally he came to my office with the worried look of a man who's convinced he has heart disease.

But there was nothing the matter with Brown's heart. A careful examination revealed that spasms of the esophagus, the 9-inch tube leading from the vocal cords to the stomach, were causing the pain in his chest.

Paul White next testified before a subcommittee of the Committee on Appropriations of the Senate on March 28, 1949. He commented in the same vein as previously: "The National Heart Institute must not be left languishing or seriously malnourished as it will be unless considerable additional money is vouchsafed by Congress beyond the inadequate amount already passed by the House. Hence our appeal to you." At one point, Paul White made the kind of unorthodox off-the-cuff comment he was apt to make which often led to headlines and attracted attention. He was talking about the need for new knowledge to prevent heart attacks among the young and middle-aged and thus empty out some of the hospital beds then occupied by these heart cases. "We may hope that the incidence of heart disease, instead of being what it is now, may someday be perhaps even a hundred percent. We have to die of something. If we can all die at, say, the age of 90 comfortably, quickly, or quietly, in bed or sitting in an easy chair, of heart disease, we will not need beds then." Senator Elmer Thomas was evidently taken aback by this testimony and probably visualizing hordes of aged persons in wheel chairs and with walkers, waiting for their 90th birthday, asked: "Do you think it is advisable to plan for everybody to live to be 90 years old?" To which Paul White answered: "I think so; yes." The Senator persisted: "Why let it end at 90?" Paul White's response was: "We may eventually want to go up above 90, but I think that is reasonable at the present time." He went on to say: "We of the National Advisory Heart Council know whereof we speak, for between us we have traveled the country over and have personally and carefully visited almost all the medical schools and teaching hospitals where research on heart disease is going on."

The House had recommended an appropriation of $7,725,000 which included $2,300,000 for research, $2,000,000 for grants to the states, $1,000,000 for construction and $950,000 for fellowships, training and teaching. This was nearly $6,000,000 less than what the National Advisory Heart Council had recommended. In good measure, as a result of Paul White's influence, the final appropriation approved by both Houses and the President was $10,725,000. This was, with the exception of fiscal years 1952 and 1953, the start of a gradual annual escalation in the Institute's budget so that in ten years, the appropriation had risen more than five-fold to $62,237,000.

Dr. James Watt has said that Paul White "found the opportunity to testify to the Congress an exciting affair; he used to enjoy it very much." The members of Congress were respectful and usually responsive, in part surely from self-interest, since many of them had and most of them would have heart trouble. However, Paul White constantly felt required to educate Congress, the administration, and the public to establish a base of adequate support for cardiovascular research. A National Conference on Diseases of the Heart and Circulation, sponsored by the National Heart Institute and the American Heart Association, was held in Washington in January 1950, and this provided useful publicity for the needs in the heart field. Paul White was chairman of the Steering Committee of the Conference which was well attended and quite successful although the number and length of the reports generated seemed disproportionate to their merit. In May of 1951, Paul White appealed to Vice President Barkley for assistance in getting more money for the Institute and received an encouraging reply which included a patient's comment for his doctor: "You will be interested to know that I now weigh what I weighed my last year in college and feel just about the same." Barkley was appealed to again for help in March 1952, and on May 2, 1952, Paul White met with President Truman and the Director of the Bureau of the Budget to press for more financial support. Then and later, the Bureau was a stumbling block, and on June 5, 1952, Paul White described a meeting with the Bureau of the Budget as "highly unsatisfactory."

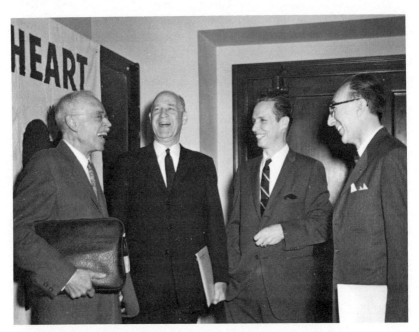

Giving a "Report to the Nation" for the American Heart Association and the National Heart Institute, U.S. Department of Commerce Auditorium, Washington, D.C. February 19, 1959.
Left to Right: Dr. Paul Dudley White, Senator Lister Hill, Surgeon General Leroy E. Burney, Dr. Michael E. DeBakey.

As rheumatic fever happily began to diminish as a major cause of heart disease, attention shifted to the frightening toll being taken increasingly by heart attacks due to coronary artery disease. Paul White spoke of this forcefully to the House of Representatives in February 1952 when, after mentioning the favorable decline in numbers of deaths from infectious disease, he testified:

> There currently remains, however, the problem of the forgotten man, the greatest challenge of all everywhere in the world, though more obviously today in the U.S.A. Who is this mysterious person, the forgotten man? None other

than you and I and hundreds of thousands indeed doubtless a few millions of professional and businessmen and leaders in government, local, state and national. These are the persons who make the world go round; yet all about us they are struck down, sometimes to die, sometimes to live restricted lives, and sometimes to recover but always with a question on their lips, "When will it happen again?" I speak, of course, of our archfoe of health, private and public, in this country in 1952, namely, coronary heart disease, the fundamental cause of which is still obscure, the treatment empirical, and prevention or at least delay not even yet begun.

More ammunition on the same topic for his supporters in Congress and for the media came in his testimony before the Senate Subcommittee on Public Health of the Committee on Appropriations in May 1955 when he stated: "It happens that the U.S.A. is one of the most unhealthy countries in the world today, in large part because of the serious threat of coronary heart disease."

Gradually, with improved financing, substantial progress was being made in strengthening the National Heart Institute, and there were also changes in the leadership. Dr. C. J. Van Slyke, the first director, became Associate Director of the National Institutes of Health in December 1952 and was replaced by Dr. James Watt, a Public Health Service officer who, like Van Slyke, had not previously been in the cardiovascular field. He proved to be extremely helpful to Paul White and their relations were eminently satisfactory. Since Watt had not yet won his spurs in cardiology and because it was important to give recognition and stature to the position of Director, Paul White early went out of his way to show his support, including having him come and sit in the front row beside him at the Cardiac Grand Rounds in the historic Ether Dome of the Massachusetts General Hospital. He also made him co-chairman of the organizing committee of the Second World Congress of Cardiology to be held in Washington in 1954. This kind of diplomatic support of an office and sensitive awareness of a colleague's potential insecurity and his actions to minimize it were characteristic of Paul White and helped to produce among his associates an attitude both of respect and of loyalty.

The Institute was meanwhile becoming besieged by applicants for support, and the appropriations for the fiscal year 1956 provided over

$8,000,000 in grants to research laboratories scattered all over the country as well as more than $4,000,000 for research going on at the Institute itself. There was an additional $5,000,000 for training and grants to state programs. These seemingly munificent sums were clearly not to be enough in an era of expensive training, technology, and construction, and much more would be required and approved during subsequent years. However, a solid fiscal start had been made, a great deal of education of key legislators and administrators and the public had been accomplished, and the machinery for reviewing and approving policy and grant applications was operating well. Paul White finished his second four-year term—and a little more—as Executive Director of the Council in 1957. He thereupon stepped down and was not replaced, and the Planning Committee chaired by Dr. E. Cowles Andrus assumed most of his duties. He turned to his many other activities, especially the international ones, leaving behind him a legacy of regard and affection.

CHAPTER NINE

The Eisenhower Case

It would appear that by the year 1955, Paul Dudley White had realized the peak of professional achievement. His many scientific papers were published in the finest medical journals. His textbook had been phenomenally successful. He was much sought after as a teacher. He was widely regarded as the premier heart specialist in the United States and indeed the world. He had been chosen as a leader of the American Heart Association, and now of the National Heart Institute and the International Society of Cardiology. Age 69 in 1955, he would seem destined for a decline in powers and popularity. Such was not to be the case.

On September 23, 1955, Dwight David Eisenhower was vacationing in Denver. Age 64 years, and to be 65 in three weeks, he was that rarity, a popular and successful president. The economy was stable, the Korean Armistice had been accomplished in July 1953, there was no immediate foreign crisis, and the unpleasant McCarthy hearing had been concluded the prior year and Senator McCarthy had been censured by vote of the Senate for conduct "contrary to senatorial traditions." The President appeared to be in excellent health, and an electrocardiogram taken at a routine medical examination on August 1, 1955 was normal. President Eisenhower had gone to Geneva on July 16 for a summit meeting with the leadership of France, the United Kingdom and the Soviet Union, then returned to Washington for several weeks to conclude discussions relating to legislation pending in Congress, and on August 14 had flown to Colorado for a vacation. Late in August, he had flown back briefly to Philadelphia to address the American Bar Association in Independence Hall.

On returning to Colorado, he went fishing 82 miles from Denver near Fraser at Byers Peak Ranch owned by his friends Aksel Nielsen and Carl Norgren. He returned to Denver on the morning of Friday, September

23, going first to his temporary office at Lowry Air Force Base. After completing some presidential chores he went out on the golf course with the golf professional Ralph ("Rip") Arnold, using an electric golf cart, but had an unsatisfactory 18 hole round (score 84), unsatisfactory owing to interruptions from telephone calls from Secretary of State Dulles. Lunch at the golf club consisted of a large hamburger sandwich with slices of Bermuda onions and coffee. Following lunch, two events occurred. One was that he played nine more holes of golf with Arnold. The second, as noted by the President in his *Mandate for Change* published in 1963, was "an uneasiness that was developing in my stomach, due no doubt to my injudicious luncheon menu." Arnold later told the press that on the 26th hole, Eisenhower who had appeared in "fine form" grinned at him and said "Boy, those raw onions are sure backing up on me."

The President and Mrs. Eisenhower were staying in Denver with the latter's mother, Mrs. John S. Doud, and he went there after his golf and painted quietly for some time. Mr. and Mrs. George Allen came for dinner and the President and Allen both declined cocktails. The Allens left early, George Allen having felt under par after dinner and having been offered milk of magnesia by his host. Eisenhower retired about 10 p.m.

What happened next was described in *Mandate for Change* by Eisenhower as follows:

> Some time later—roughly 1:30 a.m., I think—I awakened with a severe chest pain and thought immediately of my after-luncheon distress the previous noon. My wife heard me stirring about and asked whether I wanted anything. I replied that I was looking for the milk of magnesia again. Apparently she decided from the tone of my voice that something was seriously wrong; she got up at once to turn on the light to have a look at me. Then she urged me to lie down and promptly called the White House physician General Snyder. She thought I was quite sick.
>
> General Snyder arrived shortly thereafter, and gave me some injections, one of which I learned later was morphine. This probably accounts for the hazy memory I had—and still have—of later events in the night.

In retrospect, it is obvious that Mamie Eisenhower was an acute observer whose immediate instinct as to serious illness was 100% correct, and indeed perhaps more so than that of the White House physician she had promptly called.

Major General Howard McC. Snyder was born in 1881 in Wyoming and was therefore 74 years of age. He graduated from Jefferson Medical College and was an intern for one year (1905–1906) at the Presbyterian Hospital in Philadelphia. He then entered general practice in Fort Douglas, Utah, for a two year period. In 1908, he joined the Medical Corps of the United States Army, rising in rank from 1st Lieutenant in 1908 to Major General in 1943. He served as Chief of Surgery at Fort D.A. Russell in Wyoming from 1911 to 1915, had varied short-term assignments from 1916 to 1924, and then for five years was Chief of Surgery at the United States Military Academy, West Point. His early career seems to have emphasized tropical medicine to some extent as he was a member of the Research Board of Tropical Medicine in the Philippines 1909–1911, and was at the School of Tropical Medicine in San Juan, Puerto Rico 1930–1932. Another emphasis appears to have been that of administration, as he was Senior Medical Advisor to the National Guard of the United States 1936–1940, Assistant Inspector for the War Department 1940–1946, and a member of the Chief of Staff's Advisory Group 1946–1948. It appears that he first met the Eisenhowers in 1945 at a time when Mrs. Eisenhower was ill. He was retired in 1948. Doubtless as a result of friendship with Dwight Eisenhower, he was named a research associate in a project on Conservation of Human Resources at Columbia University 1948–1953 and was Senior Medical Officer to the Supreme Headquarters, Allied Powers in Europe (SHAPE) 1951–1952.

When Eisenhower became President he recalled Snyder to active duty and appointed him the head of the Army medical detachment in the White House and his personal physician, aided by Col. Walter R. Tkach. The amount of clinical experience in the latter part of General Snyder's career seems to have been decidedly limited. He did undertake graduate study at the Mayo Clinic in 1924, was at New York University and Bellevue Hospital in 1931, and was a graduate of the Medical Field Service School in 1932. He was a fellow of the American College of Surgeons but was not certified in any specialty, which was not uncommon for even very well trained doctors in that era. Whether he had ever seen or cared for patients with heart attacks is unclear, but certainly such experience if it existed must have been minimal. Since 1936, his professional life had been essentially that of a distinguished medical administrator. That the President of the United States should receive his medical care primarily from a doctor age 74 with a decidedly limited clinical exposure rather than a first class practicing physician should not occasion surprise. There was ample precedent for such an arrangement. Unhappily, our national Chief Executives have often not received the best medical care.

President Woodrow Wilson was under the care of Rear Admiral Carl T. Grayson, USN, who had also served as White House physician to Presidents Theodore Roosevelt and William Howard Taft. When Wilson first became ill in Paris in April 1919 at the time of the Versailles Conference, Dr. Grayson made a diagnosis of influenza which may well have been present as he had a cough and temperature of 103°. However, at this time the President also became suspicious of the servants, thought furniture was being stolen from the house, required that an inventory of the furnishings be made, and altogether behaved in a new and disturbing fashion suggesting cerebral disease and not merely influenza. On September 25, 1919 in Pueblo, Colorado while on a speaking tour on behalf of the League of Nations, he first developed difficulty with speech and had a severe left-sided stroke, on October 2, 1919 ushered in by a fall and unconsciousness. Grayson seems to have handled these latter episodes reasonably even though in retrospect the illness in April was not properly interpreted. He and Mrs. Wilson and those close to the White House circle stoutly refused to acknowledge the severity of the President's disability—a story fully recited by Gene Smith in *When the Cheering Stopped.*

President Warren G. Harding was chiefly under the care of Dr. Charles E. Sawyer, an old friend from his Marion, Ohio days and the doctor for his wife. Dr. Sawyer had founded the Sawyer Sanatorium for the treatment of nervous and mental diseases at White Oaks Farm outside of Marion. Harding became seriously ill with apparent exhaustion while on a speaking trip to the West Coast and Alaska in July 1923 and was forced to cancel a speech in Portland and proceed by train directly from Seattle to San Francisco where he went to bed in the Palace Hotel. Sawyer had announced that the President had a "slight attack of ptomaine" with "no serious aspect." Because he actually seemed very ill, consultations were obtained in San Francisco from Dr. Ray Lyman Wilbur and Dr. Charles Minor Cooper. Dr. Joel T. Boone, Harding's Naval Medical aide, was also in attendance. On August 2, 1923 at 7:32 p.m., he died suddenly—an abrupt ending not consistent with either ptomaine or bronchial pneumonia (which was a diagnosis which had also been entertained), but quite characteristic of a major heart attack. No autopsy was obtained but Dr. Sawyer stated that he had succumbed to a cerebral hemorrhage. It is of interest that the prominent Boston cardiologist and great friend of Dr. Paul White, Dr. Samuel A. Levine of the Peter Bent Brigham Hospital, had read the medical bulletins carefully, was convinced that Harding had a heart attack, and wished to call Dr. Sawyer and make this suggestion but had been dissuaded. Paul White's wife recalled that her husband also said at the time that Harding's problem must have been a heart attack.

President Franklin Delano Roosevelt was cared for chiefly by Vice-Admiral Ross T. McIntire, U.S.N. McIntire was not an internist but a nose and throat specialist. The President had known him when he was a cruiser doctor, summoned him to the White House to be his physician, and promoted him to Vice-Admiral and also made him Surgeon General of the U.S. Navy. Roosevelt was known to have had high blood pressure since 1937 and began to have significant difficulties beginning with an apparent attack of "flu" in December 1943. He became more tired, developed a cough and had bouts of abdominal distress. Already a candidate for reelection, he went to Bethesda Naval Hospital on March 27, 1944, where he was seen by Dr. Howard G. Bruenn, Medical Officer in the Naval Reserve who was consultant in cardiology. Dr. Bruenn confirmed the presence of very significant high blood pressure complicated by heart failure and acute bronchitis, and the President was begun on digitalis. In August 1944, he first had an episode of chest and shoulder pain while giving a speech, symptoms recognized by Dr. Bruenn as consistent with a serious lack of blood supply to the heart muscle due to coronary artery disease. He went through considerable campaigning for reelection that fall, and traveled to Yalta for the Summit Meeting with Stalin and Churchill in February 1945. He died of a sudden major stroke April 12, 1945, twelve and a half months after serious illness had become apparent. Despite evidences of significant high blood pressure and heart disease, his physicians, notably Vice-Admiral McIntire, never disclosed any of these matters to the American public. The medical findings during the last year of Roosevelt's life have been summarized by Dr. Bruenn in the April 1970 issue of the *Annals of Internal Medicine*, and the overall history of that year can be found in *FDR's Last Year* by Jim Bishop. The contrast between what a public figure has revealed when his or her health is good, and what may be revealed when the picture is unfavorable, as in this situation, is illustrated by the following quotation from Arthur Krock's *Memoirs*:

> But it was Franklin D. Roosevelt himself who first recognized in 1932—though impelled to do so as an act of political self-defense—that present and prospective health in the context of high office was a matter of legitimate public concern and should be met in a way that people would accept as objective and reliable.

Because of "mounting whispers in public, political, and medical circles," Roosevelt entrusted James A. Farley with the task of revealing in a speech given July 19, 1932 favorable reports both from a recent examination by three physicians, as well as favorable action by a life insurance company in 1930.

There is agreement that President Eisenhower had disturbing and premonitory symptoms on the golf course on the afternoon of September 23, became acutely ill at sometime between 1:30 and 2:30 a.m. on Saturday September 24, and that General Snyder was called and saw him at Mrs. Doud's home about 3:00 a.m. and administered morphine twice. Early on the morning of September 24, General Snyder told Assistant Press Secretary Murray Snyder to announce that the President was suffering from a digestive upset and this announcement was made to the press at 8:00 a.m. At noon, the press was told that General Snyder said that the condition was not serious, a "common form of indigestion", and that therefore he, General Snyder, was not going to remain in constant attendance. No electrocardiogram was taken until 1:00 p.m. on Saturday September 24 and General Snyder was the only physician in attendance until that time. This first electrocardiogram was taken in the Doud home by or in the presence of Colonel Byron E. Pollock who was Chief of Cardiology at Fitzsimmons General Hospital. Major General Martin E. Griffin, commanding officer of the hospital, also came to the Doud home with Colonel Pollock. The electrocardiogram disclosed a definite heart attack, a finding announced to the media at 2:00 p.m. The President was not transferred to the hospital until 3:00 p.m., some 12 hours after he had first received medical attention, and he traveled to it by limousine and not by ambulance.

On the afternoon of that day, Saturday September 24, Colonel Thomas W. Mattingly received a call from General Leonard Heaton, Commanding General of Walter Reed General Hospital, to the effect that the President had experienced a heart attack and that he and General Snyder wished him to fly to Denver to assist in the President's care. Mattingly was a former student of Dr. White at the Massachusetts General Hospital and had served under him on the National Advisory Heart Council and also on the Organizing Committee of the Second World Congress of Cardiology in Washington, DC in 1954. He had been Chief of the Cardiology Service, Walter Reed Hospital, and Chief Consultant in Cardiology to the Surgeon General of the Army since 1951. He had served also as a consultant in the care of personnel at the White House during the last two years of the Truman Administration and subsequently for the Eisenhower administration. Colonel Mattingly had given professional attention to some of Eisenhower's Army associates and had seen the President himself for routine cardiovascular evaluations beginning in 1953 and indeed as recently as August 1, 1955. He was respected for his intelligence, experience and good sense. Colonel Mattingly boarded a plane at the MATS Airport in Washington early that evening and in company with James Hagerty, the White House Press Secretary and Merriman Smith, United Press International reporter and dean of the White House press corps, flew to Colorado. There was a driving rain at Denver and the plane was therefore diverted from Lowry Air Force Base to Stapleton Field, arriving about midnight. Colonel Mattingly was taken at once to Fitzsimmons Hospital where, like the thorough consultant he was, he conferred with Colonel Pollock and Colonel George Powell, the Chief of Medicine, and General Snyder, reviewed the record, interviewed and examined the President and wrote a consultation report.

The entrance of Dr. White into the case was not surprising. The nation and indeed the world were shocked by the sudden announcement that the former Supreme Commander of the victorious allied forces in Europe in World War II and now the popular President of the United States was acutely and gravely ill. There was no evasiveness about the 2:00 p.m. medical announcement on September 24. It is a credit to the President that when first made aware of his diagnosis and queried as to what was to be told the public he said: "Tell the truth, the whole truth; don't try to conceal anything."

In 1955, the implications of a heart attack were very different from today. A heart attack—often called then coronary thrombosis and more commonly now myocardial infarction—was regarded as often fatal or at least a permanently disabling catastrophe. The reaction of most people was represented by that of the President's son, John Eisenhower, who had just finished a round of golf at Fort Belvoir, Virginia, when a secret service man ran up to him and told him that his father had suffered a heart attack. His first reaction was "This is curtains. This is all finished. That's the end of a career and quite probably a life." James Reston, writing in the *New York Times* dated September 25, 1955, speculated about the President's successor "if, as seems almost certain, the stricken President retires at the end of his first term." It is a reflection both of the public veneration of Eisenhower as a leader and the general reaction to his illness that on Monday September 26 the New York Stock Exchange suffered its heaviest loss in history, a loss put at 14 billion dollars and described as a "collapse." The White House reported that its offices in Denver and Washington were "flooded with telephone calls from around the world" and messages were received among others from former Presidents Hoover and Truman, Queen Elizabeth, Prime Minister Anthony Eden, President René Coty and Premier Edgar Faure of France.

That a civilian consultant should have been brought into this important case was logical. Whereas the President as a product of the U.S. Army was comfortable with Army medicine and Army doctors, many civilians including some of Eisenhower's White House Staff viewed them with suspicion. Partly this was a reflection of World War II experience in which many reserve medical officers returned to civilian life with a less than favorable impression of many of their regular Army colleagues. Partly this was the knowledge that the top medical school graduates usually avoided Army careers, although many outstanding physicians such as Colonel Mattingly and surgeons devoted their whole lives to the armed services. Partly this was attributable to the vague belief that anything done by the government is bound to be routine and undistinguished. In this instance, Army medicine was exposed and on public trial and it welcomed support from an outstanding civilian consultant.

This was especially true of General Snyder whose responsibility—and possibly blame—for the management of the first hours of the illness was absolute. It is easy today to look back and criticize his professional conduct in that span of time. Here was the President of the United States, evidently previously very healthy, suddenly becoming ill at night with chest pain and sweating—so ill that two good sized doses of morphine had to be given by injection to give relief. It would have seemed a minimal prudence for this 74 year-old Army medical officer to have sought a consultation from one or more colleagues at once. An electrocardiogram could have been taken at the very onset of the illness rather than waiting 10 hours. Why was the press twice informed that this was only a digestive upset if General Snyder knew right away that this was a heart attack, as stated in some later versions? What was the justification for not telling the family the probable diagnosis right away—Eisenhower's son did not learn of the heart attack until the afternoon of September 24th? Would it not have been judicious to have transferred Eisenhower to a hospital at once rather than waiting over 12 hours? Is it not likely that General Snyder did *not* seriously entertain the diagnosis of a heart attack until some hours after it had taken place? Searching questions regarding these matters were raised by some members of the press as General Snyder found out very promptly. The Associated Press, in its dispatch from Denver dated September 24, reported how newsmen had failed to get answers from Assistant White House Press Secretary Murray Snyder to their questions about the original announced diagnosis of a "digestive upset" and as to "why there was no announcement of the President's heart attack until mid-afternoon when it occurred at 2:45 a.m. MST." General Snyder was in an awkward spot and therefore welcomed advice and he hoped for support from an eminent consultant such as Paul White.

In fairness to General Snyder, it must be stated that a period of quiet rest provided by the morphine undoubtedly was useful. There are those who believe that a good-risk patient with a heart attack, who shows no signs of shock or heart failure or irregularity of heart rhythm, may be cared for in the surroundings of the home with results very similar to those in the hospital. The end result in terms of ultimate recovery by the President was excellent. General Snyder was also available to his patient during the rest of the night and through the next morning and he certainly did not abandon him. However, it is doubtful if many well trained medical men or women would in 1955 have behaved similarly with any patient with these symptoms.

It is likely that more than one person suggested that Dr. Paul D. White be called into the case. Late in the afternoon of September 24, Dr. Joseph T. Wearn of Cleveland received a telephone call from the White House. Dr. Wearn was professor of medicine and Dean of the Western Reserve

School of Medicine. Calling him was one of his patients, Secretary of the Treasury George M. Humphrey, who told him of the President's illness and asked for the name of the country's best heart specialist. Dr. Wearn recommended Paul White. The same suggestion appears to have been made by Robert Cutler, formerly President of the Old Colony Trust Company in Boston and Chairman of the National Security Council 1953–1955, who was based in the White House. He was also President of the Board of Trustees of the Peter Bent Brigham Hospital in Boston and knew his way around Boston medicine. That others were also considered for the role of consultant is suggested by evidence that Dr. Samuel A. Levine of Boston was alerted to go to Denver but never received a definite request.

Paul White in his notes described how he first heard of the Eisenhower heart attack over the car radio about 6:45 p.m. on Saturday afternoon September 24 while he and his wife were driving from their home in Belmont to have dinner in Chestnut Hill with Dr. and Mrs. E. Blake Dunphy. Shortly after his arrival at the Dunphys' home, he was called to the phone to answer a call from the science reporter of the *Boston Globe*, Mrs. Frances Burns, who wanted to know if he was going to Denver. Shortly afterward, he received a second call, this one from the Surgeon General of the Army, asking if he would fly to Denver to see the President. Dr. White replied that he would be glad to be of any help he could. This was followed in turn by a call from the Associated Press and later from General Snyder and White House Press Secretary James Hagerty regarding the arrangements. Dr. White was picked up at home about 8:00 a.m. the following morning and driven to Logan Airport in Boston where he, the sole passenger, boarded an Air Force DC-6 for Denver. On the trip to the airport, he received his first real exposure to the media as he was accompanied by a reporter from the Associated Press who asked him a number of questions about heart attacks and their impact, awkward to answer since he had never even met his future patient. However he did, perhaps unwisely in view of its importance later, make the general statement: "Another term for President Eisenhower is quite conceivable."

Paul White arrived in Denver at 1:10 p.m., the landing being a rough one due to a blowout of a front tire followed by black smoke which brought the fire apparatus racing out to the plane. He was taken directly to the eighth floor of the hospital where he met with the physicians caring for the President.

Dr. White's version of the start of the President's illness was written in his usual office record on the afternoon of Sunday September 25 at Fitzsimmons General Hospital and is as follows:

Always in general very well and active. Excellent findings (including ECG seen by PDW) by Dr. Mattingly on August 1st., 1955. After his strenuous visit at the Geneva Conference in July came to Denver (5,280 feet) and Fraser (8,700 feet), Colorado, in the middle of August and has been here except for two days east late in August. Much enjoyment of golf and fishing. At Fraser, leisurely September 19 to 23rd when after hearty breakfast driven back to Denver where he played 27 holes of golf enjoyably following a two hour conference except for interruptions for lunch of hamburger and raw onions and difficult phone calls to Washington. Got home at 4:30 painted till 7:30, light supper, bed by 9:30. Soon asleep. Awoke at 2:30. Complained of increasingly severe low substernal non-radiating pain for which General Snyder saw him at 3:00 and gave M.S. 1/4 gr. s.c. Second dose at 3:45. Then slept from 4:30 to 11:00 a.m. Papaverine started at 3:00 p.m. 1 gr. i.m. ev. 4 hrs. ECG taken at 1:00 p.m. showed cor. thr. Dull pain continued. Entered at 3:00 p.m. Put in oxygen tent. More morphine 1/4 gr. at 3 & 7 P.M. Good night but dull pain still present on awaking today & so more m.s. 1/6 gr. at 6 a.m. and 1:50 p.m. No dyspnea, palpitation or shock but much sweating.

Now feels well except for very dull ache high substernally and some low abdominal gas distension. Took in 3,000 cc.

Paul White followed his medical history, taken in part from the attending doctors and in part from the patient himself, with a physical examination. He reviewed the series of electrocardiograms then available and other routine laboratory reports. He agreed that the diagnosis of a heart attack was clear-cut and concurred in the medical program being followed by Colonels Mattingly and Pollock and General Snyder. He told the President about his complete support of the diagnosis and the need for bed rest except for being helped to the nearby toilet for two to three weeks, a light diet, continuation of the anti-clotting drug coumadin, and institution of the drug quinidine sulfate to prevent irregularities of heart rhythm. A more prolonged discussion was held the following morning when Dr. White examined him again.

At 4:12 p.m. on Sunday September 25, a bulletin was released to the media signed by General Snyder, Colonel Mattingly, Colonel Pollock, and Dr. White. This stated: "the President has had a moderate attack of coronary thrombosis, without complications. His present condition is satisfactory." It is significant that since the addition of Colonel Mattingly and Paul White to the medical team, the adjective describing the heart attack had been changed from "mild" to "moderate." Dr. White was also quoted in dispatches dated that afternoon saying: "Tom [Mattingly] is among the very best; calling me in is more a morale factor." In referring to his former student with generous praise, he was as he said later also going out of his way to support Army medicine which was and would be responsible for the care of the President in an Army Hospital. It was also true that Dr. White then and in the future essentially ratified the details of medical care provided by Pollock, Mattingly and Snyder. He at no time suggested any major changes of the program nor did he ever propose transfer of the patient to an elite civilian hospital. Not only was he supportive of Colonel Mattingly but he also went out of his way at a press conference to comment favorably on General Snyder's role in the case including the decision to let the President walk down stairs on the afternoon of September 25th.

Paul White's important roles were three-fold: 1. to provide the endorsement of a noted civilian consultant to the diagnosis and day to day care of Eisenhower by the Army physicians; 2. to interpret the illness of Eisenhower to the public; and 3. to provide advice as to the long term future of the President. The first role was the one most readily accomplished.

The care of a seriously ill President was a new experience for all members of the medical team. It was not surprising that Paul White and Mattingly who shared the same bedroom that Sunday night had a restless sleep, interrupted Colonel Mattingly recalls by discussions regarding the management and possible complications and outlook of their patient. Although it is desirable that the medical care of a VIP should be as nearly as possible identical to that provided John Q. Public, the fact is that it is inevitably involved with special considerations which cannot be ignored.

Paul White was to feel the full impact of the second role, that of interpreting the Eisenhower illness to the public, on Monday September 26th at 10 a.m. when a major press conference on the health of the President was held in Denver. The decision to reveal all the facts was made by the President himself, and he and his entourage including especially his Press Secretary James Hagerty were very conscious of the mishandling of reports on Presidential illnesses in the past. The conference that Monday was an historic one. This was the first time in the history of the United States that an illness of the Chief Executive had been fully described at a press conference and a free exchange with the reporters permitted. In the future it would be difficult to keep the ill health of a President a secret. The details at the time of the attempted assassination of President Ronald Reagan in 1981 and of his cancer operation in 1985 were completely in keeping with the disclosures on September 26, 1955 in Denver. Further, the event was historic in that no doctor ever before was placed in such a searching glare of publicity in which nearly every word was published and digested by millions of people not just in the United States but all over the world.

That the focus was sharply on Dr. White and not Drs. Mattingly, Snyder, or Pollock was not surprising—Dr. White was senior in experience and scientific stature if not in age (he was then 69 and Snyder was 74), he was a past master in discussing the subject of heart disease before both lay and scientific audiences, and unlike the others he clearly enjoyed and was comfortable in the spotlight. Furthermore, he soon seized upon the President's illness as a unique opportunity to promote one of his favorite topics—the relatively optimistic outlook for most patients with heart disease. All his professional life, he had been encouraging patients with heart problems to lead as normal an existence as possible; during his whole career, he had contributed enormously to the rehabilitation of those with heart disease by a combination of natural good sense, long experience and encouragement; through his native buoyancy and warmth and honesty, he had redirected the lives of many thousands of patients toward happier and more useful living.

The heart attack of President Eisenhower, its management, and the President's recovery, were to change permanently the views of many physicians, patients, employers, labor unions, insurance companies and governmental agencies on the potential for a return to useful living of patients who had suffered heart attacks. As observed several years later in the *Wall Street Journal* of January 9, 1963, the Eisenhower heart attack and recovery contributed significantly to an improved climate for employment and re-employment by U.S. corporations of individuals who had experienced heart attacks. When Lyndon B. Johnson ran for Vice President in 1960 and for President in 1964, the issue of his health and his prior heart attack were essentially non-issues. As Dr. J. Willis Hurst,

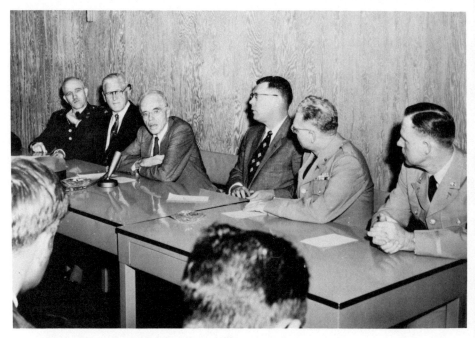

Press conference during Eisenhower illness, 1955:
Seated at table, left to right: Col. Thomas W. Mattingly; Gen. Howard McC. Snyder; Dr. Paul D. White; Press Secretary James C. Hagerty; Col. Byron E. Pollock; Col. George Powell.

a very distinguished cardiologist and teacher who was Johnson's physician and was a former student of Paul White said: "the public felt that he [Paul White] was a physician who told the truth, whom they trusted, and he communicated with them in a language they could understand."

The press conference that Monday was handled by the Press Secretary James Hagerty. It was by mutual understanding dominated by Paul White. It commenced with an opening statement by Paul White which characteristically emphasized the positive:

> I am returning to Boston today partly because the President's condition is so satisfactory and partly because he has such excellent attention here, medically and other.

He went on to say:

> There is no doubt whatsoever about the diagnosis confirmed both clinically and by electrocardiogram.

He then described some of the features of heart attacks including possible factors in their etiology, and made a point of absolving golf from any of the blame in Eisenhower's and other cases. He described the President's illness with the words "This is an average case."

Press Secretary Hagerty then read the morning progress report which included the phrase "he had a good bowel movement," at which Paul White broke in with "Now I put that in—this is an encouraging point." That there should be a description of the function of the colon of the President of the United States before a large number of reporters from all over the world—a description which was of course quoted—caused more than a ripple of astonishment. Eisenhower later wrote of his "acute embarrassment" when he read the bulletin. On reflection, he concluded: "Well in any event it's too late to object now; forget it." Some members of the British medical profession especially were offended and considered the reference to be both unnecessary and in bad taste. *Time* magazine of October 10, 1955 included the following: "A British reporter was horrified at the intimacy. After listening to Dr. Paul Dudley White's candid exegesis of a medical bulletin the Briton exclaimed: 'Imagine the BBC reporting that about the Queen!' " It was Paul White's view that this should be mentioned as favorable scientific evidence of a return from an acute illness towards normal bodily function, evidence which would be particularly meaningful to physicians reading the report. The reference did lead one exasperated New York sage to refer henceforth to Paul White as the "Boswell of the bowels."

The press conference then went on to questions, numbering 45 in all during the session. The few procedural or routine queries were handled by Hagerty and all the remainder were answered by Paul White except for a single one answered by General Snyder. In the minds of all in the room, there was a keen interest in Eisenhower's political future as evidenced by the question: "Would you give us in your own words whether you think he could run in a political campaign," to which Paul White responded: "I can't." The transcript of the session occupied nearly a full page of the *New York Times* of September 27th and a photograph of Paul White and General Snyder was on the front page of nearly all newspapers in the United States and many abroad.

This was a virtuoso performance. As Dr. Howard A. Rusk wrote on October 2 in the *New York Times:* "With his clear, easily understood statement, Dr. White did a magnificent job of interpreting for the American people and the world the physiological, pathological and emotional ramifications of coronary artery disease."

Paul White was suddenly placed in a position of both medical and political prominence. It is useful to quote from *Firsthand Report* written by Sherman Adams former Governor of New Hampshire and Assistant to the President:

> I went to Denver with my mind made up that for the next few weeks, at least, the real key figure in the government would be Dr. Paul Dudley White, a physician who was endowed with much more than the knowledge and skill that had brought him to the top of his profession. Bound together within the confines of a frail physical fortress were a doctor, philosopher, prophet, publicist of the first order, homely country man and avid bicyclist. Add to all this Dr. White's New England heritage, nurtured in the traditions and whimsies that Americans from other parts of the country are incapable of understanding, and there emerges one of the rarest characters in all my experience. I made up my mind that affairs involving the President would orbit, temporarily at least, around Paul Dudley White and his medical associates.

The return of Paul White to Boston 24 hours after his arrival in Denver was not an easy decision. There was the heady atmosphere and excitement where the action was. There was a patient, still in an acute phase, who might with every justification have been considered to require further close observation from his civilian consultant before being considered out of danger. There were the multiple and growing questions from the members of the press who quickly learned to turn to Paul White for the answers since he proved to be friendly, highly authoritative and eminently quotable. As Paul White stated subsequently, he chose not to take the easy route of staying in Denver because of his sensitivity to the confidence that the President as an old soldier had in his Army medical team, and his desire to demonstrate that he shared that confidence. The fact that Eisenhower appeared to be doing satisfactorily was a lesser but important consideration.

The next few weeks were busy ones with new obligations and opportunities thrust upon the Boston doctor whose name had suddenly become so well known. Paul White kept in touch with the Denver sick bed by phone, receiving daily bulletins as to the progress of the patient from Colonel Pollock or Colonel Powell the Chief of Medical Service.

There was a barrage of telephone calls and letters. On September 30 he appeared on the TODAY NBC television show with Dave Garroway and he collaborated with *LIFE* magazine in a large article on heart attacks which appeared in the issue of October 10. Drs. Claude Beck and Bernard L. Brofman of Cleveland urged publicly on October 10 that the President's physician consider him for later heart surgery. A letter from Boulder, Colorado advised stopping the breakfast egg, another from Los Angeles cautioned against breakfast sausages, a businessman from Baton Rouge, Louisiana wrote "I have advocated for years elimination before each meal", a chemist from Niagara Falls recommended lecithin, a man from Champaign, Illinois who had experienced a heart attack wrote "I question the advisability of keeping him so quiet", the California Prune and Apricot Growers Association mailed Dr. White a box of prunes (whether it was felt that they were needed by the patient or the doctor was not clear), a firm from Rotterdam dispatched 200 ampules of

"Vasolastine", others recommended massage, liver, vitamin E, croquet, etc. A young girl from Townshend, Vermont wrote proffering a "beautiful" puppy for the President.

Typical evidence of the pace of public interest in the Eisenhower illness and the whole issue of heart disease was shown in one paragraph of a letter from a representative of The Associated Press to Dr. White on October 14, 1955: "For every time we call Dr. White, we are the target of many more calls from individual newspapers. Give us credit for saving you from many calls even though we ourselves tax your patience! Basically it's the desire of the American people to know about their President. In addition, his case has stirred an unprecedented interest in the problem of heart trouble." Paul White's notes for his press conference of November 7 mentioned: "Acknowledge the considerable amount of advice received from a host of kind friends of the President himself or of ourselves (many of them physicians)."

On October 7, Paul White reviewed the series of electrocardiograms taken so far on Eisenhower with Dr. Eugene Lepeschkin in Newfane, Vermont. Dr. Lepeschkin, a member of the faculty of the University of Vermont College of Medicine, had a considerable reputation in the field of electrocardiography. It was agreed that the findings were consistent with the usual evolution of a myocardial infarction involving the front wall of the main pumping chamber (left ventricle), with some changes due to associated pericarditis (an inflammation of the capsule about the heart which is seen in many heart attacks).

Paul White returned to Denver and saw Eisenhower with Drs. Mattingly, Pollock and Snyder on October 8th and 9th. Things were fortunately going well, the President was an excellent patient and in good spirits, and the physical and laboratory findings were favorable. On October 9, Paul White's notes included the following:

Long conversation outlining plans for the next few weeks. 3rd week which is beginning now—continued bed rest but the bed may be rolled out on the porch. Arrange for 2 conferences with government colleagues, 1st Mr. Dulles. 4th week—begin to sit up each day and may begin to paint a little in bed or chair—some conferences. 5th week—begin to take a few steps to bathroom and elsewhere. Increase conferences and begin to have a few visitors. 6th week—walk around on the level quite freely, increasing all the other activities too. At the end of that week or after one more week, if thought advisable, he'll be ready to board plane as ambulatory patient to return to Gettysburg. The third month after the attack should be spent in complete rehabilitation and recuperation. That will be most from the end of Nov thru Dec. On good days he may even then be allowed, if he is well enough, to do some putting, see more visitors, and carry on more activity. It is hoped by the Jan. 1st he should be able to get back to the White House and to his work in Washington. P.D.W. to come again in two weeks and in four weeks. The remote future remains uncertain.

This schedule of slowly increasing mental and physical activity over three months would today be considered extremely conservative; but it represented the consensus of most medical opinion at the time.

The President was again visited by Paul White on October 22. On that occasion, Paul White awarded him a sixth star for good behavior, pinning it on his shirt collar. The President acknowledged this unusual gesture with a warm letter dated October 28:

Dear Dr. White:

I suspect you know by now of the great hit the "sixth star" has made with the doctors and nurses and members of the press corps. Of course I'm highly complimented, and trying hard to live up to the distinction conferred upon me.

Sometime I shall try to tell you, however inadequately, of my profound appreciation for all you have done. I know, as my doctor, you would not *now* approve of the effort. But permit me at least to thank you from the bottom of this scarred heart for my "good conduct star."

With warm regard,

Sincerely,

Dwight D. Eisenhower

Paul White also saw him on November 6th and 7th and then flew to New Mexico to visit his daughter and her husband and their new baby, his first grandchild. They returned with him to Denver when Paul White saw the President again on November 10th and 11th. He also introduced him to the new granddaughter. On November 11, the President flew back to Washington on the Columbine III accompanied by Drs. Mattingly,

Snyder and White. The flight back to Washington on the Presidential plane, the warm reception from the crowds in Washington, the motorcade and arrival at the White House were exhilarating to all and not least to Paul White who reacted with boyish enthusiasm and excitement. It was no secret that it had not been planned for him to fly East with the Presidential party, but he had sought it out. He also stayed for dinner that night at the White House.

The next few months were a period of an eminently satisfactory recovery by the President. Not always as completely satisfactory was the relation between the individuals in the medical troika. The President wished General Snyder to continue as his personal and White House physician. He had great respect for the professionalism and the modesty of Colonel Mattingly and welcomed him as his regular Army consultant on his heart problem. There was a lesser place now for Paul White. However, the Boston physician had served admirably in the role of civilian consultant, had fielded the public relations aspect with a high degree of success, had gotten to know and like his famous patient, and thoroughly enjoyed the whole experience. The media and the American public tended to look upon him as "Ike's Doctor" and expected him to perform in that role, including being intimately involved with the decision as to the President's long-term future. Paul White therefore continued to see the President periodically with at times the somewhat reluctant consent of his other Army medical advisors. The situation is not an uncommon one in medical practice.

It is often difficult to achieve an optimal division of responsibility between the consultant and the attending physician or physicians. It is easiest if the consultant renders an opinion and then withdraws from the case, having made a specific contribution. The situation becomes more awkward when either the consultant or the patient or both wish to have the consultant continue in an active role. At times this may be essential for the welfare of the patient, but in such situations there may be implied reflection on the competence of the patient's own physician or physicians. Further, there is the possibility of confusion from the interpretation of advice coming from two sources. Such a possibility especially existed with the President's illness and its implications for his political future.

During the President's convalescence at the White House and later at his farm in Gettysburg, the attention of all including the President himself changed from the question "will he survive?" to "will he run again?" The next presidential election was less than a year away. Eisenhower's illness surprisingly had not resulted in the development of any important negative popular view of him as an effective President. There was actually wide spread sympathy for him and a keen clinical interest in watching his day-to-day recovery. His close friends and advisors and the Republican leaders nationally wanted him to run again. After all, the party had not had an equally charismatic and successful leader since Theodore Roosevelt.

What if one or all of the doctors caring for him announced the judgement that the state of his health would not permit four more years in the White House? That would settle the issue. The person in the hottest seat in reaching a judgement was Paul White since he had become the spokesman for the medical team. As John Eisenhower stated: "There's no doubt that without White's endorsement, Dad could never have run a second time. . . . In other words, he almost had a veto power over Dad's political career."

Although Paul White was by nature endowed with a positive philosophy toward life, and although the President was clearly doing well without complications, and although Paul White had seen many men of similar age and with quite similar heart attacks return to work, he could not deny the possibility of another and possibly fatal attack within four years. It would indeed be a blow to the role of the medical expert in prediction if Eisenhower were approved by his doctors for reelection and should die in the campaign or in office. Such a happening would surely affect adversely the aura of optimism toward heart attacks engendered by the President's illness and by Paul White's remarks. It would confound the plans of his supporters and associates in the White House, the Congress and the Republican Party. It would leave the country in the hands of the Vice President, who would probably be Richard Nixon, a prospect not to be casually contemplated. These were powerful, worrisome considerations facing Paul White and he sought first a way out, one which was never publicized.

The first time after the flight back from Denver when the President was reexamined by Paul White was December 17, 1955 in Gettysburg. Colonel Mattingly drove out to Eisenhower's Gettysburg farm early that morning to take blood for a clotting test and to record an electrocardiogram and he was joined by Paul White and General Snyder in mid-morning. The findings of the examination were very favorable and were presented to a press conference that day. Paul White's notes for the conference included the statements: "The progress to date has been excellent and encouraging but he has not yet been subjected to his full load of work. Four or five weeks of exposure to that should suffice for a medical estimate as to the ability of his heart to stand it." "The future rests in the 'lap of the gods,' as it more or less does with all of us in this room. With average luck and common sense care the President can live for years and be fully active, as have many others among my patients who have recovered similarly at this age of their convalescence, but since none of them has been president of the USA I cannot speak with experience on that point. We can only advise the President medically—he must make his own decision."

At the conclusion of the press conference Colonel Mattingly and General Snyder returned to Washington but Paul White unbeknownst to them went back to the Eisenhower farm where, an unexpected guest, he was invited to lunch. That Paul White should have sought out a separate unannounced meeting with the patient, not in the presence of the Army physicians, was not received joyfully by them. The next day Paul White described in a letter to General Snyder how after lunch and a brief rest, he and the President "walked quite a long distance around the farm, not rapidly, but over much rough ground through the cornfields and up and down several gentle slopes. We went at a pace that was just suited to the ground but we didn't stop to rest. I think it took us half an hour and there was quite a cold wind." He observed: "He was not short of breath in the least nor did he complain of any discomfort, leg weariness, or fatigue." As he wrote, this was an "excellent functional test."

The "functional test" was the explanation for this visit conveyed to Drs. Mattingly and Snyder. However, there was another confidential and more important purpose. Paul White used the occasion to suggest to

Eisenhower that he forsake the idea of running again for the Presidency. Instead, he urged that he consider the option of becoming an International Ambassador for peace, using his international prestige, his years of experience with large issues, his acquaintance with foreign heads of state, and his role as an old soldier now devoting his life to a non-military cause. Should the President adopt this suggestion, it would remove the problem of an uncertain longevity of the Chief Executive. It would relieve Eisenhower of the pressures of the presidency. It would also promote one of Paul White's greatest interests, that of world peace.

Eisenhower evidently thought seriously about the proposal. Paul White had written to him on December 18, the day after the Gettysburg visit, mentioning that the proposal was an endorsement of advice given the President both by one of the President's friends (unnamed) and by a writer to Paul White, also unnamed; the letter also indicated Paul White's readiness to assist in such an undertaking using his own international contacts in science. The President wrote to him on December 27 as follows: "I much appreciate your interest in the question that is, quite naturally, paramount in my mind." Paul White wrote to him again on January 1st to the effect that the members of the Ella Lyman Cabot Trust of which Paul White was the Chairman had talked over the matter confidentially and the group would like to be "of some definite help to you in this major role." However, an essentially negative response was sent by Eisenhower on January 14th when he wrote to Paul White:

Have tried to test out my friends as frequently and thoroughly as I could on the idea we discussed on the sun porch at Gettysburg. It is astonishing how universally they have rejected the idea that an individual, no matter how well known in the world, could be reasonably effective in the promotion of peace based on understanding, unless operating from an official position of great power.

This point came up for discussion last evening with a group of my closest associates in government and the conclusions were unanimous along the line I have indicated. Nevertheless, I am not completely convinced.

With warm regard,

Sincerely,

D. E.

This letter concluded the episode. The International Ambassador for peace role was now not an option and the matter was dropped.

It was important that at the time of the December 17 visit in Gettysburg, Eisenhower made it very clear that the final decision as to his political future would be his alone and not delegated to the physicians. As Paul White wrote to General Snyder on December 18, "he does not want to be dependent on our advice for his decision unless it should be, of course, distinctly unfavorable." This theme was well known to Colonel Mattingly who had written to Paul White on December 22: "I am glad that you have learned first hand from the President that he does not desire his physicians to make decisions about his future. He will make his own decisions. He has much experience in the past in making decisions on important and vital problems in both war and peace. What he likes from his staff and advisors, medical or otherwise, is accurate and usable information, regardless of whether it is optimistic or pessimistic."

The medical team taking care of the President was thus under pressure to make up its mind on a statement on his health which would allow him to resolve the burning second term issue. Reaching a consensus proved sticky. On November 12th, Paul White had written to the President a summary of his views on his health. He concluded with the P.S.: "Confidentially, I believe that my own attitude is midway between the slightly divergent views of General Snyder and Tom Mattingly. The General's attitude is, I believe, a little more liberal than mine and Tom's a little more conservative." The three doctors had no disagreement with the obvious fact that the decision as to his future rested with Eisenhower himself. They also agreed that any statement must accept the possibility that another heart attack with or without survival could occur. They further agreed that the scientific facts upon which to base an educated opinion regarding the outlook for a male of 65 years who had endured a heart attack and who occupied the position of President of the United States were just not available. They additionally concurred that he had made a very satisfactory recovery from his attack without any of the ominous signs of further trouble such as angina pectoris, heart failure or abnormal heart rhythm. What was not unanimous was the interpretation of his current state in relation to future presidential responsibilities.

A dinner conference was held at General Snyder's apartment in Washington on January 8, 1956 with Paul White, Colonel Mattingly and General Leonard D. Heaton, Commanding General of Walter Reed Hospital, in attendance in addition to the host. Paul White's notes on this meeting included the following:

> Much debate—prolonged and from all angles concerning the hazards and wisdom re: continuing in the Presidency after this term is completed. It was obvious that all believed that the President would be active no matter what he decides about the Presidency and that the hazards to him might not be very different but he is concerned deeply about the possibility of recurrent illness or death while in office after this term is finished. . . . Dr. Snyder stated that he was giving the President all information he thought necessary about the risk of the next five years. The President realizes this. Mattingly and P.D.W. insisted that he must make it clear that the risk is great. Dr. Mattingly thinks it is even—PDW inclined to think it is less than even but also agreed that no adequate statistics are available even though they may be referred to and quoted ad nauseam. Dr. Mattingly's experience has obviously been far more unfavorable than that of PDW. . . . The impressions of some are unfavorable, of others favorable. . . .

Paul White wrote to General Snyder on January 19th thanking him for the dinner and emphasizing "that we cannot predict." However, this is exactly what they were expected to do and indeed finally did after further correspondence and discussion.

Paul White was aware of Colonel Mattingly's unhappiness both about his seemingly excessive optimism in his comments to the press, yet more conservative views when the doctors were together, and about his separate contacts with the President, especially at Gettysburg in mid-December. On February 9th, Paul White wrote to Colonel Mattingly a handwritten letter recounting for the first time the facts of the discussion at Gettysburg and apologizing: "I do believe that we can still act as a team and now that I have made this confession to you which you might tell General Snyder about. . . . My motives have been of the best (actually probably too idealistic for this rough and tumble world) and I hope that you and General Snyder (and the President too) will accept my explanation and apology for any confusion. . . ."

There was finally a reasonable meeting of the minds. The President was examined at Walter Reed Army Medical Center on February 11,

1956 by Drs. Snyder, Heaton, Mattingly and Pollock. He was checked by Paul White on the morning of February 14th. Following that last examination, there was a press conference once again presided over by Jim Hagerty. General Snyder started off by reading the favorable medical report including the findings from the laboratory studies, concluding with the statement: "Thus, the above findings show that the President has made a good recovery from the attack of coronary thrombosis which occurred last fall." A reporter, Edward T. Folliard of the *Washington Post and Times Herald* promptly asked: "Is it the judgement of the doctors that he could serve another four years in the White House without any damage to himself?" The response from Snyder was "We believe that he can serve four or five years or longer in a very active position of great responsibility." Paul White was immediately asked to make a statement, which, after commenting in a similar vein on the recovery, concluded by being even more optimistic: "Fully aware of the hazards and uncertainties that lie ahead, we believe that medically the chances are that the President should be able to carry on an active life satisfactorily for another five to ten years." When asked if he would vote for Eisenhower if he ran again, Dr. White answered: "If he runs." The *Washington Post and Times Herald* had on its front page the next day a headline extending across eight columns which said: "Eisenhower Can Run, Doctors Decide: 5–10 Years in Public Life Seen Ahead."

There it was. Despite their original intentions, a prediction had been made by the doctors. Despite the concerns of Colonel Mattingly, the statements by Snyder and Paul White were clearly optimistic. It was now up to Eisenhower to make up his mind, which he did, but not until the night of February 28, announcing the next day that subject to the decision of the Republican National Convention, "my answer will be positive, that is, affirmative." Walter Lippman commented in his column *Today and Tomorrow*, on March 2, 1956: "It was the talk of a man who has managed to say yes but is still full of doubt and misgiving."

James Reston, the *New York Times* reporter, included in his book *Sketches in The Sand* a conversation he had with Paul White which he had reported on March 4, 1956 as follows:

The President did give some reasons for his decision: the work he had set out to do four years ago was not now finished. Beyond that, he said, "I have, first of all, been guided by the favorable reports of the doctors." He went on to say, in a remark that has fascinated many observers here, that "some" of his doctors thought the dangers to his health would be "less in the Presidency than in any other position I might hold."

This, however, merely raises the other fascinating question about the philosophy of Dr. Paul Dudley White. I rode to the airport with him the morning after he made his final report that the chances were that the President could continue as he was now for "five or ten years." He is a charming man and clearly a philosopher. He explained his philosophy about advising heart patients. The primary question he asked, he said, was about the state of a patient's mind. If you could contribute to a man's happiness, he observed, you could probably add to his life.

Therefore, he continued, a man's spiritual foundation and his work were the main things to be considered. It was important to a patient to feel that he was "carrying on," Dr. White said, preferably in the work that he had been doing. Dr. White added that, of course, it was also important to see that in "carrying on" a patient did not submit himself to too much strain, but that, he concluded, was secondary.

The novelists and the historians will be interested in Dr. White and his philosophy. They will want to study, too, the role of Jim Hagerty, his influence on Dr. White, and the silence of the press and the medical profession on the merits and implications of the second term during the period when the President was making up his mind.

More than anybody else, Mr. Hagerty and Dr. White created the situation which the President recognized by saying "yes," this week. Dr. White made the reports which conformed with his honest diagnosis and his philosophy and Mr. Hagerty dramatized those reports in one of the most brilliant public-relation jobs in history.

The place of Paul White in all these discussions surrounding the political future of Eisenhower was described by Russell Baker in the *New York Times* of December 24, 1955—described with his usual wit and charm, perhaps timed as a friendly Christmas present:

Paul White, as a chief civilian consultant and spokesman on the President's illness, is a central figure in this politico-medical drama. What he says about the President's health will have a profound effect on the fortunes of both major political parties.

Yet fate can rarely have chosen an unlikelier man to carry history about in his pocket. At the age of 69, he is a short, wiry man who, on first appearance, gives the abstracted impression of the absentminded professor. The impression is reinforced by a small, unpretentious mustache and his rimless eyeglasses.

His apparent inability to posture in the spotlight, his refusal to obscure his meaning in the argot of the medical cult, his utter ignorance of political duplicity—all contribute to make him a bizarre figure to hold center-stage in the political arena.

And:

This reporter's subjective impression, from having watched the doctor since his emergence as a public figure, is of a man who has stepped out of the pages of James Thurber.

He is the innocent man in a hostile world, giving answers to questioners outraged by honesty because they expect half-truths at best and more probably lies.

It was surprising how few doubting or negative comments about the wisdom and clairvoyance of Paul White and the other physicians were evident during this whole period. Drew Pearson's column *The Washington Merry-Go-Round* of March 3, 1956, discussing the pressures put on Eisenhower by his associates to run for reelection, referred to Paul White in a somewhat derogatory fashion as "the talkative Boston heart specialist." However, this was distinctly unusual and most reporters, columnists and editorial writers maintained a respectful and generally trusting attitude.

Not all physicians were as hopeful about the President's recovery and future as was Paul White, but here too, most criticisms were muted and not expressed in public. An exception was a letter from a doctor in Newton Center, Massachusetts to the *New England Journal of Medicine* published in its August 2, 1956 issue referring to "misinformation and silly remarks" regarding the President's health. Another exception was Dr. David D. Rutstein, Professor of Preventive Medicine at the Harvard Medical School, who wrote an article entitled "Doctors and Politics" which was published in the August 1956 issue of *The Atlantic*. He stated that Paul White's optimistic statements regarding the life expectancy of President Eisenhower were "at variance with the published scientific information in the medical literature." He also indicated that while a physician's first responsibility is to his patient, the physician also has a "duty to the public;" and emphasized that: "Once having presented the medical facts and their interpretations, if the physician goes beyond this point, he then ceases to be an expert." Essentially, Dr. Rutstein found that his fellow faculty member had given a prognosis for survival of the President unjustified by the available scientific data; and had exceeded his expertise as a physician by being like "an ordinary citizen subject to political influences. . . ."

Paul White's estimate that Eisenhower "should be able to carry on an active life satisfactorily for another five or ten years" was, as he said, based on his very large clinical experience in similar cases. Paul White did, in his November 7, 1955 press conference, allude to data regarding multiple heart attacks but these did not adequately address the issue of survival. He never wrote a rebuttal to Rutstein's article, but his thoughts as expressed in various letters written at this time stress that no two patients are ever identical in regard to their illness, its cause, its complications, and its outlook, despite the fact that the diagnostic labels are the same. His prediction was only justified as being his personal judgement in this particular case. Eisenhower after all wanted and needed a definite statement applicable not to 100 other people, but to him. Whether Paul White should have publicized the more sober published facts, including some of his own, reported in 1941, covering surveys of groups of patients, and given his basis for a prediction of a more rosy future for the President than indicated by these surveys is questionable. Such a public disclosure would surely have precipitated a brisk controversy and possibly help the Democrats. It is doubtful if it would have done more than confuse the mass of voters. It is also likely that patients like Eisenhower who had given up smoking, who had no high blood pressure and who had excellent blood cholesterol levels, were unusually good long-term risks, much better than the average patient reported in the medical literature. As it turned out, Paul White's prediction was correct.

One might consider as suggested by Rutstein whether in future similar situations the medical judgement of one or more physicians caring for a president should be accepted as final. Perhaps the advice of a different physician or panel of physicians divorced from direct patient responsibility should be sought. The advantage would presumably be an additional opinion or opinions endowed with greater objectivity; the disadvantages would be a lesser familiarity with the patient and the patient's problems and perhaps the dilemma of a difference of opinion among experts. Is a split decision, as with the Supreme Court, more authoritative in a clinical case than the decision of one experienced physician? In retrospect, the Paul White approach worked well, although Rutstein's article and comments raised pertinent issues.

One odd diversion took place in December 1955 when 470 physicians listed as heart specialists by the *Directory of Medical Specialists* received a questionnaire from the American Research Foundation of Princeton, New Jersey asking two questions: "Do you think a man who has suffered a heart attack can be regarded as physically able to serve a term as President?"; and "Based on what you have read about the nature of the President's illness, and assuming a normal convalescence in the next few months, do you think Mr. Eisenhower can be regarded as physically able to serve the second term?" The questionnaire was accompanied by a self-addressed airmail special delivery envelope and no signature was required. It was reported in the *New York Times* of January 7, 1956 that the "American Research Foundation" was a blind for Benson and Benson Incorporated, a market opinion and consumer research organization. It was never known who contracted with Benson and Benson to undertake this survey. An editorial in the *Journal of the American Medical Association* condemned the questionnaire and recommended that it should be tossed in the wastebasket. Paul White wrote the Foundation on January 2, 1956 stating that the issue of the President's health was a complex enough one, and requesting that any replies from the poll not be publicized since they must represent uninformed opinions. Nothing further was heard from the Foundation.

As might be expected, a man like Paul White who had links with many groups and activities was bound to be set upon by well-intentioned friends and others to prevail upon his famous patient to endorse or otherwise help their pet cause. Paul White screened out and discouraged the vast number of these but did bring a few to the attention of the President including some on his own initiative. On the whole, over the years, Mr.

Eisenhower and his staff were remarkably tolerant and accommodating to such requests.

Fluoridation of water supplies had long been an interest of Paul White but General Snyder indicated on April 16, 1958 that the White House preferred not to comment. However, on January 28, 1959, General Snyder did write to Dr. Frederick J. Stare, Professor of Nutrition at the Harvard School of Public Health giving a personal lukewarm endorsement to the use of fluoridated water. In May of 1958, on the basis of an enthusiastic report from Paul White about the state of Civil Defense in Massachusetts, Eisenhower wrote a note of congratulations to the officer in charge. The President was kept regularly informed of the many Paul White travels abroad including, especially, those to Africa. Despite an appeal from Paul White, Eisenhower declined on November 21, 1959 to see Dr. Albert Schweitzer while on a trip to Europe, "Because my schedule for my impending trip has already been crowded to the bursting point;" but he did agree to try to say a favorable word for American-sponsored schools in Greece. The President did agree on May 25, 1960 to transmit to the proper persons suggestions coming to Paul White for securing help for Egypt in controlling the parasitic disease, bilharziasis. After leaving the White House, Eisenhower turned down a suggestion that he address the Greater Boston and Massachusetts Heart Associations, but he did, that same year after talking with the now promoted General Mattingly, agree to be Honorary Chairman of the American Heart Association. On October 29, 1963 the ex-President attended a fundraising dinner in New York for the International Cardiology Foundation, one of Paul White's pet projects and on that occasion awarded his cardiologist a gold-plated stethoscope.

From February 1955 on, the medical care of the President became more and more the province of doctors other than Paul White. Eisenhower had a check-up at Walter Reed May 10 and 11, 1956 without Paul White being present and the report was signed only by Generals Snyder and Heaton. Early in the morning of June 8, 1956, the President was awakened by lower abdominal cramps, and because of persisting symptoms was transferred to Walter Reed at 1:30 p.m. X-rays showed small bowel obstruction. A flock of surgeons soon fluttered about the problem, including General Heaton, Dr. Isadore Ravdin, Dr. Brian Blades and Dr. John Lyons. The patient was seen by Drs. White and Mattingly who found no sign of new heart trouble. An exploratory operation was performed by General Heaton and Dr. Ravdin at 3:00 a.m. on June 9 disclosing regional ileitis, a non-malignant chronic condition. A bypass procedure was performed and the President made an excellent recovery.

Eisenhower was checked by Paul White on October 22, 1956 and on January 31, 1957; but when the President had a small stroke on November 25, 1957, Paul White was not involved in his care. Paul White examined him, now an ex-President, at Palm Desert, California on February 27, 1962 and again on November 13, 1965 at Fort Gordon Army Hospital, Augusta, Georgia, where Eisenhower was convalescing from a small myocardial infarction, the first since that of September 24, 1955. These latter two were really personal visits rather than professional consultations. The next three years saw a gradual progression of difficulties resulting in several hospitalizations, chiefly for additional heart attacks including problems with unstable heart rhythms. The former president was not seen again by Paul White until February 18, 1969, when he visited him briefly at Walter Reed Hospital. Mr. Eisenhower died quietly on March 28, 1969, having lived more than 13 years after his first myocardial infarction.

The impact of the Eisenhower heart attack story was great at the time and its influences were long-lasting. Several aspects of the episode were notable.

The patient proved to be extraordinarily cooperative, poised and uncomplaining. As Paul White wrote on February 27, 1961: "The President's attitude towards his illness was ideal; he was one of the best patients I ever had." He accepted his hospitalization and convalescent period with grace, learned to live within certain restrictions, including a daily rest period, took his anticoagulant medicine regularly, submitted to the frequent blood tests required without undue fuss, did not question the professional advice or seek to find another authority with more acceptable diagnosis or treatment, and yet clearly made up his own mind on matters such as the second term issue. He was neither an excessive invalid as a result of his attack nor a person who tried to demonstrate by foolish overactivity that there was really nothing wrong. The President's

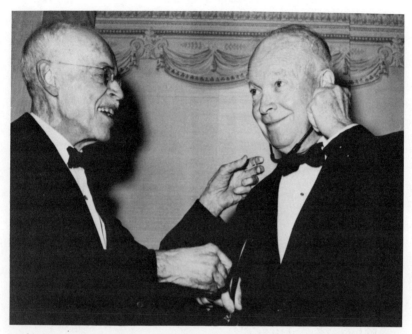

Dr. Paul D. White and former President Dwight D. Eisenhower at dinner of International Cardiology Foundation, Americana Hotel, New York City on October 29, 1963.

philosophy was well expressed in a letter to his Boston doctor from Gettysburg dated November 17, 1955:

> I am truly grateful for the trouble you took to write me such a fine explanation of what I may expect during the next few weeks. Col. Mattingly was here this morning to take a cardiogram and blood analysis, and this evening General Snyder told me that the record obtained from that examination was a good one. I understand from him that it conformed to previous findings and expectations.
>
> I think that the arrangements that you have made for my medical supervision are splendid and, of course, I shall look forward to seeing you in mid-December.

So far as a feeling of impatience on my part is concerned, I believe that I conquered that weeks ago. When I once understood what I was up against, I decided to put myself in the hands of the doctors unreservedly and to follow their instructions meticulously. These things I've tried to do—and the fact is that I am afraid that I am beginning to like the "lazy life." Anyway, it is possible that I have tried to work too hard for too many years—maybe now I will be more selective in my operations.

Today I mailed to you a book which I had inscribed to you the day I got back from Denver. This is an example of how I am beginning to practice procrastination.

Again, many thanks for your letter, and, of course, my warm regard,

Sincerely,

Dwight D. Eisenhower

The President's physicians were fortunate, therefore, in the attributes of their patient. When he did become irritated, which was not often, General Snyder as the day-by-day physician was the one who was apt to be on the receiving end. Further, the patient and his civilian consultant got along well. It was clear that Paul White developed profound respect and affection for the President and thoroughly enjoyed his visits with him. Eisenhower reciprocated these sentiments as shown by the letters quoted, and as he wrote toward the end of his life, on June 1, 1967, he viewed him not only as "one of our great medical scientists" but also "I regard him as a good friend."

The problem of having many physicians involved in Eisenhower's care was not completely solved. It is certainly easiest when a patient has only a single doctor who controls the discussions and the treatment. It is at its worst when there are multiple physicians, none of whom is recognized as the patient's doctor. With the President's illness, Paul White was recognized by the public and the press as his doctor. The President himself appears, however, to have regarded his Boston cardiologist as the esteemed consultant. Eisenhower had great respect for Colonel Mattingly who, as the leading Army heart specialist, saw the President more often than did Paul White and was more influential in meeting the requirements for the overall care. General Snyder, as a long-time friend, was useful in terms of availability and close acquaintance, but not as a source of special competence. In retrospect, what might have been a messy situation with friction and vying within the medical team was largely avoided, although differences of opinion existed from time to time. Fortunately, the physicians rose above pettiness in resolving them.

The precedent set by Eisenhower in authorizing a complete discussion of his heart attack, and by Paul White in accomplishing it was historic. No longer would it be possible to conceal for long any major presidential illness—or indeed illness of any major public figure. The advantages to the public were substantial and from this experience came others which were seized upon by press, radio, T.V. and newspapers. Later examples would be President Johnson's gallbladder surgery, ex-President Nixon's pulmonary emboli, and President Reagan's bullet wounds and colon cancer. It would be hard on the individual in public life who cherished privacy at least for his own bodily functions and health; but it also would be generally accepted that the lack of such privacy was one of the penalties for assuming a role in public affairs.

The educational value of the Eisenhower heart attack in demonstrating that an individual with a major heart attack could recover and resume useful vigorous living was tremendous. Over and over again, patients who suffered heart attacks would look to the Eisenhower illness with hope and expectation. Over and over again, physicians would quote this illness as inspiration to patients recovering from heart attacks. Over and over again, this example would help to relieve the anxiety and apprehension of families and employers and fellow workers of heart attack victims. What a heart attack was and much about its background, cause and treatment were presented in a masterful fashion.

Finally, the fact that the doctors' apparently rosy predictions for the President's recovery, return to work and survival were actually exceeded was not lost sight of by lay and professional observers. Paul White's optimism was fortunately confirmed, not just as a lucky break, but because his judgement was based on great experience, an astute scientific mind and a shrewd evaluation of the individual patient and his potential. The human computer had recorded a success.

The Healthy Life

The greatest contribution to mankind made by Paul White was undoubtedly his prescription for a healthy way of life popularized by his part in the Eisenhower case. Interested though he was in the diagnosis and treatment of heart disease, he became increasingly determined to do something to prevent illness, especially illness involving the heart, and to encourage habits conducive to good health. Beginning in his middle years, he developed a philosophy of living consonant with both mental and physical well-being, and with a useful prolongation of the life span. His ideas were based partly on what he found to be true in his own life, partly on what he witnessed in the lives of his patients and in his clinical studies, and partly on confirmation of his beliefs from the work of others. Because he appeared honest and direct and authoritative, his message made a major impact. Because his ideas seemed to make scientific and common sense, and because they were put forward forcefully but without flamboyant rhetoric, they met little opposition. He seized upon the countless opportunities afforded him to express his views both to scientific audiences and to the public at large. He clearly enjoyed speaking to and writing for the latter. And as he became nationally and internationally famous, the message was repeated again and again, became more eloquent and persuasive as it was elaborated, and evolved into a Paul White trademark recognizable around the world.

The extensive publication of Paul White's ideas on a way of life in magazines for lay audiences is one index of the exposure his views received in the media. These magazines included *Hygeia, This Week Magazine, Reader's Digest, Town & Country, Scientific American, McCall's Magazine, Parade, Vogue, Life and Health, Police, National Health Journal, Everybody's Health, Federation Topics* (Federation of Women's Clubs), *Journal of Religion and Health, The Atlantic*

Monthly, The Grade Teachers Magazine, Saturday Review, and many others. Paul White might have to decline an invitation for a lecture or interview due to conflicts with his schedule, but he usually acceded to a request for an article for a lay or scientific publication. He would fit it in by writing at night or while on a train or plane. Such articles were in addition to radio and television interviews, such as with *Meet the Press*, and interviews with reporters incidental to his many lecture tours.

Alton L. Blakeslee, formerly science editor of the Associated Press, arranged for an article by Paul White on the prevention of heart attacks to be released to the press for publication on Sunday, October 30, 1955 at the peak of public interest in Eisenhower's heart attack. He has commented that this did not appear on an inside page or in the magazine section—it was printed on *page one* of the *New York Times* and other newspapers across the country with "an audience of at least 50 million readers."

What were the elements of his philosophy, presented so widely and with such effect?

The first component which touched everything else was *optimism*—optimism as part of a positive attitude toward life. James Russell Lowell once wrote of "a nature sloping to the sunny side." This was true of Paul White who enjoyed his family and his work, relished the excitement of new adventures whether in scientific research or clinical practice or medical history or travel, and looked upon the world optimistically. He was rarely depressed, and indeed this was not to become a problem for him until the last few months of his life.

As early as 1932 he wrote a paper on "Optimism in the Treatment of Cardiovascular Disease" in which he said

> Without optimism this world would be a sorry place to live in. The natural or acquired ability to look on the bright side of things may easily mean the difference between happiness and unhappiness in any individual life.

Later in 1951, referring to attributes including optimism, he mentioned their other effects:

> It is quite certain that biologic effects also result from cheerfulness, optimism, courage, and joy. A chance to counteract the harmful effects of pain, sorrow,

and anger is possible through the inculcation of a happy disposition, which can be acquired as well as inherited. We know that clinically there are definite effects from the application of this idea. Helpful psychotherapy and the best practice of medicine depend on it in considerable part. It is probably the basis of the success for the magic temple rites in some of the treatment in the past, and also of the present popularity of such a relic as Christian Science. This situation reminds me of the current habit of the daily press of headlining and emphasizing the bad things that take place—the fires, murders, robberies, wars, and deaths—while much too little attention is paid to the good things that go on every day, every week, every month and every year.

One basis for his success as a practitioner of medicine was his recognition that even in patients with severe heart disease, the physician can almost always find some legitimate basis for encouragement and for providing hope. In 1953 in the Billings Lecture presented before the Section on Internal Medicine of the American Medical Association, he said

> The old adage of "while there is life there is hope" proves true often enough even in the sickest patients to justify its use without any overconfidence. The patient's interest in living may be supported by the attitude of those about him, and this may be the narrow margin needed for survival.

The remarkable advances in diagnosis and treatment which Paul White saw in his long career reinforced his native, cheerful and hopeful attitude. After reviewing in 1959 the records of certain of his private patients, who despite heart problems had long and useful lives, he commented: "They could be duplicated over and over again and point to important lessons, chief of which may be the need of an optimistic outlook in prognosis partly because of the rapid development of new measures of diagnosis and treatment and partly because the optimism itself has a favorable effect on the patient and on his willingness to cooperate with his medical advisors."

His attitude was summed up in May 1968 in his response to a question appearing in a Spartanburg, South Carolina newspaper which asked: "What is the cardinal rule to observe for persons who have heart trouble?" Paul White's reply was: "Just as no two persons are alike, no two cardiac patients are alike and so one cannot make set rules for all. But in the light of the medical advances in the last 25 years, the most important rule is 'be optimistic'." Happily the specialty of cardiology was rapidly developing a solid basis for this optimism, and Paul White was both an active participant in and a witness to this development.

The second component of his philosophy was the one which received the greatest attention both in the health professions and among the general public. This was his emphasis on the value of *regular physical activity*. It was indeed remarkable that a doctor in the new specialty of heart disease became a world leader in encouraging people to get physical exercise. During his early years of practice and teaching, the prevailing theme for patients with any indication of heart disease had essentially been "take it easy," and the implication often was that strenuous effort might in itself produce heart trouble in a previously healthy person. Hirschfelder, who published a textbook on diseases of the heart in 1918, suggested that one of the most important factors in producing hardening of the arteries (arteriosclerosis) in man was hard work. When David L. Edsall and Paul White joined forces in 1922 to write a treatise on "The Prevention of Degenerative Diseases," they discussed factors said by the authorities to cause arteriosclerosis and arteriosclerotic (coronary) heart disease and included long continued, strenuous physical activity (as in the heavy laborer or chronic athlete). Dr. Henri Vaquez of the Faculty of Medicine of Paris wrote in 1924: "Heart failure can be produced perfectly by overexertion and that overexertion is capable of causing the myocardial [heart muscle] changes noted after death." He suggested also that individuals suffering heart failure from physical effort must have some predisposing cause to lessen the resistance of the heart. Sir Thomas Lewis in his text on heart disease wrote in 1934 that arteriosclerosis was stated to be more prevalent in those consuming much alcohol and in those engaged in heavy manual work.

These authorities were not actually inveighing against exercise as such, but were repeating the oft-expressed view, not based on any solid evidence, that strenuous effort might be dangerous. There were few scientist spokesmen for the concept that physical exercise was actually beneficial and there was considerable bias against vigorous physical effort as being possibly dangerous even for a normal heart. Such a view was nurtured

by the increasing use of elevators, escalators, automobiles, electrical de-
vices in the home, and mechanization in the work place, all deliberately
designed to minimize the need for physical exertion.

Paul White began to write and speak about the positive benefits of
physical exercise in the late 1920's. He first emphasized its role in patients
with heart disease when he commented in 1927:

> Exercise as an aid in maintaining good health is beneficial in heart disease
> providing there is cardiac reserve sufficient to permit it. When, however, there
> is angina pectoris [chest discomfort] or dyspnea [undue shortness of breath] on
> slight exertion, no active exercise should be allowed.
>
> Walking is probably the best exercise because it is easy for anyone to accom-
> plish and easy to grade from the slowest shortest walks to the most rapid and
> longest. Golf is good exercise for cardiacs with some reserve but fast, hard,
> competitive playing over hilly holes is to be avoided. A few level holes may
> suffice. Golf has often been blamed because there is a death from heart failure
> on the links. Such deaths are to be expected when one considers the large
> number of elderly people, often with angina pectoris, who play the game and
> who would die about as quickly walking along the street. The late Sir James
> Mackenzie thought golf was a suitable game for a man with angina pectoris.

Two years later in 1929 in a presentation made before the United States
Public Health Service, he wrote more specifically about exercise as a way
indeed to prevent disease:

> You can all do something towards keeping your hearts and arteries in good
> condition. Most of you are careless of health even though you are intelligent
> in other matters. . . . Exercise to keep fit. To be indolent physically is worse
> than to be excessively athletic; there is a happy mean. To have good muscles
> and a freely moving diaphragm, not obstructed by abdominal fat, is an impor-
> tant and vital element in maintaining good health and in aiding the heart and
> blood vessels in their work. Use your arms and legs and lungs more, and your
> stomachs and automobiles less.

The scientific basis for these early statements was not of the type which
would be required later in the century by recognized authorities. Paul
White had performed no laboratory-based physiological experiments,
had undertaken no large, controlled clinical studies, and could quote little
solid work by others. Later, he did buttress his belief with limited scientific commentaries on former football players and on heart disease in

various parts of the globe where he saw populations with differing exercise patterns; and confirmation of his views began slowly to come from the work of others. His belief was founded essentially on his years of experience with patients and what he learned was helpful to his own mental and physical health.

He supported his argument for exercise with case histories of individuals whose lives bore out his views. One was that of the famous runner Clarence DeMar who had run in 34 Boston Marathons and had won 7 of them. DeMar not only ran in the Marathons to the age of 66 but continued regular exercise until his death from cancer at the age of 70. He used to run about Boston from appointment to appointment instead of walking or using the subway or taking a taxi or car. As Paul White and his associate James H. Currens reported in 1961, at autopsy DeMars' heart was found not only to be healthy but his coronary arteries which carried the blood to nourish the heart muscle were two to three times normal in size. Another case history was that of one of his patients, Charles W. Thiery, who lived to be 107½. Mr. Thiery was always very active, walking a mile or more daily even in very old age. Paul White used to ask him to come each year to his post-graduate course at the Massachusetts General Hospital as an example of mental and physical fitness in old age. This annual event delighted them both as well as the audience. White loved this kind of warm, person-to-person occasion, his eyes would sparkle, and he would ask the old man questions which he knew would result in witty answers. When, as anticipated, the audience would respond with laughter, he would join in and a good time was had by all.

The value of bicycling, which was one of his own favorite forms of exercise, was mentioned in a 1937 article written for *Hygeia*, and was repeated and expanded upon over the subsequent years:

> For a long time, observant Americans have stood by, watching the waste of health and of money by the average citizen that has insidiously crept into this country with the abandonment of simple exercise in our daily life. We are too busy or distracted or modest or lazy to intervene. Occasionally feeble or half-hearted protests are voiced, and some who should know better have said it is unimportant.

Recently, however, there has been revived an enthusiasm for hiking and bicycling trips into the country. The time therefore seems right for transforming such fads of the moment into permanent features of American daily life, not only for the sake of health but for enjoyment and economy.

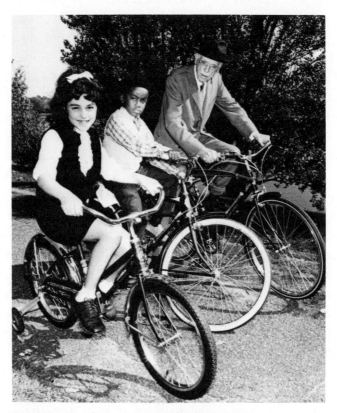

Dr. Paul White with Terry and Clement on the Paul White Bicycle Path of the Metropolitan District Commission, Boston, 1969.

There were numerous opportunities for Paul White to expound on this message, and indeed he finally became wary of welcoming committees that met him with a bicycle whenever he got off a plane.

In the same article he also referred to another of his pet themes, the value of physical effort as an antidote to anxiety and tension:

The enjoyment and pleasure of exercise come not merely in the playing of games or in exploration, if one walks or cycles, but also in the sensation of fatigue of muscles and a relaxation of mind.

Writing much later to his old friend Dr. Harold M. Marvin of Yale, who had some reservations about the Paul White emphasis on exercise, he said

> . . . I believe there is now more and more evidence that exercise, or rather lack of it, is favorable for the greater advance in earlier atherosclerosis. . . . However, I think the most important value of exercise or physical labor is as an antidote for emotional stress and nervous tension, whether or not there is an effect on the arteries per se. I myself and many of my patients and friends have found this to be true, for example, they sleep better if they are physically tired. They are relaxed. Their digestion is better. They can think more clearly. I think in many ways our strenuous ancestors thought more clearly than we do and they didn't eat three square meals a day.

One obvious target for him to aim at was middle age with its tendencies to reduced physical activity and overweight and habits conducive to heart attacks and strokes. Speaking to the Federation of Women's Clubs in 1960, he said

> Much has been said and done about youth fitness which continues to be a serious problem in this country but is now being attacked with vigor. A good deal is being done about the problems of old age, but the time of life that has been most neglected has been that of middle age which may be said to extend from 20 to 80 [when he wrote this sentence, Paul White was 73]. The former critical years from birth to 20 when infections took such a frightful toll are no longer the critical years except for the teen-agers who are killed on the road in accidents usually resulting from their own recklessness. It is at the end of youth and at the beginning of the settling down process in the early and middle 20's that danger starts. The period of 20 to 40 is a critical age, I affirm, when the rusting process in the artery walls (which we call atherosclerosis) begins. This rust piles up year by year until at the age of 45 or 50 the overnourished man of our day comes to a doctor with angina pectoris, a heart attack, or a little stroke, or he may die suddenly. This sudden death is not really so sudden. It is the end result of a long period of accumulating disease. As a matter of fact, this was pointed out by Lancisi in Rome 253 years ago. If only somebody had realized the importance of his pronouncements then, we would not be so far behind now.
>
> At 24 or 25 years of age the young man, who is the chief candidate for trouble, marries and settles down in his profession, business, or other occupation. He begins under present conditions to get fixed in his unhealthy ways of life. He eats too much rich food, he exercises too little, and he smokes too much. He is constantly harassed nervously by problems of business and family and then he blames hard work for what is due to his bad habits. No one, especially a man, should gain any weight after the age of 25 and everyone,

especially the well muscled male, should continue vigorous physical exercise or physical work all through life, reducing the tempo of it sensibly in middle age and later but never stopping. Healthy exercise is valuable not only for the maintenance of good physiological functions in the body, which include the circulation, the digestion, and the breathing, but also mental clarity and a feeling of good health. It is probably the best antidote we know for nervous tension and should be recognized as such. We certainly shall not need so many sedatives and tranquilizers if we establish such a program. Incidentally exercise in the open air is superior to exercise in a closed space. The freshness of outdoor air and a moving atmosphere are undoubtedly further aids in this program of positive health.

Thus, the type of exercise he recommended especially was outdoor activity because it was interesting and pleasurable and could be continued in some fashion to almost any age. He particularly encouraged exercise involving use of the leg muscles which act as an accessory pump propelling the blood through the circulation, and therefore he mainly championed walking and bicycling and golf. Walking he liked, as it could most easily be fitted into a person's daily schedule without need for special equipment or facilities. He vigorously endorsed bicycling, because it too was a good way to use the leg muscles and could be done out-of-doors, allowed one to enjoy a changing scene and permitted one to go from place to place quickly. He thoroughly approved of golf, but this required, of course, planning, golf clubs, a golf course, and usually a more substantial amount of time than either of the other two activities. In general, he liked all of the outdoor sports. He considered calisthenics and other similar routines better than nothing, but dull. Stair-climbing he encouraged as, like walking, it was frequently available and was good exercise.

The era of jogging commenced long after his interest in exercise had been fully developed. Dr. John D. Cantwell has published a letter that Paul White wrote in 1968 about jogging, which said in part:

I have nothing against jogging as such if it is properly done, preferably outdoors in the open air and in pleasant surroundings, begun in youth and maintained throughout life. Its older participants should be carefully checked with a physician at hand when dealing with large numbers not adequately supervised, especially with respect to coronary patients or coronary candidates among the middle-aged and elderly men who have not maintained a state of physical fitness throughout life. I have personally known of two sudden deaths of middle-aged joggers while jogging around an indoor track and of a near death in a man who became a patient of mine in an acute coronary attack, and I presume that there have been others of whom I have not heard and who quite naturally would not be publicized. Hence I would prefer walking in the fresh air or cycling indoors or out for the middle-aged or older—or swimming or other exercises that use the legs . . .

Thus you can see that I have mixed feelings about jogging.

Three years before his death, in answering a query from a 53-year-old man, which was submitted to him by a publication of the National Jogging Association, he wrote the pithy reply: "You can probably walk into old age better than to hustle into it."

Paul White was not one to give advice and then not follow it. His propensity for walking or bicycling rather than riding in a car, and of climbing stairs rather than using the elevator, became legendary. And it was these legends which promoted so effectively his belief in such a way of life. Because each of these episodes was unique, those who observed them never forgot them and they often appeared in the press.

Dr. Irving Wright has described a formal dinner at the home of Professor Pedro Cossio in Buenos Aires which ended about midnight. The host ushered Paul White to the door where the latter announced that he was going to walk the two miles back to the hotel. The Argentinians were aghast at the thought of walking alone in the dark at midnight, Paul White could not be dissuaded, and finally he had his walk, preceded and followed by a car with lights on and accompanied by a group of doctors all attired in dinner jackets.

Dr. David Freiman has described another episode in Lima, Peru, where a medical meeting was held outside the city at the fairgrounds:

There was at the entrance to the fair grounds one of those trains that are commonly on fair grounds to take sightseers around. Since it was a fair distance between the entrance to the fair grounds and the auditorium where the presentation was going to take place, the very distinguished group invited Paul White to step aboard this train which would then take him to the place of the meeting. In his characteristic fashion, Dr. White took one look at this and said, "No, we'll walk." And you've never seen such a crestfallen group! I doubt that they had walked that far in all their lives. It must have been a half-mile and to me it was a perfectly normal walk, but there was a very disconsolate group that arrived at the auditorium with Paul White leading the way.

Paul White addressed the National Press Club in Washington shortly after the Eisenhower heart attack episode. Griffing Bancroft, former Washington correspondent and commentator for CBS, has written:

> At the time I was a member of the Board of Governors of the National Press Club in Washington, D.C. Dr. White had agreed to be a luncheon speaker at the club.
>
> It was our custom to have a small reception off the main dining room where speakers could have refreshment with members of the board and other head table guests before the luncheon.
>
> The club was on the 13th floor of the National Press Building and a couple of members would meet the guests in the lobby of the building and an elevator was held to whisk them up.
>
> Dr. White was so met and one of the escorts, I don't remember who it was, remarked how nice it was to have an elevator waiting. Dr. White spied the stairway and said: "Why not walk?" With the newsmen staggering in his wake, he strode up the thirteen floors, arriving for the reception as fresh as could be. Our colleagues collapsed into chairs.

This was a bravura performance but in retrospect one of questionable wisdom for a group of men of uncertain physical training and health.*

On another occasion, he came from Boston to address the Advertising Club of New York located at Park Avenue and 37th Street in Manhattan. Dr. Theodore G. Klumpp, a long-time patient who was at the luncheon, has described the event.

> Knowing that he was a heart specialist and not knowing what his theme was to be, the members had prepared little kerchiefs to distribute with the words "Take It Easy" embroidered on them. In beginning his talk, Dr. White held up the handkerchief, thanked them for the gesture, saying, "These are very nice but there is a typographical error in the message. The word "Don't" has been omitted, and the message should be "Don't Take It Easy." Of course there was a great burst of laughter and applause that followed.
>
> Dr. White as usual made a magnificent address which was received with great and sustained applause. After the meeting and on the way out, I asked Dr. White if he were returning directly to Boston. He said that he was and the following conversation occurred: "Dr. White, I'll go ahead and hail a taxi to take you to LaGuardia Airport." "No," said Dr. White. "I'm going to walk to the airport."

---

* One member of the party declined to climb the 13 flights and died suddenly one week later.

"Oh," I said, "the airport is a long distance from here and I don't think they have a pedestrian walk on the bridge." "Yes they do," responded Dr. White, "I know because I've walked it before."

Dr. Florence Avitabile was once with Paul White at an airport, and they were walking down a flight of stairs paralleled by an escalator. As they descended, a young man passed them going up the escalator, and Paul White called to him with a twinkle in his eye: "You should be walking." The young man thus gently reprimanded turned and looked back, recognized the short, gray-haired man with rimless glasses, wearing a gray suit and the customary gray felt hat with upturned brim, and said: "You must be Dr. White!"

Yet another well-known episode occurred when, at the age of 74, Paul White flew from Boston to National Airport in Washington to see President Kennedy. It was a nice day and he was early, so he proceeded to walk to the White House wearing, as he always did, his brown Ground Gripper shoes. Apparently no one had ever before walked to the White House from the airport, and in succession the guard at the gate, Dr. Janet Travell who was Kennedy's doctor at the time, and the President himself were absolutely flabbergasted. Paul White recounted how he had been recognized by several motorists who stopped and offered him rides, all of which he declined.

He did not get exercise just on special and important occasions. Rather, this was his usual and daily preference, in the hospital in Boston, at his homes in Chestnut Hill and later in Belmont, as well as at his place in Harvard, Massachusetts. He also liked to garden, and when he could, he might bicycle, ski, skate, or swim, or rarely play golf. He maintained an active pace to the very end of his life, and bicycled for 8 miles on the boardwalk at Atlantic City when he was 83.

He opened many bicycle paths, including a pioneer one in Chicago in 1956 when he and Mayor Richard Daley joined forces on a tandem bicycle. The Mayor, who was portly, looked uneasy on this unaccustomed seat, and it appeared that Paul White, who was in the rear position and who was half his size, provided most of the motive force. He was involved in or supported various safe bicycling associations including those in Boston and Cambridge. The Bicycle Club of Homestead, Florida was named for him, and he was named Honorary President of the Bicycle Touring League of America. He was clearly a tremendous asset to the bicycle manufacturers; and while he never endorsed any one product, his influence was a major factor in greatly increased sales of bicycles starting in the 1960's. After reading a news item about the rising bicycle sales, the author and commentator Lowell Thomas sent Paul White a note in July 1969: "Looks like your dream is coming true! Many many congratulations. Even I have a bicycle, and I am much enjoying it." A Congressional Breakfast on Bicycling sponsored by the Bicycle Institute of America was held in Washington on May 1, 1964, and was attended by more than 60 members of Congress. Given wide national publicity was a photograph of a cheerful group of Congressmen on bicycles led by the smiling Paul White and Secretary of the Interior Stewart L. Udall.

A third and major part of his philosophy was the belief that people are better off in their mental and physical health if they *work*. He never encouraged early retirement unless for reasons of serious ill health, and he urged the elderly to keep involved with a job or a hobby or both as long as possible. It was his conviction that most patients with heart disease, young and old, were better off if encouraged to keep busy within the limits of tolerance, and he was a pioneer in recognizing the need for rehabilitation of heart patients—although this was not formally labeled rehabilitation at first. In the clinics at the Massachusetts General Hospital, in his office, and in his consultations, wherever they might be, it was his constant concern that patients avoid unnecessary invalidism. To this end, he encouraged, encouraged, encouraged. He and his associates, including social workers, continually maintained as a prime goal for each patient participation in some useful work—work to help the individual economically and physically and psychologically.

As early as 1921, he was writing

Heart disease and industry are not incompatible. An individual may be productive even while bedridden with heart trouble a large part of the time. The active trained mind of a cardiac cripple may be more valuable in an industrial process than a body in perfect health controlled by a dull intellect. In general we have all been inclined to shelter too much our young patients with heart disease. They can usually do more than we have permitted.

Thirty-five years later, he addressed the Harvard Medical Alumni Association on the subject "The Ways of Life and Heart Disease: A Plea for Positive Health." His remarks on work were set forth in vigorous, secure terms, with a confidence based upon decades of experience. In his address, he referred to the advice he had given to his patient, President Eisenhower, then fully recovered from his heart attack:

> Physical strain includes, of course, much of the life work of many millions of persons in the world today, but it has yet to be proved that, barring exceptions of extremely strenuous labor and accidents on the job, work per se physically ever hurt a healthy man, woman, or child. Unhappily industry and other physical occupations have been blamed (for lack of a suitable substitute for such blame in our way of life today) as the cause of many of the ills, even including coronary atherosclerosis, which in all probability are in no way associated with such physical activity. This is a serious error still currently practiced today and for the sake of the future of this country urgently demands correction. Not only is physical work not responsible for most of these ills but it is probably one of the most potent health habits which we should make full use of, perhaps most of all at older ages when too many hundreds of thousands of persons are retired to sit in armchairs and to drowse in front of television screens day after day and even year after year, both to the detriment of their own health and to that of society which could with more wise planning utilize their experience, and their accumulated wisdom often for a good many years more, though perhaps at a decreased tempo . . .

Such were the three major elements of his philosophy for a way of life: optimism, regular physical activity, and work. They clearly interrelated and reinforced each other and constituted what he believed to be a strong effective tripod—a platform for maintaining health and preventing disease.

That this message sometimes had unexpected consequences was shown by a letter he received from Iowa in 1957. Paul White was not gifted in light repartee and telling jokes, but he had an excellent sense of humor and loved to read the contents of the letter to audiences—always to their great delight. The writer indeed became a regular correspondent until his death 15 years later.

Dear Doctor:

Here I've been living the life of Riley for the past five years after recovering from a coronary. No hard work; even 84 year old grandma sees that others carry all the packages. When I do work in the garden for half hour I'm urged to sit myself in the shade to enjoy a cooling drink.

But, why did you have to tell the reporters that this was all hooey and that I could even shovel snow? What a let down! Couldn't you write the *Ames Tribune* that the reporters misunderstood you, that that was just for young healthy fellows, not for guys older than Eisenhower? You sure spoiled it, the life of Riley, what a memory. Back to the old grind.

You never lived with a woman who tried to keep you from becoming bored over the weekend. For the past forty years until the coronary deal there was a bulletin board in the kitchen of things to be done over the weekend. Now, since your newspaper statement the board is back up. Doctors can be useful, but woe is me, that a doctor of your repute should tell my wife what is good for me. Then to top it off my doctor speaks in awed tones when referring to you. That's the clincher. Doctor why did you do it, it was so nice while it lasted.

Paul White reinforced the tripod of his philosophy with several supports which in time became a part of the structure. One was his dislike of obesity because of its relation to high blood pressure and heart disease and because it limited the individual in his or her routine of exercise and imposed unnecessary work on the heart. Had Paul White been himself plump, he might have passed over this with few or no words—as some overweight physicians have done. However, being decidedly lean, he was an ideal example of what he was preaching and felt no restraint in speaking out. Writing in 1930, he spoke of the need to prevent high blood pressure (hypertension) and how important it was "to avoid over-eating and obesity . . . the obvious recommendation to make to a young, middle-aged, or even old person who wants to do what can be done to avoid hypertension." Initially he paid little attention to the type of diet aside from a restriction in calories for those who were overweight. However, in time he was exposed in collaborative epidemiological adventures to Dr. Ancel Keys of the University of Minnesota, whose career was devoted to demonstrating the hazards to our arteries (and especially the coronary arteries of the heart) of eating much cholesterol and saturated fat. Gradually in the 1950's, Paul White himself began to propound the views of Keys. Yet, he was never as much of an apostle as some, and in his own diet took considerable liberties such as drinking milkshakes for lunch and eating ice cream.

His admonitions against obesity, as well as his encouragement of regular physical activity, both seemingly aimed at the middle-aged male, at times proved hard for wives. One wrote to him in 1966 in exasperation:

> I'm sure you have saved the lives of many husbands by advising wives to protect their husbands' hearts by serving proper meals (and exercising them at regular intervals). That is wonderful. But how many marriages have you broken up in the meantime? Alas, it is a fact. You have made the wife into a tyrant. Or a nagging shrew. Or a "mother symbol."

Paul White wrote in response that she had "raised a justified challenge to me" and, acknowledging that it was "not so easy to teach an old dog new tricks," stressed the "need to educate the young to establish proper life-time habits."

Regarding alcohol, he took a middle course. He was not opposed to the "moderate" use of alcohol and would take a cocktail or glass of wine himself. He abhorred cocktail parties ("a most barbaric custom") and certainly deplored the excessive use of any form of liquor. Scientific information on the damaging effects of alcohol on the heart came after he had done most of his own important scientific work.

Cigarette smoking was yet another factor about which he gradually came to feel strongly. He had smoked briefly while in London working with Sir Thomas Lewis but gave it up, as it made him feel nauseated. It is interesting that on February 17, 1917, in answer to a letter from the chief of the medical section of the Council of National Defense in Washington asking him, as one who had recently been in the European War Zone, for the five suggestions "which you think would be of the greatest practical value to the government," Paul White listed as number four: "The YMCA's and canteens at the base hospitals did very much good work. The restriction of alcohol was wise and practical. Tobacco was dispensed to the men as rations—I do not believe in that medically." Just what he had in mind by "medically" is unclear, but the comment was clairvoyant. In truth there was at first little scientific evidence to justify a condemnation of the use of tobacco, but in time, convincing data began to be developed. In 1937, Earle Glendy, Samuel A. Levine, and Paul White together studied 100 patients under the age of 40 years with coronary heart disease and compared them with 300 individuals who had lived beyond the age of 80 years. There was a decided excess of smokers in the younger group, but Paul White was cautious in his conclusions. It was not until 1954 that the definitive study relating cigarette smoking to heart attacks was reported by Hammond and Horn of the American Cancer Society. Thereafter, Paul White, like the great majority of physicians, opposed cigarette smoking as a habit unequivocally detrimental to the health.

Finally, it should be mentioned that he made reference from time to time to the importance of spiritual considerations in a way of life. However, his spiritual philosophy was an intellectual one and presented an extraordinary contrast to the strong beliefs of his father. Paul White's father profoundly trusted in the existence and paternal love of God and of Christ as the son of God, and he found strength and comfort from a close affiliation with the Baptist Church. At least in part in reaction to what Paul White found to be at times the pervasive influence of the church in his parents' home, his own view of religious faith and doctrine was different. He was not formally affiliated with any sect and certainly was no longer a participating Baptist; he wrote in 1955 in response to an inquiry from a Unitarian minister: "It happens that I am not a Unitarian myself but I have done a good bit of work with the Unitarian Service Committee and have attended frequently the Unitarian Church in Belmont. I heartily approve of their good works."

Paul White recognized that spiritual concerns had a legitimate and proper place in completing and strengthening an individual's philosophy of life. He used the terms "soul" and "spirit" interchangeably, and said in 1951: "The spirit can be passed on by any individual during his life and can be handed on, through his inspiration at death. We physicians have the opportunity of inspiring our patients with courage, equanimity, and patience, all attributes of the spirit."

His was a practical and unemotional attitude, hardly uplifting to many people. Regarding God, a being never mentioned in his formal writings, he wrote in 1966 to one correspondent:

> In answer to your letter of September 19, I am writing to say that certainly some power greater than man must be accepted as being responsible for the world and the universe as we know it today—whatever name we may attach. Some, I believe, are likely to call such a power *nature*, others a *supreme being*, and still others with the designation that is the common one, namely, *God.*
>
> I myself am tremendously impressed with the marvelous construction of the human body in all its detail, physical and chemical, and it is not likely that man will ever be able to duplicate it, even though he can do a great deal for health in repairing damage that has been done. The brain alone is, I suppose, essentially a computer almost beyond all imagination.
>
> Certainly such a power is by no means dead, and in this sense, everyone must acknowledge that "God" is still alive. This, I think, is the best I can do in answer to your question.

In writing of Albert Einstein, Antonina Vallentin has said: "Einstein refused to admit a God who could be reached by prayer or angered by the neglect of some secular rite. But he recognized the existence of a force superior to our petty lives." Paul White seems to have had a similar recognition.

His publications on a way of life never referred to Christ but three months before his death, he did write to a correspondent:

> Yes, I believe it is the spirit that counts most but it must be fed on action, actually I think mental and physical as well as spiritual and not necessarily based on Jesus Christ, despite the fact that his spiritual value exceeds that of most other great religious leaders.

He had a utilitarian concept of prayer as expressed in a statement written in 1958 for a book on prayer:

> My experience with patients and other individuals through the years has convinced me that in many instances prayer has a favorable psychosomatic influence. It tends to counteract the physiological effects of anxiety, it favors better sleep, and stimulates one to better efforts. In fact devotion to one's work can serve as a form of prayer. This effect of prayer is personal, that is, for the individual himself or herself.

It was fortunate that the impact of his teaching on a way of life was not dependent on his references to the spiritual. He was not at ease and secure in this field, and it is doubtful if his languge or logic relating to it contributed to the mental or physical well-being of many in his audience, although they may have been educated by his views. It might have been best if he had avoided all comment regarding religious questions, but it was his nature to try to respond as best as he could to any question directed to him. Those who observed him and those who knew him were far more impressed by the example he set by his own life than by his words regarding spiritual concerns. As Mandel Cohen commented: "If there is such a person as a Christian, I think that Paul White was maybe the only one I have known, because he was so kindly and gentle."

What the public and Paul White's associates saw and heard about the healthy life might not be a reflection of his own pattern of living. Many a public figure has had a private existence which contrasts sharply with what the individual has glibly recommended for others. Such was not true here.

Paul White loved his family and liked to be with them particularly out of doors even though his dedication to the practice of medicine, to teaching and writing, and to other activities often interfered. He was already 50 when their daughter Penny came into the family, but he found the role of parent stimulating and rewarding. It was especially at Harvard in the summers that he and the children could have a solid block of time together, and he would have the physical exercise he enjoyed. The Whites dug a small pool there for the children, a walking trail through the woods was blazed appropriately with stenciled red hearts, there would be picnics, and there would be reading aloud at night.

Early in his married life, he and Ina played golf but with the passage of years, these occasions became less and less frequent. They and the children would go cross-country skiing together in the Chestnut Hill and Belmont areas in winter, and take part in informal softball and touch football games in spring and fall. In the winters, they often had a skiing vacation together in the Laurentians, and Ina and Paul White usually also took a Florida winter vacation, but without the children, several times in the company of Dr. and Mrs. Samuel Haines. Paul White particularly enjoyed working outside, and he continued this until a few weeks before his death. He was always one to cut the lawn with a hand-mower, to shovel snow, and to rake the leaves. At Harvard, he planted a vegetable garden, picked berries, pruned bushes, cut down trees, and split wood for the fireplaces. When the woodchucks found the White vegetables to be infinitely edible, Paul White himself erected a fence which extended 18 inches deep into the ground. However, he soon found that such a barrier did not outwit the woodchucks. He liked to hike for miles and could out-walk almost everyone. He was remarkably strong although his short lean build did not suggest this. James L. Jenks recalled an episode in Alaska when several of the men in their group strained to lift a cement block and Paul White went over and raised it easily.

His disposition with the family was a cheerful optimistic one despite problems of childhood and adolescence. Their son Sandy had great diffi-culties with his school work and it was found that he had dyslexia, which required extra attention from his parents and teachers. Indeed, neither child proved to be intellectually gifted in academic studies, and neither chose to go on to college. Like his father, Sandy attended Camp Becket for a month in the summer and Penny went out to a ranch in Wyoming where she enjoyed the riding.

Paul White was not the do-it-yourself type in the home, and he avoided what went on in the kitchen. When he had time in the evenings or on rainy weekends (in his early years he was often in the office Sat-urday mornings), he would be found perusing a medical book or journal, and it seemed as if he read and read and read.*

Ina White was an ardent gardener too and kept a large number of plants in the home. She also had a small greenhouse which had been built by Sandy. As the children were growing up, she managed an active life of her own, practicing the piano for two hours a day for many years and

---

* His medical reading was well organized. Dr. Joseph B. Vander Veer recalls one evening in Philadelphia when Paul White, who had just given a lecture, asked Dr. Vander Veer for the loan of the latest issue of *The American Journal of Medical Sciences* to read during his return to Boston on the train—as he always read this journal on the second Tuesday of the month.

spending several hours a week as a volunteer at the International Students Association in Cambridge, where she was head of the Art and Garden Committee and a member of the Board of Directors. She would not usually accompany her husband on his brief speaking trips around the United States but would often go with him on his longer ventures, both within and outside the country. At home, she had the major responsibility for running the household, caring for the children, and being involved in their many activities. At times, she was forced to make the major decisions, as in the summer of 1946 when Paul White was away in Czechoslovakia for more than two months and Ina White who spent much of the period with Penny with the Aub family in Rhode Island, drove to see Sandy at camp, helped to care for the vegetable garden at Harvard, sold their house in Chestnut Hill, bought a new house in Belmont, and arranged for the move with the furniture movers so as to inconvenience her husband as little as possible on his return. Yet her affectionate and slightly wistful father's day tribute to her husband was a measure of the love and admiration which made for a happy marriage:

Today's the day we say to Dad
You're the best we could have had,
You bring home honors from afar
But still to us you're dear old Pa,
You work all day and through the night
We love you Dad with all our might.
The only thing that irks you much
Is Wimpy's wicked elbow touch.
Sometimes perhaps you wonder why
The kittens over multiply
Or why the tools are all around
Or why my keys cannot be found.
We'll try and try to be like you
We love you, Pa, please love us too.

CHAPTER ELEVEN

Investigator and Adventurer

An exciting and frustrating activity was Paul White's pursuit of the electrocardiogram of a whale, which was chiefly undertaken between the years 1952 and 1957. It seems strange and unlikely for the name of the short, lean, Boston heart specialist who was certainly not a great sportsman, to become associated with whales. Such became the case, however, and the encounters and near-misses with whales received almost as much attention as did the Eisenhower-Paul White relationship discussed in Chapter Nine.*

The story goes back to 1916 when Paul White and his young associate, Dr. William J. Kerr, reported on a dissection of the heart of a young sperm whale. Then in 1920, Dr. C. Sidney Burwell and Paul White studied the heart of a 40-year-old elephant, Mollie, who had died in the Franklin Park Zoo in Boston; these findings were combined with those of an elephant Tusko in a report by Drs. Robert L. King, Burwell and White in 1938. That same year, Paul White, James L. Jenks of the Sanborn Company, makers of electrocardiographs, and Dr. F. G. Benedict, Director of the Nutrition Laboratory of the Carnegie Institution of Washington, took the electrocardiograms of nine healthy circus elephants. They had such no-nonsense names as Tillie, Myrtle, Clara, and Lizzie, and fortunately their electrocardiograms came out beautifully because Jenks had arranged to have the elephants stand on soft flannel bags saturated with salt solution enclosing German silver electrodes, which were connected in turn to a Sanborn electrocardiograph. All of this whetted Paul White's interest in the electrocardiogram of whales as he outlined in a letter written in 1939:

---

* The Japan Heart Foundation translated Paul White's autobiography into Japanese in 1980 and changed the title from *My Life and Medicine* to *From President to Whales*.

Electrocardiograms of enlarged human hearts show sometimes changes which are difficult to interpret from the standpoint of the cause of the changes; that is, we don't know for certain whether these changes are the result of simple enlargement of the heart with increased muscle bulk or size or whether they may be due to disease of the conducting tissue in the muscle itself.

An important clue was obtained from the electrocardiograms of the elephants. There, with no disease, but of course with much bulk of muscle, there was an extraordinary spread of the waves over prolonged time intervals, somewhat comparable to what we see in very large human hearts. That is, the so-called conduction time between auricles and ventricles was twice what we see in mammalian hearts of ordinary size such as that of man or dog. The duration of the ventricular complexes was remarkably prolonged.

It occurred to me, therefore, that a still larger heart, namely that of a whale, would be especially helpful if it showed still longer durations of the time intervals in the various phases of the heart beat. Thus, to obtain an electrocardiogram of a whale would be of some practical interest from the standpoint of the human heart as well as from academic interest in general biology.

This statement provided a scientific justification for the attempt to obtain the electrocardiogram of a whale. It should be acknowledged, however, that what transpired over subsequent years mainly represented adventure—nautical adventure associated with excitement and not a little hazard. As James Jenks said later: "We were willing to take risks for the sake of adventure." Involved also were a series of technical and logistic problems including selecting a site where the whales could be found, obtaining government clearance for the projects, finding boats of appropriate size and seaworthiness with capable crews, developing an accurate gun or bow and a harpoon which would penetrate the whale tissue sufficiently but not too much, investigating electrodes and leads strong enough to withstand stress, providing for a mobile accurate recording system, and obtaining sufficient funding. In the latter forays, helicopters were employed as well as boats.

The team of three heading the effort included, besides Paul White, James Jenks, who was invaluable because of his knowledge and industrial associations in electrocardiography, and Dr. Robert L. King, a prominent cardiologist in Seattle at the Mason Clinic who was well situated to facilitate the arrangements and who had participated in recording the electrocardiograms of the elephants. By the time the project got under way,

Jenks had become president of the Sanborn Company and was able to employ the expertise of his research staff.

Between 1952 and 1967, there were no less than six expeditions attempting to achieve their objective. The first one was to Bristol Bay on the Bering Sea in Alaska where in August 1952, after hair-raising adven-

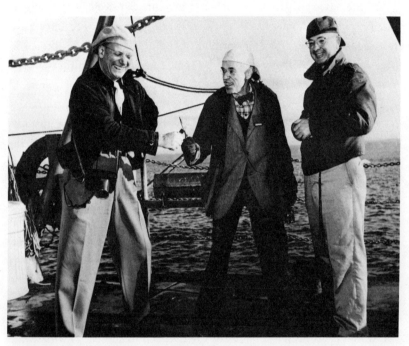

Whaling expedition, Scammon Lagoon, Baja California Sur, Mexico, February, 1956.
Left to right: James L. Jenks, Dr. Paul D. White, Dr. Robert L. King.

tures in a 20-foot open skiff, an electrocardiogram was recorded from a 14-foot white Beluga whale. The heart rate of this whale appeared to vary between 14 and 20 beats per minute, and when the whale was sacrificed, it was found that the heart weighed 2,722 grams, roughly seven-and-a-half times that of the human heart. Because the electrocardiographic recording was not satisfactory, further expeditions ensued. The next attempt was off San Diego in January 1953 where it was found that the "patient," this time a gray whale, would not allow the boat to approach near enough to fire the harpoon containing the electrode. A year later, again off San Diego and La Jolla, and despite the cooperation of the Scripps Institute of Oceanography and the U.S. Navy (including use of a Navy helicopter), there was one more failure. Thereafter operations moved farther south.

On the advice of the U.S. Fish and Wildlife Service and the Scripps Institute of Oceanography, it was decided to go early in February 1956 to the main winter breeding ground of the gray whale herd located in Mexican waters, halfway down the Pacific coast of Baja California. The area selected was Scammon Lagoon, a rarely visited body of water, 30 miles long and averaging seven miles in width, named for Capt. Charles Melville Scammon who first explored the lagoon in 1857. The auspices for this venture were indeed favorable, as the Douglas Aircraft Company and its president, Donald W. Douglas, who was a well-known sportsman, became active participants as did the National Geographic Society, which supplied a research grant, a photographer, and a writer.

A description of the expedition with excellent color photographs, written by Paul White and Samuel W. Matthews, appeared in the *National Geographic* magazine for July 1956. The plan of action was for a portion of the team including Paul White and Robert King to stay on the base ship, Donald Douglas's yacht the *Dorado*, to monitor any electrocardiogram obtained; while others, including James Jenks and Donald Douglas, would proceed in a small boat, the *Ballena*, to approach a whale and then fire into it harpoons containing electrodes. The authors wrote in the *National Geographic* magazine:

> Our plan of attack was this: by using two hand-thrown harpoons, specially designed crossbows of powerful construction, or lightweight shoulder guns, we would attempt to place two electrodes beneath the tough black hide of an adult whale, penetrating its blubber layer but not deeply enough to cause serious injury.
>
> Slender nylon-insulated wires would trail from the harpoon heads. These would be attached to a watertight sea sled somewhat resembling a midget boat, carrying radio transmitting and telemetering equipment.
>
> The harpooned whale, we thought confidently, would drag the sea sled behind it. From the instant the sled was attached, radio signals would broadcast the whale's heartbeat back to a receiver aboard *Dorado*. A few minutes would be enough to obtain a useful recording.

The auspices were favorable, the plans and the equipment seemed well designed, the whales were there, and the weather was fine, but all did not proceed as expected. Right away, the sea sleds containing the radio transmitters developed problems—one failed to work and the other gave too feeble a signal—and could not be used. Next, and not surprisingly, it was found that maternal whales do not like to be bothered while with their young. An exciting and nearly disastrous encounter with a "Mrs." Whale was described by Paul White and Samuel Matthews in the *National Geographic* magazine as follows:

> Shortly after dawn, *Ballena* disappeared up a narrow arm of the Lagoon stretching into the desert. She carried six of our party, including Mr. Douglas. Two more manned a guard-and-rescue boat; others of us kept watch and waited aboard *Dorado*.
>
> Suddenly the loud-speaker of our boat-to-ship radio blared. "*Ballena* to *Dorado*—*Ballena* to *Dorado*. A whale has hit us! We're sinking—we're sinking fast!"
>
> Our hearts sank as well, as we searched with binoculars. There was no sign of *Ballena*.
>
> Then the radio broke into sound again. "We took a hole in the bottom a foot square. The water's gaining fast, but we may be able to handle it. Here comes the guard boat. Stand by *Dorado*."
>
> Hurriedly we lowered away our one remaining skiff and attached an outboard motor. Dr. King and Paul Levesque donned life jackets to go to *Ballena*'s aid themselves. They had scarcely shoved off—and promptly stalled their motor—when the radio came to life once more. Mr. Douglas's voice boomed out:
>
> "Old Captain Scammon,
> He was sure right—
> These mama whales
> Can stand up and fight!"
>
> "We're O.K. now, *Dorado*," he reported. "We've rigged a soft patch over the hole. We're being towed in."

The story was that the hunters came upon a mother and her calf moving very slowly, *Ballena* started a slow approach and suddenly the little one leaped out of the water in fright following which the great female turned directly toward the boat and rammed it. The hull was stove in, the propeller was bent beyond use, and the rudder was lost.

There had been no chance to take an electrocardiogram that time but one more attempt was made two days later after the *Ballena* had been repaired. Two harpoons were indeed fired at a whale and at least one hit home, but in the subsequent moments of excitement and confusion, the wire leading to the harpoon was severed. Thus ended that operation.

Yet another foray took place in the same lagoon in February 1957, this time with help from the U.S. Army and an Army helicopter from which the harpoons could be discharged into the targets below. Once again, the whales outwitted human ingenuity and no definite electrocardiogram was recorded. This essentially ended the White-King-Jenks team effort although as "consultants" they did attend a gray whale expedition to the Scammon Lagoon sponsored by the Mason Research Center of Seattle in January 1967. Meanwhile in December 1959, Dr. Alfred W. Senft of the Marine Biological Laboratory at Woods Hole, Massachusetts at last obtained a very satisfactory electrocardiogram from a dying finback whale beached at Provincetown, Massachusetts. This showed a heart rate of 27 with a P–R interval of 0.74 second, approximately four times that seen in a human, and a QRS duration of 0.20 second, which was approximately twice the normal interval.

Perhaps, had Paul White been able to row up to one of these aquatic mammals and proceed with his usual careful history and physical examination he might have so charmed it that it would have floated quietly in the water to have an electrocardiogram recorded for the sake of science and the White-King-Jenks spirit of adventure.

*　　*　　*

Paul White in his later years became keenly interested in epidemiology, the study of disease and conditions associated with it as seen not in individual patients but in community or population groups. Here he was not the leader and chiefly worked with others already active in the field, learning, contributing as a cardiologist, and supporting by his energy and enthusiasm as well as by his influence in getting financial resources for investigation and training.

There was, however, in the interval of 1944–46 a significant epidemiological study in which Robert L. Levy, C. C. Hillman, W. D. Stroud and Paul White collaborated and which antedated his later work with epidemiologists. In this collaborative effort initiated early in World War II by the Subcommittee on Cardiovascular Diseases of the National Research Council of which Paul White was Chairman, the four investigators analyzed the annual medical records of 22,000 Army officers who had been followed for up to 25 or more years and obtained interesting results. It was found that transient high blood pressure (hypertension) was often a precursor of future sustained high blood pressure, as were transient rises in heart rate. Overweight showed a similar correlation, and a combination of two or all three of these factors was especially predictive of the later development of fixed hypertension, and of increased rates of retirement for medical reasons. These observations were significant in corroborating and extending similar data derived from insurance company records, and they also anticipated the findings subsequently derived from large community studies. Later Paul White was an influential and helpful supporter of the most important of these United States-based community studies, initiated in 1948 by the United States Public Health Service in Framingham, Massachusetts.

In the Hermann M. Biggs Lecture Paul White gave before the New York Academy of Medicine in 1940 on "Heart Disease—A World Problem" he said

> Heart disease is a world problem, as much as is tuberculosis or dysentery or influenza, but it has not yet been investigated as such, in contrast to many of the infectious diseases which have scourged the world, especially in the form of devastating epidemics. . . . Nature has for centuries been conducting gigantic experiments as to the effect of climate, of type of work, of diet, and of local or world-wide diseases on men, women, and children of different races, that are spread out before our very eyes for us to record and to analyze, quite readily yielding information that might never be obtainable by our own experiments on man, although certain tests could be added to enrich the findings.

In making these remarks, which sounded visionary, he was far ahead of his time.

Paul White began to share in investigating this world-wide opportunity when he became acquainted after World War II with Dr. Ancel Keys of the University of Minnesota School of Public Health who had initiated studies to identify factors responsible for the tremendous and increasing number of heart attacks due to coronary heart disease. Keys was a pioneer in his belief that the usual American diet was a prime culprit. Wanting to make meaningful comparisons between men living in the United States who were excessively prone to die from coronary heart disease and men in other parts of the world believed to be much less susceptible, Keys launched in the 1950's a series of international studies. Paul and Ina White first joined the Keys international team in Naples for several weeks in 1954 where it was found that there was indeed far less coronary heart trouble than in the United States. Similar observations were made the next year and Keys has written: "In the spring of 1955 Paul again joined us, this time at Cagliari, Sardinia, where we would find a picture much like that of the year before in Naples—a diet very low in meat, loaded with fruit and green vegetables, bread and pasta, liberally sprinkled with olive oil, providing most of the calories. Serum cholesterol, like in Naples, averaged around 165 mg per deciliter (contrasted with about 230 mg in the United States), and there was a remarkable dearth of coronary patients. The local physicians were honored to guide Paul through the hospitals and clinics of the island where he found no lack of patients with valvular disease and defects of development of the heart but coronary heart disease was rare. At Cagliari cardiologists from the University of Bologna Medical School joined us to renew their learning with the 'maestro' under whom they'd studied at Boston, proudly telling about the publication of their Italian translation of *Heart Disease*. Paul even managed to get us a sample of shepherds to examine."

The year 1956 saw a joint venture in Hawaii, and there was another in 1957 at the tip of Southern Italy. There were other forays elsewhere including southern Japan in both rural and urban settings. Margaret Keys and her daughter remember that "Paul White was always dressed in a suit with jacket, long sleeved shirt and necktie, and well polished shoes." It was repeatedly found that with his arrival all medical doors opened automatically and his name enlisted the support of local officials, community leaders and even priests. Here as on many other occasions he exhibited his natural mastery of public relations and his ability to relish every new experience which might teach him something. Despite his age—and he reached 70 in 1957—he was demonstrably young at heart and an excellent travelling companion. In May 1972, he wrote a tribute to Ancel Keys which included "special thanks for having dislodged us twenty years ago from our dedicated pursuit of the single sick man to the broader field of public health to complete the orbit of 'the individual and the common good.' "

His support for epidemiologic studies extended to others. With Dr. Frederick J. Stare, an expert in nutrition and Professor at the Harvard School of Public Health, he took an interest in a project comparing 700 Irish men living in Ireland with 700 of their brothers who had moved to the United States to the Boston area. Here he gave mainly moral support and advice although he did himself examine some of the men both in Ireland and Boston. As Dr. Stare commented, "I don't know of anyone in this general area who had as much enthusiasm. He was a great person to stimulate people to be enthusiastic about the work that they were doing and if you are enthusiastic about it then you work hard and try harder." He commented that he was also very gracious, always willing to help. This last attribute extended repeatedly also to his readiness to locate small sums of money to underwrite international graduate training programs for students in cardiovascular epidemiology organized initially by Ancel Keys with a seminar in Makarska in 1968, and carried on later by Dr. and Mrs. Jeremiah Stamler of Chicago under the auspices of the International Society of Cardiology and the American Heart Association. The interest in international epidemiology fitted conveniently into Paul White's many travels during his latter years. Although not a card-carrying epidemiologist, he as an elder statesman and cardiologist made an important contribution through his total support of what was then a new field in biological science. Fortunately, he lived to see this confidence in the epidemiology of cardiovascular disease confirmed by many studies from around the world.

CHAPTER TWELVE

International Affairs

"It is with great appreciation of the privilege and honor of representing the English-speaking peoples of North America that I acknowledge the warm-hearted welcome by the President of this Congress. We are happy and proud to be here to mingle with our colleagues and friends from all continents. Our only regret is over the absence of representatives from a few countries which we sincerely hope will join us at future meetings when the stress and strain of recent years will have abated. We who are 'médecins du coeur' would also like to perform the miracle of healing the troubled world of today by a universal bond of spiritual brotherhood and medicine from the heart."

Paul White spoke these words at the opening session of the First World Congress of Cardiology held in Paris in 1950. Thus began 20 years of intimate involvement with international organizations, following upon his most active years with the American Heart Association, and overlapping but extending far beyond his duties with the new National Heart Institute. The sentiments expressed were "vintage" Paul White. Here was the Boston cardiologist at the peak of his career, one voice speaking for North America, heralding the start of a hopefully bright new era in international relations. Paul White never considered such an event narrowly in terms of heart disease and heart specialists. His constant concern and expectation was that through the medium of scientific exchange, international good will and understanding would be created, and this in turn would contribute meaningfully to a world seeking peace.

The concept of an international cardiological organization began quite indirectly when the Mexican medical societies organized the First National Congress of Internal Medicine in Mexico City in May 1942 and invited certain foreign medical dignitaries, including Paul White, to come as guests of honor. Especially involved in this invitation was Professor

Ignacio Chavez, then President of the Mexican Society of Cardiology. Paul White found that the pressure of work in his office, in the hospital, and in other areas of obligation during wartime was such that he had to decline although he did send a short paper to be read for him. The President of the Congress, Dr. Teofilo Ortiz Ramirez, in acknowledging his letter of regret commented that when the new Institute of Cardiology was opened, Paul White's presence would be "unescapable."

The Institute was indeed inaugurated in Mexico City on April 18, 1944 with Professor Chavez as its Director; and Paul White, who had taken Spanish lessons in preparation, attended along with several others from the United States. Other guests from the United States who were prominent in the field of heart disease included Doctors Carl J. Wiggers, Louis N. Katz, Samuel A. Levine, and Frank N. Wilson. Paul White presented two papers at the meeting, and there were several reports by physicians from Mexico, Cuba, Argentina, and other Latin American countries.*

A by-product of the inaugural festivities were discussions leading to the formation of an Inter-American Society of Cardiology with Professor Chavez as both its President and Secretary-Treasurer. The inaugural program at the Institute of Cardiology was considered to have been, in fact, the first meeting of the new Inter-American Society. It was agreed that after World War II was over, another Congress would be held—also in Mexico.

The Inter-American Society was thereupon organized promptly due to the energy of its President and held its second Congress in Mexico City two-and-a-half years later in October 1946. Several foreign dignitaries were on hand including Professor Charles Laubry of Paris, founder of the French Society of Cardiology. Paul White, who had spent the entire sum-

---

* It was at this time that Paul White sat twice for Diego Rivera, the famous painter, who executed a magnificent mural for the Institute with the likenesses of 48 of the most famous men in the history of cardiology, starting with Galen from the second century A.D. Three of the 48 were from the United States—James B. Herrick of Chicago, Frank N. Wilson of Ann Arbor, Michigan, and Paul D. White of Boston. Paul White was depicted holding a curled paper in one hand surrounded by Charles Laubry of Paris, James B. Herrick, Willem Einthoven, Professor of Physiology at Leiden University, and Augustus Désiré Waller, Director of the Physiology Laboratory at the University of London.

mer on a teaching mission in Czechoslovakia, was so harassed with commitments on his return that he was again forced at a relatively late hour to send his regrets. However, he was represented by his associate, Dr. Howard B. Sprague. Howard Sprague reported back to Paul White about the events south of the border including a "moving" episode at the formal reception at the Presidential Palace when he was suddenly acutely stricken with the usual gastroenteritis, managed to crawl back to his hotel, and on opening the door to his room, announced to his wife who was recovering from a similar malady, "Take a good look at me, Lucy; this is the way I will look when I am dead."

Professor Chavez once more took advantage of the atmosphere of an international congress with the beneficent Mexican climate and much food and wine and good will to initiate discussions for the creation this time of an International Council of Cardiology with "the main purpose" being "the organization of International Congresses of Cardiology. . . ." A formal document was drawn up and signed on October 11, 1946 by 16 of the notables, providing for a council composed of five representatives of the Americas and five from Europe which was to be a self-perpetuating body, the charter Council members being appointed for life. Paul White was to be the representative from the United States; Dr. Jonathan Meakins represented Canada; Professor Chavez, Mexico; Professor Alberto C. Taquini, Argentina; Professor A. Hurtado, Peru; Professor Charles Laubry, France; Sir John Parkinson, England; Professor Gustav Nylin, Sweden; and Professor N.D. Straschesko, the USSR. One position in Europe was left vacant to accommodate a German representative at a propitious time. No representatives from Asia, Africa, or Australia were mentioned, and no officers were named although future international congresses would have presidents either coming from the Council or appointed by it. Chavez wrote later to Paul White that "the Council does not include a representative for each one of the existent National Societies of Cardiology. Instead, representatives of different cultures and even of different races were selected." That this Council constituted a small, elite, closed, European-American club was evidently not considered a problem in the warm glow of Mexican hospitality although the document did say that "the International Council may increase the number of its members if convenient or necessary."

Paul White was to find that in his absence, the group had decided that he would be the one to follow up the Mexico City pronouncement. This was the familiar stratagem of assigning the dirty work to the missing member. He was to get in touch with each member of the new Council for suggestions and advice regarding future activities. Thus was begun a long leadership involvement in international cardiological bodies, a role very different and far more complex and at times frustrating than his previous short-term international roles in which he was essentially a distinguished visiting expert giving lectures and teaching, accepting generous hospitality, and briefly exposing the local practitioners and academicians to his own particular wisdom and charm.

The correspondence which Paul White began with the other Council members soon disclosed a number of problems including sensitive personalities and delicate political considerations. It was the consensus that the first Congress should be in 1950—but where? Professor Laubry who had been present at the accouchement suggested that the first international congress be held in Paris. A bid to have the congress in Stockholm came from Paul White's old friend, Professor Gustav Nylin, who attended an organizational meeting of a European Cardiological Society in Brussels in January 1949 and acquired new international stature by becoming its first president. There was also an offer from Professors Prusik and Karasek of Prague to have the meeting there, an offer which was not seriously considered owing to the political and military events occurring in Czechoslovakia in the early months of 1948. Professor Nylin obtained a promise of financial help from the Swedish government. He thereupon seemed to believe that Stockholm had been selected for the Congress, but the offer from Paris proved to have the widest support among members of the Council, in part because Laubry, who was highly respected, was quite aged (74 in 1946) and it was recognized that this might be his last opportunity to play host. Paul White, with his usual spirit of compromise, suggested a splitting of the Congress between Paris and Stockholm, but this proved impractical. These and other thorny issues were discussed

by Nylin and Chavez when they met in Chicago on June 15, 1948, when
it was agreed that Paris should be the site with Professor Laubry as President of the first Congress.

Paul White, in writing to Sir John Parkinson on August 30, 1948,
referred more frankly than was his custom to problems which had
cropped up, constituting "a kind of emotional upset among two or three
of our fellow members of the International Cardiac Committee or Council." He mentioned "the situation in the Argentine where one prominent
man, Taquini, is viewed with some suspicion as a semi-Fascist follower
of the President [Juan Peron], and others like Cossio, one of the old line,
who feel that the Argentinian Cardiac Association isn't actually represented by Taquini"; and also "the sensitiveness of Chavez who is a considerable prima donna in Mexico and Latin America"; and also that
"Nylin has been a little upset in that we recommended Paris instead of
Stockholm for the 1950 meeting."

The Argentine issue was finally handled in Paris at the time of the
Congress when Cossio was elected a member of the Council, displacing
Taquini. Taquini later became Vice Chairman of the Research Committee
of the new Society. Another difficulty was getting a response from Professor N. D. Straschesko, named to be the Council member from the
USSR. He either did not answer his mail, or was not allowed to, or was
just plain not interested. Finally, because of lack of contact except for a
report that he had retired, he ceased to be a member of the Council, and
his place was not immediately filled. Paul White did endeavor to have
other Russian scientist representation at the Paris Congress, but his
friendly overtures to Moscow were ignored.

The British cardiologists were accustomed to a democratic process and
found this whole business of a small, self-perpetuating, international
committee suggested by Chavez most distasteful. Sir John Parkinson, on
further reflection, despite being a member of the Council himself, wrote
to Paul White on July 28, 1947 asking, "Would it not be well to reconsider its constitution, allowing the Cardiac Society of each country to
nominate its representative and also a deputy?" Subsequently, the British Cardiac Society expressed its unhappiness with the Mexico City state-

ment on membership in the Council, and its Secretary, Dr. Kenneth Shirley Smith, wrote to Paul White that the Society held that its continued participation after the Congress in 1950 would depend upon acceptance of an amendment regarding the self-perpetuating principle. Parkinson stated that in any case he would withdraw from the Council after the 1950 Congress. It was clear that the membership of the International Council would have to be altered to be acceptable to the existing national cardiac societies. Dr. F. Van Dooren, the Secretary General of the European Society of Cardiology, expressed similar reservations in a letter to Dr. Louis Katz in which he complained that a member of the committee nominated for life would assume perpetual control over the activity of the Society. Paul White again sought a way out by compromise, writing on August 1, 1949 to Dr. Charles Conner of the American Heart Association to suggest that the International Cardiac Council, originally elected in Mexico City, might be allowed to remain as a permanent, honorary, lifetime body on an academic basis relieved of official duties after the Congress in Paris next year. "There will be no harm in that rather than to advise its abolition, and people like Chavez, Taquini, and Nylin, among the members I know, would be a little offended if we should vote for its complete abolition." However, he seemed to accept the inevitable as he concluded, ". . . It may be that an entirely new active International Cardiac Council should be selected to help in furthering international relationships." Meanwhile, each national Cardiac Society was asked to appoint an official representative for the Paris Congress.

The contentious and sensitive issues did not end with that. Paul White received word that the Egyptian heart specialists felt left out and wanted to be invited to send a representative to Paris. The Inter-American Cardiac Society was upset that the letterhead of the new Congress, prepared by Laubry and his staff, made no mention of the membership of the International Council. A few arms had to be twisted to obtain small grants of money from the National Heart Institute, and the American Heart Association to help finance the Congress. Papers for presentation in Paris had to be arranged for and selected by each of the national societies. In January 1949, Taquini reported to Paul White that the Argentine

Society of Cardiology declined to work with him as a member of the International Council, and the Society was grieved that it had not been consulted in the first place when a representative from Argentina had been selected. There was opposition from the Secretary General of the European Society of Cardiology, Dr. F. Van Dooren of Brussels among others, to the idea of continuing the existing Council even merely as an honorary body. These and other vexing matters were resolved or in some cases not resolved but merely postponed for the Congress itself.

Paul White and his wife and two children had decided to have a six-week European tour prior to the meeting and so left New York on July 19, 1950 on the *Caronia*. The voyage was a smooth one, and Paul White played shuffle-board, ping pong (he lost to a lady passenger in the tournament), and deck tennis. He also worked preparing various talks. The Whites first visited England and Scotland for three weeks, mainly visiting friends and sightseeing. Paul White then went to Finland by himself on August 12 where he went fishing with poor results, and lectured three times at the University in Helsinki. As was often the case, he developed an upper respiratory infection which developed into sinusitis, but he plugged along. He rejoined the family in Stockholm where Professor Nylin first took them to his summer place and then back to Stockholm where Paul White gave a lecture. This was followed by brief visits in Norway, Germany and Holland. The family finally reached Paris on September 1, and at once Paul White was immersed in Congress activities.

The Council met on September 1 and 2, and the Congress itself officially opened on the 3rd in the main hall of the Sorbonne. There were speeches by Robert Schuman, the Minister of Foreign Affairs, Laubry, Chavez, Nylin, Parkinson, and Paul White. The Congress was a large one and 486 papers were presented and, not surprisingly for a first international endeavor, more a tribute to quantity than to quality although the caliber of some of the presentations was remarkably high. Paul White who was the official delegate of the American Heart Association himself gave papers on international cardiovascular research and the use of radioactive iodine in heart disease (in which he was presenting data from the Beth Israel Hospital group in Boston headed by Herrman Blumgart). The usual international congress wining and dining took place including two banquets and a reception by the President of France at the Elysée Palais followed by ballet at the Palais de Chaillot.

The crucial issue of the form of the new international organization was hammered out, and new statutes were adopted on September 8 by the official national delegates to the Congress. Gone were the original provisions for a comfortable small club with lifetime tenure and right of selection of successors. Even gone was Paul White's idea of an honorary council composed of the founding members. The fervor of national interests predominated in a new International Society of Cardiology (ISC), which was to have its headquarters in Geneva. Its purposes were set out

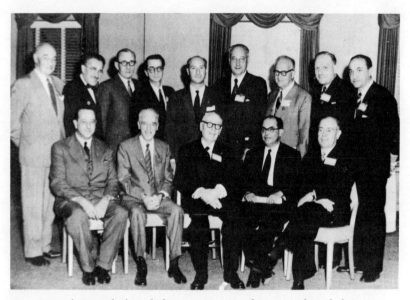

International Council of Cardiology, International Society of Cardiology, Washington, D.C., September 12, 1954.
Front Row, Left to Right: Pierre Duchosal, Switzerland; Paul D. White, U.S.A.; Charles Laubry, France; Ignatio Chavez, Mexico; Gustav Nylin, Sweden.
Back Row, Left to Right: J. Hepburn, Canada; Louis N. Katz, U.S.A.; Evan Bedford, United Kingdom; Eduardo Magalhaes Gomes, Brazil; Vittorio Puddu, Italy; Hernán Alessandri, Chile; E. Wolheim, West Germany; Pierre Rijlant, Belgium; Pedro Cossio, Argentina.

with appropriate rhetoric including stimulation of cardiology in all its aspects, the improvement of scientific exchange, assistance in scientific development of its members and the maintenance of ethical standards, the preparation and support of courses, conferences and publications, and organization of congresses every four years. Members were to be representatives from national and continental societies of cardiology, and there was to be a General Assembly composed of two delegates and the president from each national society. A Council was to be continued, elected by the General Assembly, which would be the Executive Committee of the Society with seven members from Europe, seven from "the American continent," and one each from Asia, Africa, and Oceania. The Assembly was also to elect officers of the Council including a president. Official languages were to be English, French, and Spanish.

The critical area of finance was handled in a gingerly fashion with reference to a "periodic subscription from affiliated societies" with later reference to annual dues to be "in accordance with the economic status" of each country. No expressed amount or formula was stated, and there was no penalty for failure to pay. There was no mention of any staff except for two auditors of accounts. The statutes were signed by four from Europe (Laubry, Parkinson, Duchosal and Nylin), two from the United States (Paul White and Louis Katz), and one from South America (Cossio). Laubry was elected President of the Council, Paul White First Vice President, and Chavez, Second Vice President. It was also agreed that the congresses would be held every four years (instead of every six years as originally planned by the now defunct Council) with the next one in 1954 in Washington, D.C.

Thus a mechanism was launched for holding international meetings and for facilitating the exchange of information. An Assembly was created with the national heart societies as a controlling force. A corps of distinguished cardiologists left over from the Chavez-inspired Mexico City era continued in the top posts, but this group could no longer be self-perpetuating. The touchy area of money was not faced up to and was to continue vexing, tending to keep the Society weak in action and quite unable to fulfill the expectations expressed in the statutes. Such a posture was not viewed unfavorably by many who felt threatened by the prospect of a rich and powerful international agency, especially if money contributed by one nation might be spent beyond the borders of that nation without its control. The accomplishments at Paris, however, were considerable, particularly in creating the mechanism for the congresses. It would, however, take another 25 years to confront the fact that the Society was living from year to year in a chronically impoverished state.

Sandwiched in between the large quadrennial international congresses of the International Society of Cardiology were to be the regional ones— Inter-American, European, and later Asian-Pacific. Paul White attended nearly all of these as an invited speaker and guest of honor, and in the process always fitted in lectures in neighboring countries, reunions with former students, sight-seeing ventures, and consultations with illustrious private patients. These consultations were often thrust upon him unexpectedly by his local hosts; and with his kindheartedness and willingness to work long hours, he almost invariably managed them in his usual, thorough fashion. These frequent visits to foreign countries, these meetings with friends, new and old, these conversations with key political figures, these teaching exercises, even these patients, all had their place in establishing Paul White's role as the foremost spokesman for international cardiology and for the international societies.

The Fourth Inter-American Congress of Cardiology was held in Buenos Aires, Argentina in September 1952, and Paul White's itinerary and involvement during that period were very typical of his style. He left New York on August 18 on a 6:00 a.m. flight and arrived at Bogota, Colombia late that afternoon, being met by one of his old graduate students. There, over the next two days, he lectured at the National Academy of Medicine, saw a series of patients including the President of Colombia and the mother of the Minister of Health and was taken on a tour of the salt mines and the cathedral. On August 21st he took a flight to Caracas, Venezuela where he met with a group of doctors, was driven about the city, and saw a number of patients at the Vargas Hospital Clinic. He reached Rio on August 23rd and the next day flew on to São Paulo where he visited a hospital and a coffee plantation and gave a lecture at the Academy of Medicine. On August 26, he flew to Montevideo, Uruguay where he met with a former student, again visited a hospital where he gave a talk and toured the local sights. In Buenos Aires from August 28 to September 7th, he participated in the Inter-American Congress, gave the Battro Memorial Lecture, presided over a session at the Congress and spoke on pulmonary embolism, visited various medical facilities, and attended many luncheons and dinners.

There were two meetings with Juan Peron, President of Argentina. The United States representatives had been distressed to find that Peron had arbitrarily removed some of the most eminent Argentinian scientists, including Nobel laureate Bernardo Houssay, from their laboratories and positions of reponsibility in the University of Buenos Aires because of political differences. Dr. Irving Wright recalls how a small group including himself, Louis Katz, Howard Sprague, Carl Wiggers and Paul White had coffee with Peron. "There were four big husky men one in each corner of the room of Peron's residence, Casa Rosada. Peron began to boast and asked, 'What do you think about our wonderful new medical school?' There was silence. I have forgotten who made the first statement but we all backed him up. 'A medical school is only as good as the people you have in it—the teachers, and we have learned that you have dismissed your great Nobel laureate and other professors.' We didn't know whether we were going to be beaten up by those four big men or not but we couldn't stand the idea that Peron thought he had created a great medical school out of bricks and mortar." Paul White wrote about this encounter: "It was, I think, a productive event for shortly afterwards I saw as patients the Minister of Health and the State Minister and they told me that they thought something worthwhile would come of this conference." Perhaps the blunt comments of the doctors from the United States made some impact as, in time, Houssay was reinstated as Professor and Director of the Physiological Institute of the University of Buenos Aires.

After the Congress, Paul White vacationed briefly at Mar Del Plata, a seaside resort, and also visited the lake country in northern Patagonia. He then took a plane to Santiago, Chile ("a rather shabby city with pleasant people") where he again lectured, conducted a conference and was asked to see four private patients. He made a side trip to Valparaiso and then left on September 13 for Lima, Peru. In addition to a lecture there at the local Academy of Medicine, and another to the 4th year medical students and rounds at the hospital, he saw in consultation a friend of President Ibanez and made a side trip to Cusco to visit the ruins, which was an especially thrilling experience. He finally arrived back in Boston on Friday September 19th at 4:30 p.m. Far from exhausted he went in to the hospital the following morning for a research conference and cut his lawn with a hand mower in the afternoon.

The Second World Congress of Cardiology in Washington in September 1954 was headed by Paul White. Fortunately, his position as President of the Congress was greatly buttressed by a team of dedicated assistants. Dr. L. Whittington Gorham was the Secretary General and with his wife, took care of a large portion of the correspondence and scheduling details. Also very helpful were Dr. Bernard Walsh of Washington, one of Paul White's early residents, and his wife Agnes Donovan Walsh, who had been Paul White's first secretary at the Massachusetts General Hospital. Colonel Thomas W. Mattingly, also a former Paul White student and now Chief of Cardiology at Walter Reed General Hospital, was on the Organization Committee as were representatives from the National Heart Institute, the American Heart Association, the United States Navy and the Air Force, the Veterans Administration, and a cadre of seven top civilian cardiac specialists from around the country.

Colonel Mattingly described an unusual episode which occurred in the course of the preparations:

In the midst of all the preparations and his visits to Washington, in association with details which he, as President, had to accomplish, I was amazed at the demonstration of his enthusiasm in a single event such as a sandlot baseball game. I had made all the necessary arrangements for the use of the Pan American building for the opening reception—a choice location in the District of Columbia. The only item remaining which I desired P.D. to decide on personally, in addition to visiting this beautiful building and grounds, was to arrange for the receiving line and especially who was to be in it and where we would have an alternate line in case of unsuitable weather. I picked him up at the

Mayflower Hotel where he was staying for the night and as I did so, he informed me that he must be back at a certain time as he had an important appointment. Our visit with the building superintendent was prompt, P.D.W. toured the building and garden and was well pleased and we proceeded to walk to my parked car in good time to return him to the hotel. A few yards from the car, he spotted a sandlot baseball game in progress. He stopped, for what I thought would be a few minutes, but before I could get him away, he pitched and batted and ran the bases. He finally gave up and we reached the hotel an hour later than his appointment.

The eminent President of the Congress clearly had a wonderful child-like quality which was a vital part of his optimistic view of life.

The summer of 1954 was a busy one with "much work on Congress," as he noted repeatedly in his Memindex, especially busy since the Congress was to be simultaneous with the Annual Scientific Session of the American Heart Association. On the night of September 9, he and his secretary Helen Donovan worked at the Mayflower Hotel in Washington until 4:00 a.m. on last-minute problems including the seating at the banquet. Another last-minute need for him was to arrange an exhibition of his old books on heart disease at the National Guard Armory, where most of the sessions were held. The opening ceremonies of the Congress on September 12 were attended by Vice President Nixon, and were followed by a distinguished program of scientific presentations over the next five days. Over 3100 people were registered, two-thirds of whom were physicians representing 50 nations, and the papers were simultaneously translated into French and Spanish. A high point was the Laubry lecture given by Sir John Parkinson on "Leadership in Cardiology" in which he spoke with grace and affection of his friend Paul White as follows:

> When one speaks of unity and of leadership, your thoughts will go at once to our President himself, Dr. Paul White. Friendship for a country rests largely on personal friendships with its citizens. On that basis, though not solely, I would pay my tribute to the lead taken by the United States in the realm of cardiology, and also give thanks for the close friendships which have bound me to this great country. I have been blessed by a long and firm friendship with Paul White. We spoke earlier of hero worship, and he remains one of my abiding heroes. A counterpart to Osler in medicine, he has been an ambassador of goodwill and good hope to cardiologists all over the world. He has made many original contributions, and by means of his famous book, he has proved a trusty, unseen consultant to countless doctors. In it he has reverently com-

bined a choice of the past with the best of the new. By kindly understanding and enthusiasm, he has inspired men wherever he has gone. His qualities of character and judgment place him high in our esteem; and that extends to his wife, whom we all admire. Paul White has gained the favor and affection of us all, and in him, we possess an ideal leader in the world of contemporary cardiology.

The Congress went extremely well and Paul White was particularly exhilarated by the presence of two Russian doctors, Professor E. M. Tareev, a physician, and Professor B. V. Petrovsky, a surgeon and later Minister of Health of the U.S.S.R. They were accompanied by Mr. Y. I. Gouk, cultural attaché at the Embassy, and security men. Paul White had been trying for years to lure Russian scientists to a meeting in Europe or in the United States, and now he had finally succeeded. The State Department was quite astonished at their presence, and Secretary of State John Foster Dulles even had a meeting with the National Heart Institute staff to lecture them on how to be proper but not too friendly with visitors. The two Russian professors initially appeared grave and unsmiling and stayed together, but Paul White did have a separate meeting with Professor Tareev at his exhibit of old books and managed to converse in French, which started a more friendly relationship. The surgeon, Professor Petrovsky, also had his opportunity for more personal attention when, at his request, he was taken to the Walter Reed Army Hospital. He was to witness an operation for coarctation of the aorta, a congenital anomaly associated with a block in the large blood vessel leaving the heart leading to the development of high blood pressure. The surgical procedure involved removing the area of obstruction, something which fortunately was accomplished without incident, and which resulted in a much improved circulation of blood to the lower portion of the body. One of the Army surgeons escorting Petrovsky later wrote in his report: "Professor Petrovsky manifested reserved interest during the procedure; however, at its conclusion, on palpation of a bounding dorsalis pedis pulse, he became warmly enthusiastic and this warmedly unreserved attitude characterized his contacts with the undersigned from then on."

Paul White was elected President of the Executive Committee of the ISC by the General Assembly, and Dr. E. Wolheim from West Germany was chosen to occupy the vacant seat on the International Council. The conclusion of the Congress did not actually end the Whites' obligations as it had been arranged to have a series of four post-congress medical tours which would visit major medical centers including Boston. Thus on September 26, the ever gracious and hospitable Ina White provided lunch for 32 foreign guests—including the Russians—at their house in Belmont, with 16 also for dinner two days later.

The final congress in which Paul White was to have a major part was held in Brussels in 1958 at the time of the World's Fair. As was his wont, Paul White traveled to Corsica, Poland and Czechoslovakia for two weeks before the congress. At the congress, in addition to his opening address and his role with the scientific sessions, he had dinner at the Palace, sitting between ex-King Leopold and Prince Albert and on another occasion returned to the Palace for dinner with Dowager Queen Elisabeth. His official duties at this congress were not heavy compared with the previous one.

Dr. Florence Avitabile recalled an entertaining episode which occurred two years later when Paul White attended the European Congress in Rome, where he was staying with Professor Puddu. It revealed him to be both ingenuous and determined. "He arrived and he had a very bad cold; you know he was subject to colds. As usual, he had lost his suitcase. It seemed a habit with him. Wherever he went, he returned without a suitcase. He arrived at an airport, everybody would be there to greet him, there would be so much confusion that he would put his suitcase down and never think of it again. So he arrived in Rome, and he had lost his suitcase, and he had a fever; but the following day, he wanted to go to the inauguration of the Congress to give a welcoming address and meet the Russian delegates. He was going around in Puddu's house in his underwear because he wanted to save his suit since it was the only suit he had. The doctors were saying 'you should not go to the Congress if you really have a fever; it's too dangerous.' So he went and took an ice cube from the refrigerator—his host found that out from the cook—and he put it in his mouth and then he put in the thermometer and announced that he did not have any fever. And he went to the inauguration and he did not get pneumonia. The determination of that man!"

Such international scientific organizations are created to encourage communication between professionals from different parts of the world, and the ISC undoubtedly achieved this to a considerable degree. The quadrennial congresses were clearly enjoyed by Paul White and the other leaders in cardiology, and the reaction from attending physicians was decidedly favorable. Nevertheless and not surprisingly, the enjoyment was in some measure offset by the awareness by the leadership of the financial poverty of the new Society. Essentially it had money from registrations and a few other sources related to the congresses but no assured regular income. Contributions from national societies were varied, small, and unpredictable. Its committees usually operated without budgets which meant that at their infrequent meetings, they talked about what they would like to do. Paul White, as an international traveler and the most visible leader of the ISC (and chairman of its Research Committee), was repeatedly exposed to situations in both developed and underdeveloped countries where there were opportunities for valuable scientific research and for a unique experience in professional education which were jeopardized or lost because of a lack of financial support. As he demonstrated in the National Advisory Heart Council of the National Heart Institute, he believed that it was important to encourage the search for new knowledge with seed money even if the caliber of some of the investigators and investigations was marginal in comparison with studies from sophisticated laboratories in the United States and Europe. He thought it especially important to foster a climate favorable for research in heart disease in regions in which research had been previously unknown. His own experience convinced him of the enormous value of a partnership of scientists and lay men and women in meeting such a challenge. How could all this be done?

He had a vigorous ally in his thinking in Dr. Louis N. Katz of Chicago who was the assistant treasurer of the ISC 1950–1954 and then treasurer from 1954 until 1962. He was born in Poland and had his scientific training in the United States at Western Reserve University under the eminent physiologist Dr. Carl Wiggers. He had become Director of the Cardiovascular Department of Michael Reese Hospital in Chicago in 1930 and acquired a distinguished reputation as an investigator, especially in the areas of arteriosclerosis and electrocardiography. He had served as President of the American Heart Association and of the American Physiological Society. A highly intelligent, articulate leader, he was not reluctant to make his views known in a forceful manner which tended to intimidate the faint-hearted but which often served to illuminate and resolve issues. As contrasted with Paul White, he was a physiologist rather than a clinician, was interested in basic rather than clinical research, and was of a rather formidable mien whereas Paul White was characterized by charm and warmth of manner.* Both were involved in the ISC as officers, both were painfully conscious of its financial stringencies, and both were dedicated to the proposition that international cardiovascular research needed more support. Also and most important, both had witnessed in the American Heart Association and the National Advisory Heart Council how lay men and women had made valuable contributions to matters of policy, organization, administration, and finances without interfering with scientific issues. Paul White and Louis Katz resolved to do something together.

The fateful step was taken on January 29, 1957 when the International Society of Cardiology Foundation (ISCF) was incorporated in the State of Illinois as a not-for-profit corporation. There was a board of eight directors which included White, Katz, Ignacio Chavez of Mexico, Evan Bedford of England, Pierre Duchosal of Switzerland, John Palmer of Canada, and legal counsel headed by Frank D. Mayer of Chicago. Frank Mayer was soon to be replaced by Hugo J. Melvoin. Paul White became president of the new Foundation and Louis Katz was the treasurer, thus duplicating their current roles in the ISC. It was these two who were to

* Dr. Howard Sprague spoke at a testimonial dinner to Louis Katz arranged by the American College of Cardiology in Chicago on February 3, 1966, and said in part: "I must have met Louis about forty years ago. My first recollection of him is seeing him charge down the aisle at a meeting of the American Heart Association to discuss a victim's paper. He reminded me of the description given by the marine patients in my hospital in New Zealand to a medical officer, who always came into the ward with his boilers at full pressure. They called him 'The Saratoga' because he reminded them of that famous aircraft carrier which used to steam into the harbor with all her planes in the air ready to dive-bomb any intruder . . . Behind Louis Katz's belligerence, his willingness to meet challenge, his upstanding personality and his upstanding hair, there is a very warm and sentimental being."

operate the Foundation in its early years. Its purpose was to provide a tax-free depository for contributions to support research and education in the field of cardiovascular disease anywhere in the world, with the specific aim of thereby helping the ISC and its councils to be more effective. However, it was a legal and administrative entity distinct and separate from the Society, and monies were not usually granted by the Foundation to applicants through the Society. This was in part because the Society was comparatively puny with a minuscule permanent office staff and budget and a shadowy committee structure. The main initial link between the ISC and the ISCF was through the existence of a common leadership.

The first five years of the ISCF were relatively tranquil. Paul White exercised his charm and wide acquaintance and public stature to obtain small grants of money to the Foundation from patients, admiring friends, and, to a limited extent, the national heart societies including the American Heart Association. However, the amounts received were modest indeed, only $19,000 being listed in the first two years and only $12,000 for the whole year 1962 when the Foundation had been in existence for five years. Necessarily, therefore, the sums granted for research were small, and decisions on these were made by White and Katz with the approval of the Board of Directors. An Advisory Committee was set up to make recommendations when larger sums were involved. Limited travel allowances were made to permit a few foreign investigators to visit laboratories in the United States, and likewise for United States research- ـ ers to visit foreign centers. Typical were grants made to a physician in West Germany to help establish a research laboratory, to an Argentinian investigator to buy equipment, to a community hospital in India to purchase a heat exchanger to be used in heart surgery, and to a doctor from Nigeria who received money for purchase of an electrocardiograph to be used in clinical research. Small as these sums were, they encouraged the recipients by recognition of their efforts, and they had the inestimable advantage of being made speedily—something impossible for most large granting agencies. The overhead of this undertaking was nonexistent as it was operated without charge from the offices of Paul White, Louis Katz, and the Chicago lawyers. Beginning in 1960, the American Heart Association assigned Dr. John H. Peters to be administrative officer and to handle the paperwork of the grants from its New York office, and the Association also covered this expense.

In comparison with the burgeoning National Heart Institute and the American Heart Association, the ISCF was indeed "small potatoes," both in program and in budget. Two steps were taken to try to assess and improve the situation. At a meeting in Chicago in January 1962, it was agreed that the ISCF would hold a conference in Houston that October, just prior to the Fourth World Congress of Cardiology in Mexico City, to discuss the future of the Foundation with the leadership in cardiology from around the world. Secondly, a lay committee was organized by Albert Baer to assist in procuring funds for the Foundation, a project first discussed in 1961 and implemented the next year.

Baer was to play a pivotal role in the affairs of the Foundation. He was a New York businessman, Chairman of the Board of Imperial Knife Associated Companies, Inc., who first met Paul White when both were members of the Board of American Youth Hostels. Albert Baer found "that he was just mesmerized by him;" and when White, aware of Baer's international connections, asked him to take an interest in the ISCF, he accepted with alacrity and became its foremost volunteer fund-raiser. For the next eight or more years, he was extremely dedicated to his new philanthropic project, working in and out of the United States, suggesting and planning and carrying out fund-raising events, and contributing quite generously from his own funds. He also became intimately involved with the administrative and organizational aspects. His devotion to Paul White and to the Foundation was unquestioned. It is unlikely that the Foundation would have survived without him. It was not surprising that this energetic, and to some viewers, brash, businessman, who liked to foster a spirit of camaraderie by singing and playing on his banjo after dinners and liberally handing out small penknives, did not suit everyone. To a few, including some Europeans, this involvement by a layman in matters hitherto restricted to physician members of the ISC was unwelcome and was considered ill-advised meddling.

The meeting in Houston October 5, 1962 was courtesy of Dr. Michael DeBakey, the prominent surgeon, and was an amiable one, with a friendly and free discussion concentrating on the ways in which physicians and laymen could work together to raise funds for the conquest of cardiovascular disease. It was a tribute to Paul White and Louis Katz that physicians and, in many cases, lay leaders from all around the world came to discuss the affairs of such a small foundation. In many ways, the atmosphere of good will which characterized the meeting represented the high point in the life of the Foundation. From it came considerable education for all the participants in the history and accomplishments of the ISCF (which shortly after the Houston meeting changed its name to the International Cardiology Foundation—ICF). There was broad agreement on the desirability of the continued existence of the Foundation as well as rambling presentations with suggestions for the future. The underdeveloped countries particularly stressed the value to them of travel funds. Dr. S. Padmavati of India commented: "Perhaps most of you here coming from the United States and other countries with high standards of living do not realize what it means for a person from an underdeveloped country to travel, because most people, even professors, have very small salaries and it is often not possible for them to pay their own expenses." Overall, this exhibition of moral support for the ICF was heartening, but with it came no pledges of financial assistance.

A happy event also occurred in October 1963 when the first of a series of six, formal, fund-raising dinners took place. This event, under the aegis of Albert Baer, was held in New York City and honored Paul White who was presented with a gold stethoscope by his patient, former President Dwight D. Eisenhower. The occasion was attended by much favorable publicity. It netted approximately $60,000 for the Foundation which was sorely needed as the ISC, hard-pressed itself for funds, was to begin regular and urgent appeals to the Foundation for support to keep its office and small program running. Subsequently, over the next six years, five more fund-raising dinners were to be held.

Not so happy, however, was the first of a series of changes in the cast of characters, changes which were to take place over the next ten years.

Louis Katz, burdened with his duties at Michael Reese Hospital, resigned as treasurer of the Foundation and was replaced by Paul White's valued Boston colleague, Dr. Howard B. Sprague. Further, Dr. John H. Peters, who had been the administrative officer, left his position with the American Heart Association and the Foundation; and as a result, the administrative center shifted from New York to Paul White's office in Boston where it was placed under the direction of Dr. Florence Avitabile. Dr. Avitabile had been working under Dr. Vittorio Puddu, Secretary of both the International and the Italian Societies of Cardiology and a well-known cardiologist in Rome. She had moved to the United States in 1960 and promptly went to work for Paul White, first in clinical research but shortly afterwards in relation to his international obligations. She had an acute informed mind, excellent judgment, knew the personalities on both sides of the Atlantic, seemed indefatigable, and was precise and responsible with committee and financial reports. She was an invaluable asset to Paul White. Her special usefulness became increasingly apparent as Paul White became older and the issues more tangled.

Others also entered from the wings, some to disappear from the scene, others to persist. From Boston was Dr. Allan L. Friedlich, a fine cardiologist trained under Paul White, who became active as secretary of the ICF and was extensively involved in the protracted negotiations in the United States and abroad. He was relied upon heavily by his former chief because of his complete personal loyalty, good sense, and warm personality. Later he was to become Paul White's personal physician. Also from Boston were, successively, John Cancian and then Jesse R. Fillman, distinguished lawyers whose legal advice in the affairs of the Foundation was repeatedly sought and obtained. From 1968 until 1970, Rome A. Betts, the notably successful and thoroughly experienced former Executive Director of the American Heart Association, took over as the paid fund-raiser for the Foundation, and the administrative office in that two-year period was moved to New York. Betts soon found vigorous opposition from the affiliates of the American Heart Association to his efforts to obtain funds within the United States for the Foundation, no matter how gingerly and tactfully he approached the problem, and he was forced to retire defeated. The office then was moved back to Boston once more under Dr. Florence Avitabile's wing. Beginning in 1969, Dr. Lewis E. January, a former president of the American Heart Association and Chairman of its International Committee and a professor at the University of Iowa, assumed an increasing leadership role on behalf of Paul White and was chosen Vice President of the ICF. As a surrogate for White, he worked devotedly for a decade to unravel the various complexities.

From 1962 on, there were attempts to give the ICF an identity satisfactory to the various national leaders, societies, and foundations and at the same time to provide a reasonably secure financial backing which would in turn buttress the ISC. Meanwhile donations from patients and friends of Paul White dwindled, any dependable income from foreign heart societies and foundations was not at hand, and it was clear that one could not go on living on receipts from annual $100-a-plate dinners as their novelty and attraction were wearing off. At an exhausting ICF meeting in New Delhi in 1966, a frustrated Paul White even lost his temper, which almost never happened, and sharply told the surprised Albert Baer: "And Albert, it is high time you stopped playing the banjo at these meetings." He almost at once regretted his irritation and wrote a note of apology that night.*

The ISC continued in an impoverished state although the exact condition of its finances was usually difficult to ascertain as the accounting procedures could be charitably described as adolescent. At a meeting in Geneva in June 1966, Dr. Pierre Duchosal, President of the ISC, realistically acknowledged the financial help of the ICF without which the Society "might well have collapsed before now." Soon after this, the administrator of the Society reported to the Foundation that "we are poor, the balance being approximately $530 . . . we need at least $4,000 to see us through June 30, 1967." The American Heart Association at

---

* Although often frustrated by the organizational and financial difficulties, Paul White was usually tolerant and patient, writing in 1966 to Florence Avitabile: "My sentiments and dream world are much the same as yours but, being older, I am more hardened to the buffetings of fate."

this time generously agreed to support one-half of the budget of the ISC through a grant to the ICF for the years 1967–70 with the ICF somehow to provide the rest. The 10-year-old United States-based program of making small research and travel grants essentially ended at this time. Grasping for money, a 10 million dollar Paul Dudley White International Fund was launched in 1968 but with only very modest results. As it was considered desirable to remove the ICF from the taint of its United States location, finally in 1969 it became incorporated in Switzerland with its central headquarters in Geneva with the ISC, and its United States office in the American Heart Association.

Meanwhile, more than a dozen countries had created national heart foundations, stimulated and assisted greatly by Paul White who time after time made foreign pilgrimages to encourage and often initiate these endeavors. These included Australia, Belgium, Canada, Finland, India, Ireland, Italy, the Netherlands, Norway, Portugal, Sweden, Switzerland, and the United Kingdom. Dr. Allan Friedlich recalls how in May 1965, White, Dr. Howard Sprague, Albert Baer and he went to Israel to launch the Israel Cardiology Foundation. Publicity for the Foundation was going to be difficult to get due to the competition from urgent foreign news, and ingenious Paul White had Friedlich plant a question in the press corps. The question was popped in the middle of White's interview with the reporters—"Dr. White, how do you like matzot?" That gave Paul White the opportunity to dilate on the good qualities of matzot—low in fat, sugar and salt—which in turn resulted in a front-page article in the *Jerusalem Post* on both matzot and the Foundation.

The logical idea of making the ICF into an international federation of these foundations was repeatedly considered, particularly to ensure its survival when White was no longer able to be its leader. Finally, at Geneva on May 8, 1969, the name of the International Cardiology Federation was registered with this happy possibility in mind. A definite formula for financial contributions from the national foundations to an International Cardiology Federation proved elusive, however, and to avoid controversy, the ICF agreed not to seek donations from individuals or corporations in countries having established foundations without their approval.

A solution to all these difficulties was proposed at Geneva in September 1969 at a two-day conference of the ICF chaired by Paul White with 32 representatives attending from 14 countries. There would be an assembly of national heart foundations at the time of the Sixth World Congress of Cardiology in London in September 1970. At this time, a set of by-laws would be adopted to activate the new Federation of foundations, officers and directors would be elected, Paul White would retire as leader, and a budget developed including "estimates of the proportion of the total budget to which the national foundations would be expected to make contributions." The old ICF would be phased out, its United States activities remaining the responsibility of the American Heart Association. An international program in cardiology would be considered, aiming to achieve an eventual union between the ISC and ICF. Hopefully, the ISC and its officers would begin to share responsibility for the ICF lay-physician branch of international cardiology, and an assured fair formula for long-term financing from national federations would be obtained. This was ambitious, almost euphoric language in view of the past history; indeed, it was too ambitious to succeed.

The preliminary discussions and correspondence prior to the September 1970 London assembly, indicated that all was not going well. Paul White had been aware of reservations held by his British colleagues regarding the existence of the ICF, reservations which had prompted him to refer, as early as May 1969 before the September 1969 Geneva meeting, to the "isolationism of the British." These concerns seemed lessened but not resolved at the Geneva meeting which had been attended by Professor Sir John McMichael, Chairman of the Council of the British Heart Foundation who, at the conclusion of the meeting, had uttered some apparently conciliatory words. The distinguished Professor Sir John McMichael was a key figure, not just for Great Britain but also for Europe and the whole British Commonwealth. He had held the very important post of Director of the Department of Medicine of the Royal Post Graduate Medical School in London for 20 years, was a top investigator in cardiovascular and lung physiology, was Director of the British Post Graduate Medical Federation, and was a trustee of the Wellcome Trust. He was also a Vice President of the famous Royal Society and furthermore, he was the President of the London World Congress at which the ICF's future was to be solved. He now became increasingly distressed and distrustful of the plan proposed for the London meeting. Correspondence between Great Britain and the United States became brisk and testy as a consequence—Paul White referred in a letter dated August 14, 1972, to "Brickbats passing in both directions."

Sir John's concerns were several. Why not have just one organization, the ISC, to reduce administrative costs and simplify channels of communication? How could an international group function as well as a national one in judging the validity of grants for travel, research and education? Were not the people nearest the scene best qualified to judge these matters? Great Britain was no longer a rich country and how justifiable was it to siphon away from its own British Heart Foundation funds for vague international undertakings—and how much would it cost? In truth these concerns were not so very different from those of the affiliates of the American Heart Association which refused to let Rome Betts solicit funds for the ICF in their own local areas. Sir John prepared and mailed out a six-page summary of his views, in essence recommending abolition of the ICF and perpetuation of a small, efficient ISC which would receive annual dues from national cardiac societies to take care of its modest budget.

The London meeting proved a disaster for Paul White. He opened the meeting at the Britannia Hotel at 3:00 p.m. on September 8, 1970 with representatives from 26 countries on hand. He made a brief speech and thereafter said very little. There followed a keynote address by Mr. Adrian Pelt of the Netherlands and there were four panels. The following day saw the real action when it was moved that the proposed International Cardiology Federation be established to "cooperate in every way possible with the Society and that a joint body be created to work towards merger." On a point of order, Sir John McMichael indicated that the British Heart Foundation had decided not to become a member of the new ICF. A vote on activation of the new federation was then taken, with 12 votes in favor, four against, and two recorded as abstaining. Countries voting against the motion included Denmark, Iceland, Norway, and the

United Kingdom; Japan and Australia abstained and eight countries remained silent. What appeared a victory was thus a hollow one, as less than half the national representatives present supported the motion. The United Kingdom and Australian members of the ICF nominating committee, Sir Michael Perrin and Sir Kempson Maddox, then proceeded to resign from that committee, an especial blow since Perrin was its chairman. Sir John McMichael once again rose and voiced his regret that a unity of opinion could not be achieved, he seemed to have been excommunicated he said and added that "the international machinery was in a powerless state and his suggestions aimed at giving it a new look and securing financial support from the British Foundation had not been accepted." The British delegation thereupon walked out.

A depleted and unhappy assembly then voted to approve new officers and a board of directors. Mr. F. C. Collin of Belgium replaced Paul White as the ICF president. It was symbolic of the state of affairs that after being elected, Mr. Collin left for the airport, leaving Dr. Lewis January, the new Vice President, to preside over the remainder of the meeting. Two more defeats were yet to occur. The American Heart Association proposed a resolution for the appointment of a committee "to work on effecting the unification [of the ICF] with the ISC as soon as possible," but this was voted down eight to one, being supported only by the U.S.A. Thus the new Federation was created but without a viable base of support. The idea of planning for union with the ISC was soundly rejected. Paul White received a final blow when, at the election of officers for the ISC, the name of the nominee for president-elect, a former associate of Paul White in the U.S., was put forward by the ISC Executive Committee, only to be defeated when the name of Professor Puddu from Italy was placed in nomination from the floor.

The whole unhappy episode was referred to later by Paul White as "the holocaust in London." Had he been 64 years of age instead of 84, perhaps he would have taken a vigorous leadership role with successful results. However, regardless of age, he was not a political person, and the situation required a skillful, behind-the-scenes negotiator, comfortable in the atmosphere of international prejudices and political and philosophic differences. He was not that sort of person, and he was ill at ease when faced with controversy. As Florence Avitabile said, "He thought that everybody was as simple and direct as he was, but they weren't." Sir John McMichael's objections were not only influential but had validity and had to be met with some type of compromise. The lack of experience of European and other foreign scientists in working with lay members in a health movement had to be recognized and their wary often behind-the-scenes negative attitude understood. The vigorous approach of the American Heart Association's representatives needed to be muted even though that association had been paying much more than its share of the ISC budget.

The epilogue was no less an unhappy story during the remaining three years of Paul White's lifetime. No longer actively involved, he witnessed a continuation of bickering and interminable ineffective maneuvering. Without the help of Paul White and Albert Baer, the financial situation worsened, if that was possible, helped by the unwise decision to have separate offices and staffs in Geneva for the ISC and the ICF which doubled administrative expense.

It was not to be until five years after Paul White's death at the World Congress in Tokyo in September 1978 and under the skillful and patient leadership of Professor John Goodwin who came from the same country and city and medical school and hospital as Sir John McMichael, that the two organizations were at long last dissolved and merged into a new and viable International Society and Federation of Cardiology (ISFC). With this accomplished, there came extraordinary progress. In 1983 at the end of yet another five years, the ISCF included representation from 44 national heart foundations. Dr. January recalls how, on his death-bed, Paul White spoke sadly yet still hopefully of the ICF and pleaded with him, "I have to depend on you. Don't fail me, please." That failure was finally turned into success, that the concept of an international partnership of scientists and lay people was accepted, was a tardy memorial to his 1957 vision.

CHAPTER THIRTEEN

Citizen of the World

Beginning after World War II during the last 25 years of his life, Paul White was a frequent traveler around the United States and overseas. Indeed, the word "inveterate" is probably more appropriate than "frequent" since travel became a persistent feature of his life. In 1958, for example, he took 36 separate trips away from Boston, mainly without his wife, although she did, of course, accompany him on his vacation in Florida and on his visits to Europe and Australia.* That year was by no means unusual—it was typical of his schedule.

Why did he travel so much? Most of his journeys about the United States were to give lectures on heart disease with especial emphasis on prevention, to attend committee meetings of the National Heart Institute, American Heart Association or International Cardiology Foundation, and sometimes to see patients in consultation (often fitted in when he was going to a city for another purpose). His trips overseas were ostensibly in relation to activities of the International Cardiology Society and International Cardiology Foundation, and for lectures and teaching, or for participation in medical research teams. However, underlying these foreign journeys was his abiding belief that science could not be viewed in purely national terms and that by promoting friendship and understanding between scientists in all parts of the world, he might contribute usefully to a better climate for global progress in medicine as well

* Twelve of these were only brief visits to New York for meetings and consultations, four were to Montreal or Toronto, four were to Washington, four to various cities in Pennsylvania, and there were others within the United States to Atlantic City, Baltimore, Florida, Chicago, and the West Coast. In addition there was a brief trip to Mexico City and another similarly short one to Bermuda. Much more prolonged was a two-week trip to New Zealand and to Australia to help the new Australian Heart Foundation (which included stops with receptions, lectures and press conferences in Auckland, Sydney, Adelaide, Melbourne, and Canberra). Yet another and even longer itinerary encompassed Brussels, Paris, Warsaw, Cracow, Prague, Zagreb, Venice, Rome, Corsica, Madrid, and Lisbon.

as for the maintenance of world peace. As he wrote to the State Department in 1952, he felt he was qualified to serve in this role:

> I've had a great interest in international medical affairs over a good many years because of many travels to various medical centers abroad, the visits of a good many young and older medical men to my clinic for periods of time up to two years of graduate study, and because of many patients that have come to me from foreign lands. Thus, with the lapse of time I have accepted a kind of role of medical ambassador for the U.S.A. medical profession and for the people at large. This I say without any desire to boast but simply because it is a function that I think can be served by doctors like myself who have had a great deal of relationship with foreign physicians.

That Paul White thrived on a heavy schedule of travel was testimony to his amazing tolerance and indeed enjoyment of it. He was in many ways ideal for it. Clearly he was often ready to leave his home, family, patients, office, and the obligations they imposed, as well as the comforts they provided in order to fulfill what he saw as his mission in life. His wife and children were justifiably proud of his achievements; however, such frequent absences imposed hardship on them, as well as on his patients, who would be cared for by his associates—consequences he and they had to accept. He did not seem to be significantly disturbed by changes in the time zones. His energy rarely flagged. He could get along on minimal sleep and was able to get a lot of work done on a plane, ship or train. Dr. Irvine Page recalled how once in Russia Paul White was going strong at 2 a.m. ("he was the life of the party") despite having just arrived on a long flight from India where he had met with Prime Minister Nehru and had arisen at 4:30 a.m. While he abhorred cocktail parties, he accepted the hazards of long receptions, dinners and speech-making with little, if any, complaint. He was exhilarated by new sights and new faces as well as refreshed by renewing old acquaintances. He seemed able to find interesting topics to talk about before a wide range of audiences and was ready to function as an expert cardiologist in clinics all over the world. He rarely fussed about poor food, uncomfortable beds, noisy hotel rooms, nagging reporters, or the inevitable photographers. He handled the many requests for consultations on patients with extraordinary patience, considering the impositions on his time and energy. He did not require a special diet or bedtime hour in order to be happy.

Most of all, his warm, friendly, honest personality was appealing to doctors and lay persons in all parts of the world, and his integrity and motives were accepted without hesitation. When there were disagreements with him as in some of the proposals relating to the International Cardiology Foundation, these disagreements never involved a dislike or distrust of him as a person. A charming anecdote related in 1967 by Professor Ignacio Chavez, Director of the Cardiology Institute in Mexico City, illustrates beautifully how this attractive man captivated the imagination and the respect of so many.

I first met Paul White many years ago, when we were both young men. It was in the summer of 1938, to be more precise. Since then our paths have crossed on a number of occasions over the years, in many corners of the globe. During these brief encounters, I have always felt the same sense of joy and it is because I have found the same man, a fundamentally simple man, an essentially good man, a man whose spirit is always open to the claims of friendship.

We Mexican cardiologists gave Paul White a cordial welcome [in 1938]. What with dinners, visits to hospital and excursions, everything was done to ensure his stay with us would be agreeable. In company with him we penetrated the old, colonial quarters of the city, visited the murals of our great painters and admired the archaeological treasures of our Pre-Columbian past. Standing before the great Pyramid of the Sun, neither he nor I could resist the temptation to climb to the very top. Once standing upon the highest point of this great temple, there lay before our eyes the sacred city in all its splendor. While I lost myself in historical and mythological explanations, two little Indian children drew near to listen until, tired of not understanding us, they settled down to play marbles. Seeing them, we both succumbed to the same impulse, an impulse which took us back to our infancy. We asked the children to lend us their marbles and, squatting down in the approved manner, played a game . . .

If he had any limitations as a traveler, one was that he was not a natural linguist. Wherever he went, he tried to learn enough of the language to make a few introductory remarks in the appropriate native tongue as the start of a formal lecture or after-dinner speech. Because he would not be fluent, the brief remarks might sometimes be painful to hear. Professor Alvin Pappenheimer recalled how once in Rome, at a very formal banquet, Paul White gave his brief speech in halting Italian, which unfortunately was followed by the distinguished British chemist, Sir Cyril Hinshelwood, whose Italian was, if anything, better than that spoken by

most Italians. His other limitation was a tendency to acquire upper respiratory infections. All his life this was a problem, and hardly a trip of
any length was completed without some comments in his daily record of
sneezing or a congested nose or perhaps coughing and fever. He rarely
gave in to these infections totally, but might be slowed down briefly from
his usual brisk pace.

Of all of the places beyond the borders of the United States he visited
over 60 years, five shall be mentioned for special reasons. To review all
of Paul White's travels would not be productive. The first to be mentioned is England, where in 1913 he received his baptism in cardiology
under Sir Thomas Lewis, and developed what became life-long bonds
with the Lewis family as well as with Sir John Parkinson and his wife and
children. Over the years, Paul White frequently visited these and other
British colleagues, their clinics, and their laboratories and found these
occasions warm and rewarding. The details of the 1913–1914 experience
have been described in Chapter Two. A second area was Czechoslovakia,
the site of a successful 1948 teaching mission. This experience was crucial
in kindling in Paul White excitement about the potential for other exchanges between scientists from different lands. A third country was the
USSR, where in 1956 Paul White was a pioneer in bringing United States
cardiology to the Soviet Union and in establishing friendly relations with
Russian physicians. A fourth geographic area to be mentioned is Lambaréné in Gabon, West Africa, where Albert Schweitzer had established
his hospital. The two brief Paul White visits (the first in 1959) to Lambaréné are included, not because of their significance per se, but because
they illustrate how, as with many of his other foreign travels, a visit by
Paul White to a new region was not an end in itself but was followed by
a series of entanglements. Finally, there was the journey to the People's
Republic of China in 1971—an historic event.

*   *   *

Early in 1946, Paul White was asked to be Chairman of a medical
teaching mission to Czechoslovakia under the auspices of the Unitarian

Service Committee. Czechoslovakia had been occupied by Nazi forces during World War II, although a government-in-exile had existed in London under Edward Beneš. With the winding down of the War, the Nazi troops had been replaced by Russian military and political forces which had created yet another foreign presence. However, a fragile, independent Czech government was temporarily in power as a result of the election of a Constituent Assembly in May 1946, with the Czech communist leader Klement Gottwald as Prime Minister and non-communist Jan Masaryk holding the portfolio for foreign affairs. The Czech medical profession had undergone a most difficult and debilitating six years during the Nazi occupation. It had been separated from all the newer scientific developments and thus looked forward keenly to the prospect of a visit by medical experts from the United States.

An outstanding team of 14 doctors from academic centers from all over the United States was organized by Paul White. The group included an anesthesiologist, microbiologist, pharmacologist, neurosurgeon, cancer surgeon, pediatrician, physiologist, biochemist, obstetrician, orthopedic surgeon, internist, two dentists, and Paul White as cardiologist. One of the dentists, Joseph Peter Rudolph Lazansky, was of Czech origin and spoke the Czech language, which proved extremely helpful. Although sponsored by the Unitarian Service Committee, the mission was actually under the umbrella of the United Nations Relief and Rehabilitation Agency (UNRRA). It is a remarkable tribute to American medicine that such an outstanding faculty was recruited for a mission which lasted nearly two months and which paid the participants almost nothing. Indeed, Paul White took out a loan to cover his family expenses at home while he was away. The wives were not invited and Paul White who had travelled first to England wrote to his wife on June 28: "Ina Dearest, It was 22 years ago this evening that we walked up the aisle together. Just think, half your lifetime and a large share of mine. The only thing about this summer's expedition that I really don't like is that you are not taking part in it; in fact, this is the longest time we have been separated since June 28, 1924. But it will make my return in September all the happier."

The group, which was the first major medical mission to reach Czechoslovakia after the ending of the war, arrived in Prague on July 3 having had an unsettling trip crossing the Channel by ship from Newhaven to Dieppe, then by train to Paris, and thence by train to Prague. In order to keep track of the many aspects of such an undertaking, Paul White had assigned members of the mission to various duties: Joseph Aub as historian, Otto Krayer as accountant, Leo Davidoff for transportation, and Joseph Volker and Joseph Lazansky for luggage. These assignments were especially necessary as the transportation system in Germany and Czechoslovakia, badly damaged during the war, was only just beginning to recover. Despite this planning, all did not start off well, as Paul White wrote to his wife on July 2:

> Now for the sake of our records and for your own amusement too, I must tell you the saga of our impedimenta, the 20 or more (at the moment 21) boxes, crates, and footlockers containing our precious instruments, drugs, and books which we laboriously collected to use for demonstration in Czechoslovakia this

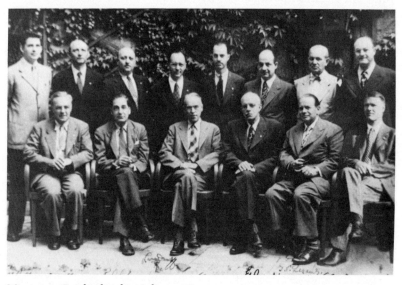

Mission to Czechoslovakia, July, 1946.
Front Row, Left to Right: Drs. Milan A. Logan; Joseph C. Aub; Paul D. White; Everett Dudley Plass; James E. M. Thomson; L. Emmett Holt, Jr.
Back Row, Left to Right: Drs. Joseph F. Volker; Otto Krayer; Ralph W. Gerard; Leo M. Davidoff; Colin M. MacLeod; Emery A. Rovenstine; Joseph P. Lazansky; Alexander Brunschwig.

summer and to leave in Prague when we depart. Constantly we have counted and recounted the individual boxes as we have also, of course, our personal luggage (2 or 3 bags apiece). We've bonded them and registered and even paid for their overweight on occasion. . . . These sums came out of our own pockets, UNRRA being quite unprepared or at any rate unwilling to assume the charge which seemed a bit odd at least to us. . . .

When we got on the train in Paris last night all this valuable freight of ours was nicely stowed away in the baggage car on the train and we were repeatedly assured by all we asked, UNRRA, railroad men, and others that our troubles were over and that the teaching equipment would arrive in Prague with us tomorrow morning. We were suspicious—it was too good to be true and sure enough our fears have been confirmed. We watched the baggage car occasionally but at one unguarded moment before we pulled in to Stuttgart where we planned to inspect the train again, without warning the train was split and ten minutes later when we were proceeding around a curve I put my head out of the window to admire the countryside and to my consternation saw no baggage car fore or aft. My first inclination was to pull the emergency cord, but then I realized that the rest of the train with the baggage car was doubtless on its way too, towards Munich—we were en route to Nürnberg without stopping at Stuttgart at all, of which we'd had no warning. A hurried Council of War decided us to phone with the help of our German conductor (a cooperative man) and the station master from the first station of any size to Munich to hold the baggage car there or at least to take out our stuff so that it would not go on to be lost forever in the Balkans, and at the same time to have Joe Volker and Joseph Lazansky (who knows well both German and Czech) leave us at Nürnberg and commandeer an UNRRA or Army car to drive south to Munich in order to rescue our things and get them in some way or another back to us in Bohemia.

The episode ended on a bright note as Volker and Lazansky sat up all night in a dark, crowded and windowless train compartment from Nürnberg to Munich, where they had the luggage (which had already reached Salzburg in Austria) removed and shipped back to Munich, finally were able to commandeer an Army truck in Munich, and drove over the mountains to Prague arriving at 4 a.m. on July 4.

Thus began a busy and successful mission.

The next eight weeks were exceedingly full. The members of the mission visited clinics, hospitals, other health facilities, the medical school in Prague and its new satellite at Hradec Králové, made ward rounds, gave lectures, attended countless luncheons, dinners and receptions and did some sightseeing. Especially in the cities, they saw extensive evidence of damage from aerial bombing, but they found the morale of the people good despite their ordeal. The Czech doctors, some of whom had been in concentration camps, welcomed them with open arms and gave them a heavy work and social schedule. Paul White wrote on July 5:

> We have been received most royally everywhere—it has been actually embarrassing and I'm running out of expressions of appreciation of their hospitality . . . I am again in bed writing this at midnight with Joe [Aub] gently snoring in the next bed.

Paul White with the help of Dr. Lazansky learned a brief speech in Czech which he used repeatedly to acknowledge the kind words of greeting from their hosts and to introduce the group. After about three weeks in Prague and the adjoining region in Bohemia (which included a visit by Paul White to the YMCA-operated Camp Masaryk 60 miles southeast of Prague directed by a Camp Becket alumnus), the group headed east and travelled from place to place by bus in Moravia and Slovakia. Books and reprints were given to help restock the medical libraries devastated by the war, as well as a limited amount of equipment.

Joseph Volker, who was one of the two dentists on the mission and who later became Chancellor of the University of Alabama, has commented

> He [Paul White] worked longer hours than any of us, and we all worked very hard. He was always attempting to see how we could have the maximum effectiveness in our presentations and at the same time to establish with the Czechs the understanding that we were there to help them, to bring them up to date with what had happened in their fields during the period of time of the German occupation, and to go beyond that to indicate our willingness to help them after we had gone. . . . We met with everyone from the students to the faculty to the staff of the hospitals to practitioners in the region, nurses, laboratory chiefs and radiologists. . . . We were beset with newspaper people who knew the Americans were coming and wanted to know about America. They wanted to know what we were doing there. I guess there were some who suspected us of ulterior motives. But Paul was so disarmingly frank and friendly. Even those who suspected that we were a political group, which we certainly weren't, quickly became convinced that we were "for real."

Professor Pavel Lukl of the new Medical School at Hradec Králové found that one of the most useful parts of the mission was the demonstration of teaching methods. Hitherto, most of the European instruction in medical schools including in Czechoslovakia had been by lectures. However, the members of the Unitarian Service Mission not only gave lectures but conducted ward rounds—that is, walked about the hospital wards in small groups and saw and discussed at the bedside the problems of individual patients. Professor Lukl said that as a result of this demonstration, the Czech medical schools tried to reform their teaching to include this more intimate teacher-student-patient relationship. The mission finally ended on August 28 when the group had an audience with Prime Minister Gottwald and were informed by the Minister of Health that they would be decorated with the Order of the White Lion.

This long mission had a major impact not only on Czechoslovakian medicine but on Paul White himself. Here really for the first time he saw in action the happy and broad consequences of a well organized program for the exchange of scientific information and for the promotion of friendship between two very different countries. Fortunately the time was ripe for the mission, the Czechs were eminently receptive, and the group from the United States was exceptionally qualified and congenial. Paul White began to visualize other similar opportunities and on July 13 wrote after a meeting with the Russian administrator of UNRRA of the possibility of "following up this pioneer experience with medical missions of this type elsewhere, as for example in Russia itself . . ." He had a relatively favorable impression of the Russian presence in Czechoslovakia in 1946, particularly in comparison with the Nazi regime which had preceded it, noting that "this country has been treated well by the USSR." He tended to view the Czech communists as "essentially socialists." The Unitarian Service Committee mission was such a great success that it created expectations of similar successes elsewhere in the world, expectations which were not to be fully realized. For example, a similarly constructed mission to Greece in 1948 also headed by Paul White was much less rewarding, largely due to the narrowness and self-interest of the leaders of the Greek medical profession. Indeed, Paul White never took part in any other undertaking which equalled this one in Czechoslovakia for constructive dialogue and good will.

There was to be one unexpected and unhappy aftermath of the 1946 mission. In February 1948, the political picture in Czechoslovakia abruptly changed when the leaders of the non-communist parties resigned from the multi-party cabinet and the communists, aided by police brought into Prague from other areas and workers' militia, took complete charge of the government. Jan Masaryk, the non-communist Minister for Foreign Affairs, was found dead on March 10, of uncertain cause but possibly murdered by communist agents, and President Beneš, who had been ill, resigned on June 7. The relatively tolerant atmosphere changed abruptly, and most of the non-communist leaders fled the country. In the midst of this uncertainty, Charles University in Prague was to celebrate its 600th anniversary and Paul White had been invited to be present to receive an honorary degree. It was also arranged that he would go as the official representative of Harvard University to bring its greetings to the occasion. However, while in Paris en route to Prague, he received on March 28 a cable from President James B. Conant of Harvard:

OUR INQUIRY TO STATE DEPARTMENT IN WASHINGTON RESULTS IN INFORMATION LEAVING NO DOUBT THAT DRASTIC GOVERN-MENT ACTION HAS STARTED PURGE OF CHARLES UNIVERSITY PRAGUE THEREFORE HAVE CABLED RECTOR WITHDRAWING ACCEPTANCE OF INVITATION PLEASE DESTROY GREETINGS FOR YOUR INFORMATION PRINCETON YALE AND COLUMBIA HAVE ALREADY WITHDRAWN IF YOU ATTEND PLEASE DO SO IN PURELY PERSONAL CAPACITY SUGGEST YOU CONTACT AMERICAN AM-BASSADOR PARIS FOR COMPLETE INFORMATION.

Paul White did call on Ambassador Jefferson Caffrey in Paris but decided to proceed to Prague anyway without Harvard's blessing in the company of Professor J. Serrail, Rector of the Sorbonne, and others because, as he wrote

I did desire to pay tribute to the fine medical accomplishments of Czechoslo-vakia of the past with no desire to condone the present status . . . I wish to show the vast liberal majority of the faculty that still remain in their posts that there is a friendly interest in their future welfare from across the seas and in our hope of the restoration of their academic freedom . . . and . . . I desire to tell the host of friends whom I had made throughout the country in 1946 that I had not forgotten them. . . .

The impressive formal ceremony was held in Prague on April 8th, and Ina White recalled the beautiful medieval stone hall with trumpeters high in the clerestory announcing the colorfully robed academic procession. The high point came when the frail President Beneš spoke of the strength and continuity of Charles University over the centuries despite political upheavals every hundred years, a reminder which had the great audience in tears.

Paul White's presence and his remarks were interpreted by most of the faculty as he had hoped, and his brief speech included the following expression of faith:

> Charles University has been through many troubled times and today is no exception. It is disturbed outside and in by the political changes of these times but I have confidence in its future when it will again return to complete academic freedom which is so vital to the healthy life of all institutions of learning and for which Charles University has been a champion during its long and glorious past.

Paul White found Prague much changed from his earlier visit. This time he had a different view of the communists and he wrote that it was clear Czechoslovakia was "now a police state" and "friendly interchange of visiting teachers and students to attend meetings, to study, and to teach is now next to impossible, and such prohibition has been recently and abruptly imposed under the guise of various inadequate reasons." Ruefully, he wrote on April 9 on a postcard from Rome to his mother: "We must stop the communists—you were right!" While he did return to Czechoslovakia in later years, he would never again experience the warm democratic atmosphere of 1946.

*   *   *

While the sobering Prague visit for the Charles University ceremonies might have deterred some from pursuing a scientific rapprochement with Moscow, this was not the case with Paul White. If anything, it may have spurred him on. Despite the constraints of the Cold War after World

War II, he was persistent and hopeful in seeking an active dialogue with cardiologists in the USSR. As usual with him, this was partly for the benefit of science but also partly from his deep-seated hope to be able to contribute to a better understanding between peoples.

His friendship with Russian scientists had begun in 1926 when the distinguished Professor Alexander Samoiloff of Kazan University, a pioneer in physiology and electrocardiography, came to Boston, met Paul White, and gave a lecture at the summer course in cardiology. Professor Samoiloff got to know Paul White still better on a subsequent visit in 1929, when Samoiloff and the great Professor Ivan Pavlov attended the International Physiological Congress in Cambridge, Massachusetts. The White and Samoiloff families became intimate over the years, and when Russian physicians came to Boston they tended to gravitate to Paul White's office and often were entertained at his home. However, the war years and subsequent cool relations between the US and the USSR discouraged and indeed prevented visits by American scientists to their Russian counterparts. With the inauguration of world congresses in cardiology, there was clearly an opportunity to encourage more meaningful relations with Russian heart specialists; and Paul White, having failed to get their participation in the 1950 Congress in Paris, was finally successful at the Second Congress in Washington in 1954. A small Russian delegation attended the meeting as described in Chapter Twelve. Thereafter, the ice of the Cold War began to break gradually as far as science was concerned, and a series of medical missions visited the USSR.

In 1956 Paul White received at last an official invitation from the Soviet Minister of Health, Professor Maria Kovrigina, to visit Russia for 10 days with a group of other scientists. He had been hoping for such a bid for years. This was the first invitation for a US team involved with cardiology, and he as the leader chose a small broadly based group including Dr. James Watt, Director of the National Heart Institute; Dr. Herman Hilleboe, Commissioner of Health of New York State, who was interested in chronic disease including heart disease; Dr. Ancel Keys, specializing in nutrition and its relation to coronary heart disease; Dr. Howard Rusk, the head of the New York Rehabilitation Institute; and Dr. Mark Field, a sociologist with the Beth Israel Hospital in Boston with training in Russian at the Harvard Russian Center.

This was to be very different from the mission to Czechoslovakia. The group arrived in Moscow at 1:15 a.m. on August 30 on a delayed flight from Helsinki and spent the next ten days there except for one trip to a regional hospital 40 miles south of the city. However, one member of the group, Dr. Watt, flew to Sukumi on the Black Sea to inspect the monkey colony. There were visits to the First Medical School and Clinic of Moscow, two medical institutes, and to two hospitals as well as a meeting with leaders of the National Academy of Medical Sciences. A few lectures were presented and some patients were seen and laboratories visited. There were also the usual dinners including a final banquet given by the Minister of Health, evening entertainment, a press conference, and a brief broadcast over Radio Moscow. Unlike the experience in Czechoslovakia, Paul White noted that the Russians "made little effort to learn from us and asked surprisingly few questions. Almost all of the time was taken up by telling us of their ideas, research and plans. It was obvious that they wanted us to know about them and their work, to appreciate their efforts and their accomplishments."

This brief mission, while not a rousing success, helped to open the door for future exchanges. Paul White referred to it as a "successful preliminary effort in the reestablishment of closer medical relationships." The Russian hosts were very courteous and hospitable and reasonably forthcoming, and clearly wished to show off their brand of science. The Americans in turn were impressed that many of the Russian scientists were highly capable and that it would be well worthwhile to have further meetings and in greater depth.

There were two specific achievements. One was that the members of the group for the first time got to know several of the top Russian doctors. In particular, Paul White had several sessions with Professor Alexander Myasnikov, head of the Institute of Medical Practice, a specialist in high blood pressure and the leading Russian cardiologist. Myasnikov was a formidable individual described by Paul White as a "very dynamic person with strong convictions, not very receptive of the ideas of others which do not agree with his—the old type of German geheimrat who can do no wrong." As a result of their meetings and despite their decidedly different personalities, they developed an acquaintance which ripened over the next few years to a close friendship. This relationship culminated at a dinner of the International Cardiology Foundation in Geneva in 1965 when Paul White presented gold-plated stethoscopes to Myasnikov of

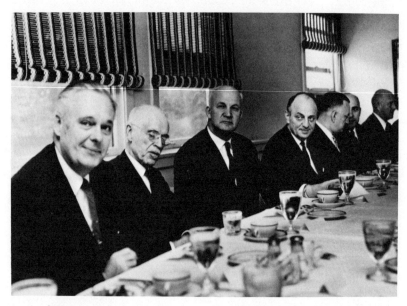

Dr. Paul White meeting with Professor Alexander Myasnikov, Bethesda, Maryland, September 25, 1962.
Left to Right: Dr. James Watt, Chief, Division of International Health, U.S. Public Health Service; Dr. Paul White; Professor Alexander Myasnikov, Director, Institute of Medical Practice, Moscow; Dr. Luther Terry, Surgeon General, U.S. Public Health Service.

Russia, Parkinson of England and Lian of France as symbols of leadership and achievement in international cardiology. Myasnikov was clearly moved by this tribute and this evidence of acceptance as an equal by Western heart specialists. Indeed, after his sudden death from a heart attack in November 1965, this same gold stethoscope was incorporated into the burial marker. Of course useful friendships were also established with other Russian leaders which were renewed on subsequent visits to the USSR. From these contacts, Paul White acquired a special under-standing of the Russian attitude, of their privations and terrible experi-ences in World War II, of their pride in their own scientific achievements, and of their basic desire—often poorly promoted—to be accepted as equal participants in the world of medicine.

The other significant achievement was a presentation by Paul White and his group to the National Academy of Medical Sciences of the USSR of an invitation both for joint US-USSR work in rehabilitation and car-diovascular epidemiology, and for several Soviet physicians to come to the United States for 6 to 8 weeks to observe the activities in several of the leading research centers. The offer was politely received at the time and later became a reality. Myasnikov himself visited the United States in 1958 as did many others on different occasions including several of the younger scientists. The United States in time sent other groups to Russia, and joint research projects were organized by the National Heart Institute.

Thereafter Paul White made six more trips to the USSR between 1961 and 1966. Two were missions similar to that of 1956, and one was for a joint attendance at a World Congress for General Disarmament and Peace and at an International Cancer Congress, one was for a visit to Professor Nodar Nikolaevich Kipshidze in Georgia regarding some of the report-edly very aged residents of that area, and one was as a member of the elite Fourth Dartmouth Conference held in Leningrad in 1964 to further communication and understanding between private citizens. The final trip at Christmas time in 1966 was the result of an invitation to attend as "our dear guests" the first All-Union Congress of Cardiology in Moscow. Paul White was the only physician present from west of the Iron Curtain. On this occasion, as a signal evidence of his personal good will, he as-signed any royalties coming from the Russian translation of his short book *Clues in the Diagnosis and Treatment of Heart Disease* to the sup-port of young members of the Soviet Society of Cardiology. This last visit was also memorable for Paul and Ina White for a Christmas Day on which they had a festive meal in a dacha in a birch forest, and were taken on a fairy-tale troika sleigh ride in the country. When they signed the

guest book in the dacha, their names immediately followed a bold signature with the familiar name Fidel Castro. That Paul White was invited
to make so many trips to Russia after the ice had finally been broken in
1956 was not because of his scientific eminence alone. More than anything, it was as Joseph Volker had remarked regarding the mission to
Czechoslovakia because he was "so disarmingly frank and friendly." He
was trusted. As Norman Cousins, former Editor of the *Saturday Review*,
has commented about Paul White's role at the time of the Dartmouth
Conference:

> He was a very popular member of the American delegation, especially with the
> Russians, largely because he did not feel it necessary to play it close to the
> chest . . . He was conciliatory and constructive and was a good bridge builder
> psychologically. He was also a little bit of a pixie. He had a good sense of
> humor and a twinkle and was a good story teller . . . If the Russians like you
> and trust you, even though you may have strong disagreements with their
> position, you can go far.

That the Russians did indeed like and respect him was demonstrated
best in 1961 when he became the first American to be elected to the
Academy of Medical Sciences of the USSR. This was a truly unique
honor, and an extraordinary testimony to the respect he had won by his
keen intellect and his warm personality. It also was a tribute to his persistence and faith in personal encounters which "will eventually break
down the barriers" as he wrote to a correspondent on March 7, 1961.
That these efforts were appreciated was also shown by a 1964 letter he
received from the Permanent Mission of the Union of Soviet Socialist
Republics to the United Nations expressing gratitude for "everything
you have already done and are still doing for the development of medical
science, for practical application of this achievement for the health of the
people, for international cooperation in the field of medicine and for the
better mutual understanding between American and Soviet peoples."

The rate of progress made through these friendships and scientific
meetings was not, however, always satisfying or significant. Thus in
1963 after the third scientific mission to Moscow and doubtless recalling
the more constructive Czech mission of 1946, Paul White expressed frus-

tration, writing "what has been happening in the last few years has been simply an annual repetition of talk talk talk, very tiresome and really getting nowhere . . ." However, this was not his usual reaction.

There was only one occasion when he tried to intervene in a political matter, and that was in Washington in August 1972, at a meeting with the then Soviet Minister of Health, Boris V. Petrovsky. Paul White had been prevailed upon to raise the issue of six Jewish prisoners held in the Moscow area who were said to be in poor health. No sooner did he mention this report to the Minister, whom he now regarded as an old friend, when there was "an almost instantaneous change in the atmosphere," the Minister denied the charges, and there was "a considerable cooling of our relationship on the spot." It turned out that the Minister had just been given a hard time by the American press on the same subject and was very touchy in that area. Paul White wrote that "in the future, I think I must continue to be doctor first and politician way down the list."

His most eloquent statement of what he had learned from his international activities—and particularly those involving Russia—was made at the Fourth Dartmouth Conference held in Leningrad in July 1964. This was a meeting of important private citizens of the US and the USSR to discuss international issues of concern to the two countries with the aim of making a contribution to a better understanding and thus it was hoped to world peace. The US delegation was a select one including besides Paul White, Norman Cousins, Charles Frankel, R. Buckminster Fuller, John Kenneth Galbraith, James Michener, Franklin Murphy, David Rockefeller, Marshall Shulman, Norton Simon and Shepard Stone. After reviewing his own experience and interest in preventive medicine and commenting "that I truly regard myself as a citizen of the world," he said

The lessons of the past and of the present too should teach us more actively than we are doing now the need of discovering and applying constructive preventive measures for this sick world of ours, without displacing the programs of the United Nations but rather supplementing them and probably moving faster and with more initiative. Why can't the USSR and the USA sign further agreements, as they have already done with at least some success for health and some of the arts and sciences, though often too meagerly and too slowly, against other common enemies in the world which can lead to war which include hunger, poverty, ignorance, and unhappiness without forcing ourselves on peoples who do not need or want help? I believe that if we could do this open heartedly and adroitly, even for China, we might very well save the world years and years and years of Cold War and worse, and if it could be done open heartedly and accepted as such, how really marvelous it would be.

He concluded with a quotation from Sir William Osler from a 1902 lecture given in Montreal—a quotation representing for both Osler and White a mixture of impatience and frustration as true in 1964 as in 1902.

There is room, plenty of room, for proper pride of land and birth. What I inveigh against is a cursed spirit of intolerance, conceived in distrust and bred in ignorance, that makes the mental attitude perennially antagonistic, even bitterly antagonistic to everything foreign, that subordinates everywhere the race to the nation, forgetting the higher claims of human brotherhood.

*   *   *

It is not surprising that Paul White met Albert Schweitzer—after all, he met in his lifetime most of the great men and women of the world. What was remarkable and fascinating to observe was that from a first brief visit came a vigorous continuing interest on the part of the aging Boston doctor and a muted but appreciative response from the legendary and aged Lambaréné physician. That an active and overall productive relationship would develop would not have been expected partly because Paul White at that time had, even more than usual, an overfull schedule and appeared unable to take on any new projects and interests. Further, there was a striking contrast between the two personalities.

Paul White first met Albert Schweitzer in 1959 when he was 72 and the latter was 84. Schweitzer, like Paul White, was a direct, warm, simple and generous person, was a doctor of medicine and was dedicated to the search for world peace and international understanding, but there the similarities end. A native of Alsace, Schweitzer had two other degrees as a doctor of philosophy and as a doctor of theology and had served not only as a minister of St. Nicholas Church in Strasbourg, but also as Professor of Theology at Strasbourg University and Director of the

Seminary. Further, he was a world famous student of organ music and had written a book on organ building as well as an important treatise on Johann Sebastian Bach. He had essentially put these activities behind him when in 1913, he chose to dedicate his life to service for those in need and left Europe to establish a small general hospital situated on the equator in Lambaréné in Gabon on the west coast of Africa. There he lived for the rest of his life, with the exception of the periods 1917 to 1924 and 1927 to 1929, and occasional visits back to his old home in Günsbach in Alsace. He came to the United States just once in 1949. Albert Schweitzer became famous not so much for what he accomplished even though that was major—indeed his hospital cared for 137,000 patients between 1924 and 1966 and 18,500 operations were performed in that period. Rather, he was admired throughout the world for his manifest selflessness, dedication to serving others, and his profound reverence for life. By turning his back on the more comfortable opportunities for recognition and success in Europe, he had chosen a career which many would have liked to emulate had they possessed the fortitude.

Unlike Paul White, he avoided travel. The great figures of the world came to Lambaréné, rather than he to them. Unlike Paul White, he was suspicious and wary of new approaches in science and was reluctant to accept change until it was clearly demonstrated that change was necessary. Many considered him stubborn and backward in his reluctance to accept modern innovations in his hospital—and indeed it was *his* hospital—which existed like a small tropical village to which patients came with their families and animals, and received diagnosis and treatment without the benefits of toilets and a sewage disposal system, electricity (except in the operating room) or a telephone, and with only limited running water and refrigeration. Whereas Paul White was a promoter of teaching young people of all national origins about medicine, Schweitzer was regarded disapprovingly by many because of his failure to help to train young Gabonese men and women in the health field. He sincerely believed such an attempt in Gabon to be unpromising and a serious diversion of scarce resources and energy away from the care of the sick. Paul White had become an enthusiast for organizing and working vigorously with groups to ráise money to underwrite research, education and service; whereas Schweitzer was wary of large fund-raising efforts on his behalf and preferred contributions from individuals.

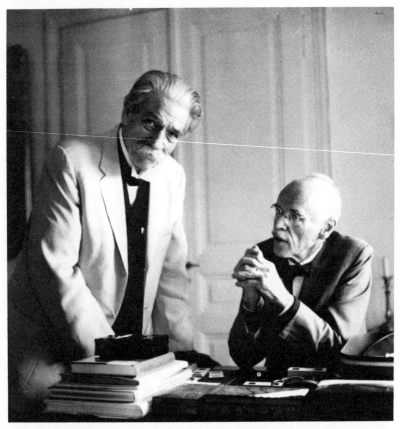

Dr. Paul White with Dr. Albert Schweitzer, Günsbach, Alsace, September, 1959, photographed by Erica Anderson.

Paul White actually saw Albert Schweitzer very little, which was unfortunate, as Schweitzer and his world represented a complex inter-action of elements not easy to absorb and place in perspective. In April 1959, Paul White and his wife visited Schweitzer in Lambaréné for three days. Stimulated by that meeting, he saw Schweitzer for a few hours five months later in Günsbach. The only other personal encounter was in August 1963, when Paul White again saw Schweitzer at his hospital for a three-day period. In addition, Albert Schweitzer wrote about a dozen letters to Paul White over the years until his death in 1965.

It was clear that Schweitzer liked Paul White and respected him and appreciated his interest in the hospital. This interest would not have been entirely to Schweitzer's liking had he known about it, as Paul White's initial reaction—like that of many others—was to admire what the hospital in Lambaréné and its leader represented, but also to think how it could be made far more effective; and to face up also to the question—after Schweitzer, what?

On his return to the United States after his first visit, Paul White had written: "I felt that I had been transported several hundred years back to the middle ages to some secluded monastic institution with great devotion to the ideal but not as practically useful in this day and age as certainly it could and should be." He also prepared a summary of his observations which included the following striking word picture:

> On one's arrival at the hospital all seems to be utter confusion and uproar but after a day or two it settles into a quite orderly bedlam. The entire area is overrun by animals, many of which have been brought by the patients themselves as food, such as hens, ducks, sheep, and goats, but the staff and management and Dr. Schweitzer himself have their own animals including not only innumerable hens and chickens, woolless sheep and milkless goats, but also dogs, cats, pet antelopes, parrots, and a chimpanzee or two. Added to the noisy throng of animals and birds is the mass of patients and their families often talking shrilly in their native tongues and now and then crying out in pain during treatment or from their illness. I found it extremely difficult to auscultate heart and lungs and blood pressures; certainly a quiet examining room or two would be highly desirable. The humidity is also a considerable handicap, at least to those not used to it; everything is wet all the time, clothes and towels and sheets. However, it was not so intensely hot as I had feared. One result of the inadequate sanitation, heat, and humidity is the universal more or less fetid odor to which we gradually became accustomed. The most memorable experience of our short visit, like that of many others (e.g., three women from a mission in Nigeria visiting for a few days), has been the long table after dinner with 35 to 40 staff members and visitors listening to Dr. Schweitzer reading and expounding the scriptures and playing the piano for the group singing of a hymn, all by the light of oil lamps.

It was Paul White's conclusion that if the hospital was to have a future, there would have to be several changes: a larger and permanent staff (including possibly several American blacks), a broad program of hygiene and preventive medicine for the hospital and surrounding area, and improvements in the hospital itself including sanitation, refrigeration, lighting, animal control, and a library-conference room for the staff.

Because Paul White respected Schweitzer and was fully aware of his dislike of change, he moved with care in proposing these ideas. He started with a series of inquiries to people in the United States and Europe who were knowledgeable about the Lambaréné situation. Most of these persons were delighted to learn of his interest, but their views as to any concrete proposals were few because they too were reluctant to upset an individual whom they profoundly admired. Paul White talked to the authorities at the National Heart Institute, especially Dr. James Watt, and with Schweitzer's blessing arranged to have two young doctors, David C. Miller and Steven S. Spencer, assigned to the Lambaréné area for six months to study cardiovascular disease in that region. He got in touch with the Sanborn Company which donated a battery-operated electrocardiograph to the hospital, equipment it had never had before. He wrote to MEDICO to obtain assistance in sending medical books and journals. As there was understandable concern regarding the old man's health, he prevailed upon him to have a physical examination and electrocardiogram done in Strasbourg in the fall of 1959, and he examined him himself in Lambaréné in 1963. He got in touch with the Department of State to get the views of the American ambassador and the government of Gabon toward the hospital and its future. In 1963, he arranged a meeting in Libreville with the Gabonese Minister of Health and the Deputy Minister of Education, as well as with Rev. James Robinson, of Operation Crossroads Africa, and the American Ambassador, Charles F. Darlington, to explore the possible creation of an Institute for Public Health Research and Development at Lambaréné. When Paul White later mentioned this possibility in a cautious fashion to Albert Schweitzer, Schweitzer rebuffed him and appeared "largely indifferent to the future of the hospital."

Two years later in 1965, Paul White also arranged to have the International Cardiology Foundation finance in the amount of $14,000 a six-month survey of high blood pressure in the Lambaréné region. After

Schweitzer's death, Paul White was elected to the Board of Directors of the Albert Schweitzer Fellowship which, with other agencies, accomplished many of the changes in the hospital that had been considered in the past but never started. He agreed to sign a number of letters to well-known personages asking for their support, and spoke at a fund-raising luncheon in New York in 1972—an event which Schweitzer himself would have regarded without enthusiasm. The extent of Paul White's involvement can be gleaned from the fact that his files contained 88 folders of correspondence and other material relating to Schweitzer and his hospital.

That Paul White did as much as he did considering their different personalities and styles and their geographic separation was due, Paul White wrote in 1963, to his "love of Dr. Schweitzer himself." However, as Paul White grew older, it became apparent that he was frustrated at having his well-intentioned efforts largely rejected by a strong willed man who disliked being told what to do. In 1970, when asked to prepare a foreword for a biography of Schweitzer, Paul White wrote:

> I appreciate greatly the kind invitation so to do. Since, however, I would, as a physician and teacher, be expected quite naturally to write of Schweitzer's medical career, outside of his spiritual and intellectual contributions to mankind, I would hesitate to say publicly in such a volume what I have said so often privately, that his work in medical science, public health, and hospital administration, was of such a low order that I would be embarrassed to write of them.

Along the same lines was his sentence written in 1971 when he himself was 85:

> . . . we were good friends and he was, as emphasized, too much of a hero.

One cannot help wondering if these seemingly uncharitable comments would not have been phrased differently or perhaps not written at all had Paul White gotten to know Albert Schweitzer better; and if their expression did not represent to some degree the same aging process in Paul White which he had found so difficult in Albert Schweitzer.

For the young doctors David Miller and Steven Spencer who spent six months with Schweitzer in 1960 had found it took considerable time for a United States trained physician to acquire a balanced view of "le grand docteur," his philosophy of life, and the lot he had chosen for himself in such "medieval" surroundings. Spencer wrote to Paul White on November 2, 1960 after his return to the United States:

> As you can probably surmise from my earliest letters to you my feelings about Dr. Schweitzer's hospital underwent a period of evolution from an initial disillusionment and disapproval to a final quite favorable impression based on an understanding of the reasons for some of the shortcomings and an appreciation of the some of the intangible values that are manifested there. I came to realize that much of what I initially would be inclined to change was actually worthy of preserving as an expression of his philosophy of Reverence for Life, and that some conditions there do not really compromise good medical care as much as it would have first seemed. And I adopted a more charitable attitude as I learned that Dr. Schweitzer many years ago had concerned himself with problems such as isolation of contagious cases, privies and improved sanitation. That the hospital has had incomplete success with these problems may be to a considerable extent the responsibility of those who are at present more actively engaged in medical care and hospital administration than is Dr. Schweitzer.

David Miller on January 12, 1961 wrote to Paul White in a somewhat similar vein:

> Considering these aspects of the man, and remembering further the trying equatorial conditions, the geographic and professional isolation, and the many endeavors other than medicine which he pursues, it is, in a way, remarkable that the hospital is as good as it is. For despite the serious shortcomings which you and I have seen, it has performed a great service . . . and irrespective of quantity and quality of medical and surgical care, there is no question whatever that Dr. Schweitzer and the hospital are held in high esteem and trust by a great majority of the patients who have been served there. It will obviously be a pity if this service and this spirit cannot be continued there after Dr. Schweitzer's death.

One happy consequence of Paul White's interest in Albert Schweitzer was that Dr. David Miller, whom he had arranged to go to Lambaréné, met there and later married Schweitzer's daughter Rhena. Rhena Schweitzer Miller has written

> I had the distinct impression that there was mutual respect between the two men, though not mutual understanding. Dr. White saw the shortcomings of the hospital from his extensive experience, but did not realize that for my

father the hospital was mainly a concrete realization of the principle of Reverence for Life, applied to humans and animals, and offered to people who could live there as they did in their villages. An important point in my father's organization of his hospital was his concern to adjust to the customs and life style of the patients who came there to seek help. He knew, what Dr. White did not, that if they had not felt comfortable in his hospital they would not have stayed and so could not have been treated. Given these fundamental differences, I doubt if a more prolonged visit would have changed anything.

I very much enjoyed Dr. White's visit, his stimulating presence and challenging conversations. However during our long walks at brisk pace in the equatorial heat and humidity, I could hardly keep up with him! When somewhat exhausted, I had brought him to the airport, his last words were: "I don't think I could live in Lambaréné, there is not enough opportunity for exercise."

And in the words of Norman Cousins who had also stayed in Lambaréné and who knew Paul White:

The point about Schweitzer is that he brought the kind of spirit to Africa that the dark man hardly knew existed in the white man. Before Schweitzer, white skin meant beatings and gun point rule and imposition of slavery on human flesh . . . He has supplied a working demonstration of reverence for life.

In retrospect, Paul White accomplished and attempted so much for Albert Schweitzer and Lambaréné that it was sad he could not have paused to comprehend more fully its real successes and its disturbing challenges as well as its unquestioned limitations.

* * *

In September 1914, Paul White received a letter from Dr. Frank P. Gaunt of the Methodist Hospital in Nanking, China, who had been a classmate at the Harvard Medical School. He wrote: "In all China, I believe there is no pure pediatrician. Come out and start things going. The possibilities for service are unlimited . . ." Paul White declined the invitation, not only because he had just returned from his period of training in London, but also because pediatrics was no longer his field of interest. However, in subsequent years, he often envied the easy access to China offered to him in 1914. For as he traveled about the world in

the 1940s, '50s and '60s, there was one large geographic area—China—
to which he was never invited. Everyone else, even the Russians, loved
him and wanted him, but not the Chinese, who regarded him not as Dr.
Paul White, but as a citizen of the United States whose imperialist government did not recognize the legitimate existence of the People's Republic of China.

With relations with Russian cardiologists on a satisfactory footing, he
commenced a protracted and for nine years unsuccessful campaign both
to wangle an invitation from some authority in the People's Republic of
China to visit that country and to obtain a visa from the U.S. State
Department should the invitation by chance come through. He wanted
to meet Chinese doctors, to make friends of them as he had in every other
country, to observe and understand their work with their 800,000,000
citizens, and to get them in turn to visit the scientific centers in the US.
What a breakthrough for science and perhaps world peace if he could
accomplish this!

The long scenario began in Moscow in 1962 when at the VIII International Cancer Congress, an old friend Professor Huang Chia-ssu of
Peking informally and orally invited him to visit the People's Republic
as guest of the Chinese Academy of Sciences, of which Professor Huang
was the president. This certainly appeared a favorable omen and attempts
were made to obtain a *bona fide* official invitation. After some months of
correspondence, Dr. Huang finally wrote that a visit by Paul White was
unfortunately out of the question owing to the "reactionary" attitude of
the US government toward "New China." Paul White was not daunted
by this refusal, and from 1962 on, he pursued a variety of approaches,
hoping finally to find the key which would fit the lock which would open
the door. Involved in various capacities was a long list of scientists, dip-
lomats, and others who might be able to be helpful and who were repeatedly approached on a confidential level so as not to disturb the
sensitive Chinese authorities. Fortunately, the issue of the US State Department's permission to visit China was resolved in 1965 by a change in
regulations affecting doctors and other scientists, but the necessity of an
official invitation to visit the People's Republic remained.

A person who was an intimate part of this China operation from 1962 until his death in 1967 was Grenville Clark. A distinguished and charming retired New York lawyer, and spokesman for world peace through the application of world law, he was a friend and patient of Paul White's and acted as his advisor and confidante in the delicate and frustrating negotiations. It was Grenville Clark who introduced Paul White to the author Edgar Snow. Snow knew China well and had written sympathetically and informatively about the People's Republic (*Red Star Over China* was his most quoted book) and was therefore *persona grata* in the highest echelons of that country. In May 1963, Snow wrote to Chairman Mao Tse-tung "to urge the People's Republic to cooperate actively with Dr. White's desire to visit China." The seemingly excellent introduction came to naught. Over the next eight years, Paul White pursued his quest, corresponding with Secretary of State Dean Rusk; meeting with Under-Secretary of State Averill Harriman; exchanging letters with Dr. Wilder Penfield of Montreal and Prof. Alexander Haddow of London, who as a Canadian and a Briton might have better credentials as intermediaries; writing to Marshall Ayub Khan of Pakistan for his help; enlisting through Albert Baer of New York the aid of the Belgian Ambassador in Argentina; twice sending letters to President Lyndon B. Johnson; and appealing directly to Premier Chou En-lai. Edgar Snow also made discreet inquiries again. All these overtures were played to an unresponsive audience.

Success finally came suddenly in 1971, the result of an abrupt thaw in international relations preceding and leading to the Kissinger mission in July of that year, which was followed shortly by the famous Nixon visit. The door at last began to open. An American table tennis team visited China in April 1971 followed in May by Professors Arthur Galston of Yale and Ethan Signer of MIT, the first American scientists to visit that country since 1949. On September 1, 1971, through an introduction from Prof. Galston, Dr. Victor Sidel, a specialist in community medicine, and his wife Ruth, who was a psychiatric social worker, of Montefiore Hospital in the Bronx, New York, received an invitation from the Chinese Medical Association to visit China. At the same time, an invitation was extended to Dr. and Mrs. E. Grey Dimond as well as to the Paul Whites. Grey Dimond was the son-in-law of Grenville Clark, having married his gracious and talented daughter, Mary D.; he was a former student of Paul White's and a prominent cardiologist, and was Provost for Health Sciences at the University of Missouri in Kansas City. The Dimonds' invitation came through the efforts of their friend, Edgar Snow; and at Grey Dimond's urging, Snow's efforts once again involved Paul White, this time successfully. Also asked to visit China at the same time and under yet different auspices were Dr. and Mrs. Samuel Rosen of New York. Dr. Rosen had developed a highly successful operation for hearing loss and had received an abortive invitation to visit the People's Republic in 1964. The four couples, representing three different areas of interest, were asked to come to China for one month commencing on September 15, the first American physicians to do so in more than 20 years.

That such a long-sought opportunity was to be realized and realized in approximately two weeks caused both delight and consternation. Trips had to be made to Ottawa to obtain visas; the Dimonds flew on short notice to Switzerland via a medical meeting in Helsinki to get a briefing from Edgar Snow. Paul White mowed his front lawn on September 11, visited a patient in the hospital, received an injection of cholera vacciné and gamma globulin, and with his wife departed that evening for Los Angeles. After an overnight stay there, they flew to Hong Kong, arriving at 10:00 p.m. and meeting the Dimonds. The Rosens had already arrived, but the Sidels, who were delayed by family obligations, met them four days later.

Thus began a hastily arranged and exciting journey, momentous and successful for the four couples. For Paul White it was a dream finally come true. The only drawback was that because he and Prof. Alfred V. Boursy of Holy Cross College were to have an audience with the Pope on September 29 to give him a special presentation of the translation of *De Subitaneis Mortibus* by Lancisi, the Whites were forced to reduce the length of their stay in China to 12 days. Grey Dimond had promised the Chinese that he would watch over the health of the 85-year-old Paul White, and he and his wife on that account also cut their trip short. The other two couples remained for the entire month.

The mission of the four doctors and their wives came while the Great Proletarian Cultural Revolution, started by Chairman Mao, was still very much in force. As Grey Dimond wrote in the *Journal of the American Medical Association* of December 14, 1984, the results of the 1965 aggressive policy were that "all medical schools were closed, all students declared graduated, all specialty societies closed down, all medical journals stopped, all medical meetings banned, and many faculty and new

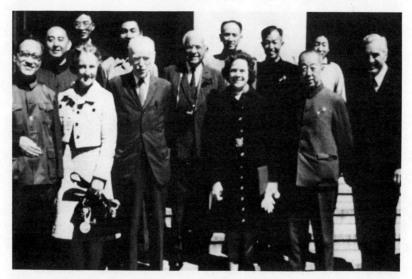

Mission to People's Republic of China. In front of Peking Hotel, September 20, 1971.
Front row, left to right: Dean Chu, Mrs. Ina White, Dr. Paul White, Dr. Samuel Rosen, Mrs. Mary D. Dimond, Professor Wu Ying-kai, Dr. E. Grey Dimond.
Back row, officials of Chinese Medical Association.

doctors were sent to live in the countryside." When the eight Americans arrived, the medical schools were just beginning to reopen after a five-year lapse but were still subservient to the drastic egalitarian teachings of the Chairman.

An incident early in the trip underlined the political instability of the time. The flight of the party from Canton to Peking was supposed to take place on September 16, but the group was told that weather problems interfered and it was not until late afternoon on September 18 that the

flight was actually accomplished. It later developed that the reason for
the delay was not the weather but the presence of a precautionary ban on
all flying over China owing to an attempted revolt within the Central
Committee of the Communist Party. The uprising was quickly quelled,
but in the process the second-in-command of the Committee, Lin Piao,
with his wife and child, the Army Chief of Staff, the leader of the Air
Force, and the chief political officer of the Navy all suddenly disappeared,
presumably while attempting to escape in a plane which was shot down
over outer Mongolia.

Aside from this delay, the 12-day trip went busily and well, although
for the Whites and the Dimonds, it was limited to three hot days in
Canton and nine in Peking. The Canton portion had been hastily arranged and there, for the first time, the group saw major surgical procedures being performed under acupuncture—including an open chest
operation on a surgeon who talked with the visitors during the procedure
and even sipped tea. There was a formal reception at the Peking airport
including a greeting by the Minister of Health, an interview with the
President of the Chinese Academy of Sciences, and a dinner at the Peking
Hotel given by the Chinese Medical Association. On this last occasion
the statement by the head of the Chinese Medical Association included:
"Dear American friends! You have crossed vast oceans to come to visit
China. This manifests your friendly feelings towards the Chinese people
and your good desire for the restoration and development of the friendship between the Chinese and American peoples." There were many
activities in between, including hospital rounds with observation of
acupuncture, library visits, inspection of a commune and a kindergarten,
a tour of the reopened Peking Medical College, and sightseeing. Patients
were seen who had a variety of surgical problems and types of heart
disease, including coronary heart disease. The telephone was busy
with overseas calls from the media because of an erroneous announcement over the BBC that Paul White's visit to Peking was to treat Mao's
heart disease.

Paul White, who as the senior member present always rode in the first
car with his wife, escorted by Dr. Chu Hsien-i, Dean of the School of

Medicine at Tientsin, was called upon to respond to toasts, and ask the first questions at briefings. The Chinese doctors, as might be expected, regarded his age favorably and respectfully. As Professor Tao Shou-chi of the Cardiovascular Institute and Fu Wai Hospital in Peking wrote: "The presence of Dr. White, because of his eminent international position and his age, greatly enhanced the importance of their visit." Grey Dimond has commented that for him, the high point was Paul White's "sense of excitement . . . he was just like a kid . . . he was animated, not missing a simple opportunity to see, talk, make propositions, propose exchanges, not in the least daunted by any of their propaganda." His health was good, and he exhibited no undue fatigue despite a full schedule. He was in no way inhibited from congratulating the Chinese on their widespread use of bicycles as well as chastising them for their equally widespread use of cigarettes. At one point, Ina White did demur at signs depicting Americans as running dogs. Her husband, meanwhile, was highly impressed by what was being done in public health and by the warmth and the hospitality of the Chinese physicians, and he said so. His laudatory comments were appreciated by the Chinese hosts; and Victor Sidel, speaking of the visit, said, "I don't think that there is any question that it played a major role in what followed later. The further exchanges that developed indeed were based on that first visit. It was seen by the Chinese as very successful." Following this success came a veritable flood of visitors including, shortly, thousands of tourists.* Later, the Whites would repay the hospitality they received by acting as hosts to a Chinese medical delegation visiting the United States.**

---

* Subsequently the Dimonds and the Sidels visited China on other occasions and building on the experiences gained with this first visit have published several books including *More Than Herbs and Acupuncture* and *Inside China Today* by Grey Dimond; and *Serve the People* and *The Health of China: Current Conflicts in Medical and Human Services for One Billion People* by the Sidels.

** There was an interesting episode when the first group of Chinese doctors came out to Belmont to have dinner with the Whites, and as was his custom, Paul White announced after dinner, "Let's go for a walk."; and so they did, very pleasantly in the moonlight. However, this was not so pleasant for the security force assigned by the apprehensive authorities in Washington to guard the party which had never expected this potentially hazardous outing and whose members uneasily and warily accompanied the expedition.

The arrival back across the border on September 27 was an extraordinary scene with the Whites and the Dimonds besieged by "many, many" newspaper, radio and television reporters who wanted the scoop on Chairman Mao's supposed heart condition and wanted to hear about the trip. With the bedlam of the press, radio, TV conferences behind them, the Whites departed by air for a one-night stay in Iran en route to Rome and the audience with Pope Paul VI.

That was the last major journey Paul White took. Not that he just stayed home in Boston and Belmont. He continued to take short trips within the United States, often to speak enthusiastically about his experiences in China. In the spring of 1972, he visited Paris and Milan briefly, and in the fall flew to Madrid for one more medical meeting. However, the trip to China was really the happy grand finale to his world travels; he died two years later.

In the back of his daily record for the year 1973, the last year of his life, he had copied the following stanza by R. L. Sharpe:

Each is given a bag of tools,
A shapeless mask, a book of rules;
And each must make, 'ere life is flown,
A stumbling block or a stepping stone.

Paul White regarded his international travels first as such a stepping stone to a better understanding between peoples, and second as rewarding personal adventures. The record indicates that in a considerable measure, he achieved both these goals, although success with the former was limited by what one remarkable man could accomplish, and by the political realities of a complex world.

CHAPTER FOURTEEN

Winding Down

> The want of energy is one of the main reasons why so few persons continue to
> improve in later years. They have not this will, and do not know the way.
> They never "try and experiment" or look up a point of interest for themselves;
> they make no sacrifices for the sake of knowledge . . . hardly anyone keeps up
> his interest in knowledge throughout a whole life.

This quotation from Benjamin Jowett describes most men and women
as they approach the age of 70, and for some even earlier. Paul White in
his mid 80's appeared an exception. To those observing him, he had inexhaustible energy almost until his death at 87. There seemed to be no
"want of energy." He maintained an eager curiosity for the world around
him, relishing new scientific reports and new knowledge, enjoying new
patients and new friends, and inviting new adventures, many of them
overseas. In his later years, he once told Louise Wheeler that it was the
things which he had *not* done that he regretted. He was not one to complain in public that doing all this carried with it a strain. Yet there are
clues that suggest not only his increasing awareness that he was pushing
his human machine too hard, but also his inability to do anything about
it.

As early as November 1952 when he was 66 years of age, he wrote to
Ashton Graybiel suggesting that he might start to slow down a bit:

> Thank you for your congratulations on the number of events which I fear come
> with increasing years and indicate that I'm beginning to get superannuated.
> However, there is still a good deal of life in me yet and for a few more years I
> hope to keep going, not quite at the pace I've had in this past year for I have
> covered a good deal of ground in nine months . . .

There was of course no slowing of his pace. In March 1964, he wrote
of his "customary annual fatigue at this time of year from Heart Association barnstorming." Two years later in August, 1966 he wrote that he

could not take on anything more, "no matter how vital," and a month after this he described his program as "too strenuous." On May 2, 1968 he complained that he did not have "a minute to myself" and on February 21, 1969 wrote that he was "too much on the move as usual." Again on May 15, 1971 he was in his own words "working too hard." It was following his first stroke in May 1973 that he wrote that it was "largely I believe the result of much overwork."

Paul White's demanding schedule which was lifelong and which he continued despite these comments had several explanations. He enjoyed almost everything he was doing and the scientific and public recognition he achieved. He felt that he had a unique mission: to promote the prevention of heart disease and to bring the world of scientists together. He was generous in helping others and found it hard to turn down requests from patients, former and current associates, and friends. Like the aging star in the theater, his act had become a lifelong habit and he liked being welcomed on the stage. Not a rich man, he found that his children and grandchildren continued to need his financial support into his old age. Thus, responding in March 1965 to an appeal from a friend for a contribution to a fund-raising dinner, he declined with the partly jocular comment ". . . someday before long someone will have to have a $100 a plate for me. Meanwhile I am just scraping by." Finally, he was practicing what he preached, for it was he who had said in 1956: "Hard work, physical or mental, never killed a healthy man"; and also "the one most important means to improve and to maintain the health and happiness of our oldest citizens is to keep them working both mentally and physically."

It was unfortunate that Paul White never expressed for himself and for others in similar roles the wisdom of a judicious graded step-down in responsibility and physical and mental demands of work with increasing age. While he would refer briefly and loosely to a decreasing tempo, he never spelled out any guidelines. His emphasis in the advice he gave was to avoid the mental and physical deterioration often seen following retirement. It is possible that he believed to propose guidelines would weaken the impact of this message which he was preaching. Because he had retained his own remarkable good health into his 80's, he was reluctant to change his pace (or recommend changes for others) even though he was conscious that the pace was increasingly excessive for his strength.

Especially appropriate for his latter years was his one real hobby, which was his collection of old medical books, which he kept at home in his library. His classical education had given him a background for enjoying the past, and this was apparent very early in his medical writings. Unlike most physicians, he could read Latin and Greek and was able to translate some of the earliest medical treatises. As early as 1928, while in Paris, he had spent three hours going over a fine, private library of old and modern French medical books, and this collection seems to have made quite an impression on him. Later, while in Vienna that same year, he began to purchase old medical books, an intellectual hobby which was to continue for the rest of his life. Subsequently, as his library grew, he often brought one or two of his old books from home to the hospital and while teaching, would show them to the students with obvious enjoyment. In his collection were 15th, 16th and 17th century volumes including a particularly fine copy of the first edition of *De Fabrica Humani Corporis*, published in 1543 in Basel, Switzerland by Andreas Vesalius. This volume was purchased by Paul White in 1938 from a London dealer who in turn had bought it in Vienna from an Austrian monastery. It had an especially beautiful white tawed velum binding which was in perfect condition as it had been protected by an outer leather jacket. There were also works by Benedictus (1493), Fernal (1554), Columbus (1559), Harvey (1645), Bonetus (1675), Leeuwenhoek (1695), Auenbrugger (1761) and many others, most but not all relating to the heart. In the introduction to the 4th edition of his textbook *Heart Disease*, Paul White wrote: "Not only is the history of medicine of importance culturally in the education of a physician and a source of pleasure and interest through the lifetime of anyone who has once fallen under its spell, but it has a practical value in revealing clearly the gaps in our knowledge and in presenting occasional clues or discoveries long forgotten and needing revival." Dr. Paul David of Montreal, one of his former students, has told how when he and his wife were loaned the use of the White's home one summer, the only request was "to take good care of the library and see that nothing was disturbed."

One major effort late in his life involved the translation and publication with Professor Alfred V. Boursy of Holy Cross College of *De Subitaneis Mortibus* by Giovanni Maria Lancisi. Paul White was much interested in this manuscript which, written in 1707, had never been properly translated from the Latin. The story behind this work was that Pope Clement XI had become greatly concerned by a veritable epidemic of mysterious sudden deaths which were occurring in Rome in the first years of the 18th century; and in 1706, instead of forming a committee as would have happened in the 20th century, he asked his doctor, Lancisi, who was also a professor of anatomy, to study the problem. Lancisi's report, *De Subitaneis Mortibus*, discussed the chief findings on autopsy of these cases, many of whom showed enlargement of the heart and disease of the heart valves, of unknown origin. Paul White and Professor Boursy presented the first copy of their translation to Pope Paul VI on September 29, 1971 in the Vatican.

As Paul White grew older and he and Ina White in 1962 moved from Marsh Street into a smaller house on Juniper Road in Belmont, he began to give parts of his collection to the Countway Library. In the years 1957–1962, he gave the library 124 books, and he donated 135 more in 1963. There was another major gift in 1966. These donations, added to the other volumes accumulated over the years, gave Countway Library a marvelous historical resource on heart disease. It was typical of Paul White that although by no means a rich man, he chose to give away his books to individuals and to a great library rather than sell them to a dealer, as was the choice of many collectors who clearly regarded their accumulated treasure more as an investment than a source of perpetual pleasure to themselves and to others.

Not appreciated by many, and perhaps not even by himself, was the extent of his other activities and commitments. Sandwiched in between seeing patients, teaching, writing medical papers, and traveling were a host of other activities. Some of these were local Boston affairs, such as membership in the Saturday Club; the St. Botolph Club; The Examiner

Club; the Roxbury Society for Medical Improvement; the Ella Lyman Cabot Trust, of which he was the chairman; and the YMCA, where for a time he was chairman of the Camp Becket Committee. Some were obligations to major national and international bodies, such as the American Heart Association, the International Society of Cardiology, and the International Cardiology Foundation. Some were in relation to other local, national and international organizations and committees which often persuaded him to join in some limited, but very visible capacity, so that they might benefit from his reputation. They always had the hope, which was usually not mentioned in the letter of invitation, that he would play an active role, such as writing a statement or a leaflet for the cause or speaking at an annual dinner. Especially in his later years, he seemed to find it hard to say "no" to such invitations, which mainly involved worthy causes. However, aside from the use of his name, he was clearly capable of making a contribution to only a few.*

In time, there was, as there had to be, a gradual winding down of such a performance, even though on the surface much remained the same. As was true for most aging men of science, his publications and his lectures tended to be repetitious of the same Paul White themes so successful when first introduced but now no longer novel. He was inclined to talk

---

* A partial list of organizations to which he gave tacit or active support includes: The American Bicycle Hall of Fame (honorary president); The American Farm School, Salonica (national committee); the American Middle East Rehabilitation, Inc. (honorary director); American Youth Hostels, Inc. (honorary president); Anatolia College, Salonica (trustee); Cardio-Pulmonary Research Institute (honorary trustee); Committee for Safe Bicycling, Inc. (president); Elbanobscot Foundation (honorary chairman); Executive Health (chairman, editorial board); Massachusetts Council of Churches (sponsor); Medical Committee for Civil Rights (national advisory board); Medico, Inc. (board of directors); Mended Hearts, Inc. (advisory council); Museum of Science and Hayden Planetarium (medical advisory committee); the National Council on Drug Abuse (scientific advisory board); National Council for Youth (director); National Jogging Association (consultant); National Youth Science Foundation (board of directors); New England Citizens Crime Commission (advisory membership committee); Physicians for Social Responsibility (sponsor); Praying Hands Charitable Trust (honorary advisor); President's Council on Youth Fitness (citizens' advisory committee); Preventive Heart Reconditioning Foundation, Inc. (honorary president); Resuscitators of America (sponsor); Smith College (counselor and friend of infirmary committee); Sex Information and Education Council of the United States (sponsor); Thomas A. Dooley Foundation (fund raising committee); Unitarian Service Committee (sponsoring committee); World Law Fund (sponsor).

more about himself. His patients would find that visits to his office educated them more on Paul White's recent itinerary than on the details of their own health. He was restless if he could not dominate a conversation. On occasion he even appeared fatigued, which was something new. Dr. Lewis Dexter recalls a dinner party when as the guests were standing about before leaving, Paul White who had just returned from a trip was seen to be asleep on his feet "just like a horse."

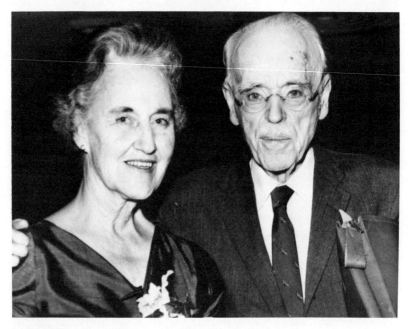

Paul and Ina White in Boston October 17, 1970.

Meanwhile the family circle, which had never been large, had been shrinking over the years. His sister Miriam had died in 1932, his mother in 1949, and then in 1959, his brother J. Warren White, died suddenly of a heart attack. J. Warren White, who was a distinguished orthopedic surgeon and at one time was president of the American Orthopedic Association, had lived for many years in Greenville, South Carolina, where he was Chief of Surgery at the Shriners Hospital for Crippled Children. In 1949, he moved to Honolulu where he held a similar post. He and Paul

White were close despite their geographic separation, and his death from a heart attack left Paul White as the sole surviving member of that generation of the White family.

There were other difficulties in his immediate world which complicated his last years. His daughter Penny who had been married at 19 was severely injured in an automobile accident in December 1956, was comatose for more than 10 days and never completely recovered. Divorced, she subsequently remarried and had two children. In 1969 her two daughters, aged 4 and 7 years came to live with Paul and Ina White which, while in many ways rewarding, was also a financial as well as a physical strain. The burden was especially felt as the older granddaughter Jennifer, a lovely little girl, was not well, having both Down's syndrome and congenital heart disease. She died in 1973 shortly after her grandfather. Paul and Ina White's son Sandy had been challenged by the circumstances of his sister's accident. He did not go to college and instead became interested in emergency medical service and founded a small company, the Massachusetts Medical Service which engaged in rescue work.*

These family and other problems Paul White shared with his wife whose companionship, support, and affection were always there. No longer young and under great strain at times, she wrote to her husband a heartwarming note:

Dearest Paul:
I don't often tell you how much I love you—how much I need and depend on you. Lately especially I've been touchy and horrible—I'm sorry. You have given me the best and most interesting life possible with high ideals fulfilled and motives and work one can deeply respect. Again, I love you.

Paul White had always been able to rely on his young associates to carry the load of his private practice when he was away. However, as he became increasingly separated from the world of the MGH, this dependable expert assistance was no longer always available, for his former associates and their young successors were themselves heavily involved in

* On January 10, 1979 at the age of 39, he died suddenly while at a Civil Defense training program.

their own obligations. This introduced yet another complication. In November 1972, now age 86, Paul White sent out a sad letter to the chairmen of medicine in several of the Boston hospitals seeking help:

> As I grow older and seem to get busier despite any efforts that I feebly make, I recognize that the time is coming when I must begin to retire. I would like to do that gradually, perhaps in the next year or two, with the help of some young but able and personable cardiologist or internist largely concentrating on cardiology.

Possibly reference to the uncertain timing of retirement was a deterrent, but in any case no suitable young cardiologist could be obtained. Six months later an advertisement was prepared for publication in a medical journal which began "Senior cardiologist in planning his retirement seeks affiliate with mature cardiologist or internist." After a period of uncertainty, he was able to obtain the much needed part-time help of Dr. Warren Strauss. The office at 264 Beacon Street was thus able to continue to function during the last few months of Paul White's life, both with Dr. Strauss' assistance and the experience and wisdom of Dr. Florence Avitabile. There was, however, now no regular secretary, which was a handicap, but Mrs. Margaret Thayer was at hand to take the electrocardiograms.

Several writing projects were clearly in Paul White's mind for the future, but they were never completed; time began to run out. One consideration, raised in 1968, was for a book on *Dramatic Episodes in the History of Medicine*. A manuscript was written and he did discuss the topic in a talk in Boston in 1968 but no publication resulted. He began in 1972 a book to be titled 60 *Years of Medical Writing* but this too was never finished, partly because of a negative response from two publishers. He then considered altering the emphasis with titles such as *The Evolution of Preventive Cardiology* and *Growing Older* but these projects were not finished. Yet another book was one he proposed to write with Alton Blakeslee, Science Editor of the Associated Press, on lifestyle and the prevention of heart disease. An outline of the contents was developed but further work was interrupted in 1973 by the first stroke.

Although these and other problems complicated Paul White's last years, he kept on, buoyed up by other rewarding events. His 80th birthday was happily celebrated on June 6, 1966 with Ancel Keys and his group in southern Italy. The occasion was recognized again that year at the World Congress of Cardiology held in New Delhi in November with a profusion of congratulations from around the world. Perhaps the British expressed the sentiments best when in a letter signed by their leading cardiologists, they wrote:

> To Paul White, in respect and admiration. We, your friends in Britain, acclaim your enduring achievements as a pioneer and teacher in cardiology, as a humanist, and as a commanding figure in World Medicine.

A volume titled *Hearts, Their Long Follow-up* by Paul White and his long-time secretary Helen Donovan appeared in 1967. This documented the course of many of Paul White's patients whom he had followed for periods of up to 50 years. It was a book which no one else could have written.

Also published in 1971 was his autobiography, *My Life and Medicine.* Several publishers had asked Paul White to write his memoirs 10 and more years earlier at the peak of public interest in his career as a result of his role in the heart attack of President Eisenhower, but he had been too busy at that time. It would have seemed as if now, in his mid 80's, he would have had the opportunity to go over his letters and speeches and scientific writings at leisure, enjoy the recollections of events and personalities, the successes and the failures, and put together a volume reflecting his eight decades of wisdom and experience. Such was not the case, and the fact that the autobiography appeared at all was a tribute to his persistence and that of others.

In undertaking this, Paul White to some extent made use of his previous writings, but most of the autobiography was new material or revisions of earlier efforts which he wrote out long-hand over a period of more than two years. This time he had substantial help from a professional writer, Margaret Parton, who rejected his ideas for including "Dramatic Episodes in the History of Medicine," badgered and cajoled him for material, pruned, revised and edited. Writing was an effort. Because he had no regular secretarial help in the office, he turned to his two former secretaries, the sisters Helen Donovan (now retired in Swampscott) and

Agnes Donovan Walsh, living with her husband in Washington. If ever there was a time when an unbroken period of writing in Boston and Belmont making use of his library and files was needed, this was it. But that did not happen. Believing that he needed the money from his travels (although it is likely that a similar income would have been generated if he had stayed and seen patients in his office), and seemingly unable to turn aside requests requiring him to be away, he was forced to write the chapters on the run.

On July 19, 1969, driven and harassed, he wrote to Margaret Parton breathlessly:

> . . . it is obvious that I must establish at least one or two weekly sessions to get on with the book despite my hectic schedule which has trapped me (in part because of the need of our financial support of our children, a heavy burden still requiring my earning a maximum amount fortunately possible by my being able to receive fairly liberal honoraria on most of my speaking engagements in other cities of the U.S.A., and a good-sized fee during the early part of this very week from an emergency call to see a patient in the Far East which included two sleepless nights in the air, from which I am now recovering at the end of my two week vacation—on that trip of four days I had to catch up on mail and three manuscripts (now out of the way). This pressure for income I hope will subside).

And again on November 11, 1969, he wrote

> I need time and at least some leisure to think and this year that is about to end has been the busiest and most complicated of my entire life.

And further on May 25, 1970:

> Despite Japan, Denmark, Chicago, New Orleans, Washington, Princeton, and way stations in the last few weeks I've been checking and correcting the first four chapters (45 pages) . . .

The book started in 1968 was finally published in 1971. It combined personal history and accounts of the problems of some of his patients with his views on healthy living including the prevention of heart attacks. It was an extraordinary summary of a long, full and productive life, but called almost no attention to the roles of others including his family and associates. Barely mentioned was his wife, an omission commented upon by the reviewer in the *Boston Globe*. Paul White planned to correct this deficiency, should there be a second edition, with the following two sentences:

> Happily for me and for my medical career, my wife has played a vital role in her ceaseless support of our family and social life together. Although keenly interested in the arts, especially music and sculpture, she has sacrificed much of her time during these many years in aiding me in my medical travels abroad, most of which she has done with me, in my contact with my absorbing and demanding private practice, and helping my literary efforts and in officiating as the charming hostess in entertaining in our home our many guests, teachers, colleagues, and students and their wives from all over the world.

Favorably received by reviewers, the autobiography was not a publishing success. Perhaps the modest sales implied a recognition by some that they had heard a portion of the message before. Perhaps another handicap was the fragmented and unsatisfactory composition.

The travel schedule continued much as before. For example, on May 6, 1972 Paul White talked in Park City, Utah, on May 9 and 10 in New York City, on May 24 in Chicago, and on May 25 and 26 in Los Angeles —and May 1972 was in no way unusual. He continued to see patients in the office several days a week and was active at home. On Saturday May 26, 1973 three days before his first stroke and now nearly 87 years of age, he taped an interview for the Voice of America, saw a patient in consultation at the Lemuel Shattuck Hospital, went to his office for the mail, took a walk with his youngest granddaughter, mowed the entire lawn of their house in Belmont with a hand mower, and in the evening played dominoes with the family. The following day, a Sunday, saw him raking his lawn, working on letters and journals, and going to Randolph as well as to their house in Harvard. Thus up to five months before his death, he continued active physically and mentally and was leading a productive life.

As Paul White subscribed to the view that details of illness should not be concealed from the public, it is appropriate to discuss briefly the course of his own health problems.

He was blessed with excellent health until late in life, except as mentioned for respiratory infections each year. His friend Dr. Samuel Levine is said to have commented once: "Look at those small wrists. He will live forever!" His blood pressure in 1946 was 135/80 and in 1958 122/78, his electrocardiograms were normal, and his blood cholesterol levels were 156 in 1957, and 169 in 1964—all eminently satisfactory values. His first distressing illness came on August 30, 1963 when 12 days after being exposed in Istanbul to a young girl convalescent from chicken pox (the daughter of the American Consul) he contracted shingles (herpes zoster) in the right upper chest region. This produced a protracted upset of his intestinal tract. He saw his colleague Dr. Chester M. Jones and others, had studies of his colon which were unrevealing, and over many months gradually got over the problem. Chester Jones wrote to him on December 3, 1963 suggesting "see how you can keep reasonably and happily active and still avoid the continuous overdoing that has been characteristic in recent years".

On December 31, 1964 then age 78 Paul White wrote in his own medical record with apparent satisfaction and pride the events of his life during the last half of 1964, making it clear that the advice of Chester Jones had not been heeded:

> Meanwhile, although not feeling in tip-top shape PDW was able to continue hard work professionally and physically with four additional round trips to Europe (following his visit to Iceland, Poland, and Japan in May and that to Canada (Montreal and Ottawa) in June); to Leningrad in July, to Prague and Ireland in early August, to Helsinki in late August, and to France in December. Also in October there was a trip to Chile and Peru, and there were many domestic travels—Chicago twice, NYC, North Carolina, Portland (Oregon), Birmingham (Alabama), and local travels in New England including a climb of Mt. Monadnock.

It was in 1964 that his physician Dr. Guillermo Sanchez first observed evidence of a slight leakage of the aortic valve of his heart, "confirmed by PDW himself on September 23" as Paul White wrote in his own medical record. This was not to be a problem but on April 16, 1967 Paul White wrote:

> Two new developments in the past ten days—mild angina pectoris [chest discomfort associated most often with coronary heart disease] on effort (e.g. fast

walking) and blood pressure is up to 165–180 systolic and 85–90 diastolic several times.

The "effort" which first produced his angina was hurrying to see the finish of the Boston Marathon. A year later on June 6, 1968 he noted his angina "has continued, occasionally on effort but never at rest and easily controlled by nitroglycerine which I have taken prophylactically as well as in treatment—total number of tablets of 1/200 gr averages about five a week. There have been no severe attacks."

Paul White's first major illness occurred at the age of 84 on December 20, 1970 when while resting in bed prior to going to sleep, he experienced 3½ hours of chest pain which this time was not relieved by nitroglycerine and was accompanied by nausea but no sweating. Dr. Allan Friedlich promptly saw him at home and drove him to the MGH, but not directly, as the patient insisted on stopping first at his office on Beacon Street to collect a briefcase full of work. He was hospitalized for 10 days and it was determined that there had been no actual heart damage but abnormalities did develop in his electrocardiogram. The diagnosis was a mild heart attack which he referred to later as "a smidgeon of coronary trouble."

He was back in his office briefly on January 4 and despite his recent illness and the fact that Ina White was in the hospital with pneumonia, on January 19 he flew to New York and then to Mexico City where he addressed the new Mexican Heart Foundation on January 21, returning on January 22.

Paul White was fortunate and made an uneventful recovery from this mild heart attack and thereafter did well except for some fatigue and a tendency to imbalance until May 29, 1973. On that date when in the office he had a mild headache, loss of coordination, and confusion. He was again hospitalized at the MGH.* A diagnosis of a stroke possibly due to an embolus (a blood clot which travels in the circulation) was made but he gradually improved and even talked at cardiac rounds on June 12

---

* Paul White was in the hospital on his birthday June 6, 1973. That evening in Symphony Hall, with Arthur Fiedler conducting, the Boston Pops Orchestra played in his honor "Where Is Your Heart" from "Moulin Rouge" by Auric.

on the new and exciting subject of coronary spasm. He was discharged on anti-clotting medicine on June 16 to be quiet at home. He and Ina White had a happy time over the next few weeks but he was again admitted to the MGH on August 13 due to increasing incoordination. It

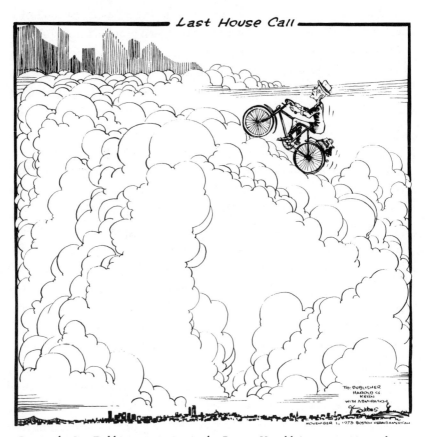

Cartoon by Jim Dobbins, appearing in the *Boston Herald American*, November 1, 1973, reprinted with permission of the *Boston Herald*.

was found that he had something new, a large collection of blood pressing on the brain (a subdural hematoma) which had to be relieved by an operation. He also now developed a persistent irregularity of his heart (atrial fibrillation). The hospital course was further complicated by signs of blood clots in his lungs and the anti-clotting drug which had been stopped had to be resumed. He was able to be discharged from the hospital on September 18 but for the first time was quite depressed.

He returned to the MGH for the last time on October 15, 1973 having had an abrupt turn for the worse with the onset of heavy breathing and inability to speak. A new stroke on the other side of his brain possibly due to another embolism was diagnosed and he slowly went down hill and died October 31, 1973 at the age of 87.

A simple and moving memorial service was held in the Memorial Church in the Harvard Yard November 13, 1973. Three quotations read at the service stand by themselves as eloquent testimony to the life of this great man.

The first was written by Paul White's long-time associate, Howard B. Sprague, whose remarks intended for presentation at a meeting of Paul White's former students on October 17, 1970 were never actually presented as he himself suddenly became fatally ill. They were later found in his coat pocket and were quoted at the Memorial Service by J. Willis Hurst:

> It is not the accumulation of years alone that has built the image of Paul Dudley White. His industry, his unconquerable optimism, his ability to induce his patients to take heart, his gift of serving as an example. His friend, Albert Schweitzer once said, "example is not the main thing in life—it is the only thing." He has been able to convince men that what Sir William Temple recommended is probably true—"The only way for a rich man to be healthy is by exercise and abstinence, to live as if he were poor." But Paul's reputation has the solid foundation of his labors as a teacher, for in the incubation of his laboratory under Ward G and in the basement of the Bulfinch Building were hatched the birds, you in fact, who have flown out to inhabit the roosts of cardiology throughout the earth. This is the stuff of a man's immortality; for as Henry Adams wrote, "A teacher affects eternity; he can never tell where his influence stops."

The other two quotations, read by Bishop Henry Knox Sherrill, were selected by Ina White. They speak of that infinite world of which Paul White had finally become a part.

The first was by Rabindranath Tagore in his volume "Gitanjali";

> Where the mind is without fear and the head is held high;
> Where knowledge is free;

Where the world had not been broken up into fragments by narrow domestic
walls;
Where words come out from the depths of truth;
Where tireless striving stretches its arms towards perfection;
Where the clear stream of reason has not lost its way into the dreary desert
sand of dead habit;
Where the mind is led forward by thee into ever-widening thought and
action—

The second quotation was an excerpt from William Faulkner's speech
delivered in 1950 in Stockholm on the occasion of receiving the Nobel
Prize for Literature:

I decline to accept the end of man. It is easy enough to say that man is immortal
simply because he will endure; that when the last ding-dong of doom has
clanged and faded from the last worthless rock hanging tideless in the last red
and dying evening, that even then there will still be one more sound: that of
his puny inexhaustible voice, still talking. I refuse to accept this. I believe that
man will not merely endure: he will prevail. He is immortal, not because he
alone among creatures has an inexhaustible voice but because he has a soul, a
spirit capable of compassion and sacrifice and endurance.

APPENDIX

White Family Lineage

I. THOMAS WHITE. Born in 1599, died August 1679. Name of wife unknown. Settled in Weymouth, Massachusetts and was made a freeman of Massachusetts in 1635. Was Deputy to the General Court of the Colony. One of his sons was

II. THOMAS WHITE. Died April 11, 1706 in Braintree, Massachusetts. Married Mary Pratt of Braintree. Lived in Weymouth and Braintree. His eldest son was

III. THOMAS WHITE. Born in Weymouth, died 1765 in Weymouth. Married 1st Mehitable Adams on July 21, 1697 who was born November 23, 1673 and died October 21, 1713. Married 2nd Mary Bowditch on April 29, 1714 who was born February 17, 1686/87 and died February 8, 1723/24. Married 3rd Abigail Penniman on July 17, 1725 who was born July 13, 1685. Thomas White lived in Braintree. His tenth child was

IV. MICAH WHITE. Born December 10, 1721 in Braintree, died 1802. Married Susanna Yeager on September 10, 1746. Lived in Randolph, was representative to the Massachusetts General Court and was Speaker of the Massachusetts House of Representatives. His fifth child was

V. MICAH WHITE. Born March 10, 1758 in Braintree, died November 1841. Married Sarah Mann on December 15, 1783, who was born July 11, 1762 in Randolph and died June 2, 1852. A Micah White of Braintree served as a Minuteman April 28, 1775 to October 6, 1775. A Micajah White of Braintree, a fifer, served for 4 days at the time of the "alarm of April 19, 1775" under Capt. Seth Turner. He was a selectman in Randolph. His eighth child was

VI. WARREN WHITE. Born July 12, 1801, died April 17, 1878. Married Lorena Mann, his first cousin, March 13, 1828. She died January 4, 1900. He lived in Randolph, Cambridge, and Boston Highlands and was one of the owners of the Blue Hill Turnpike. His second child was

VII. EPHRAIM MANN WHITE. Born March 7, 1830 in Randolph, died July 4, 1869 also in Randolph. Married 1st Mary Frances Niles on January 14,

1855. She was born October 6, 1835 in Randolph and died September 15 or 16, 1859, in Randolph. Married 2nd Carrie E. Richards on April 21, 1861, who was born September 13, 1836 in Charlestown. They were divorced. He served in the Union Army 1862–63. Was associated with his brothers in C.W. White and Company, Boston. His son was

VIII. HERBERT WARREN WHITE. Born November 12, 1858 in Charlestown, died November 21, 1929 in Roxbury. Married Elizabeth Abigail Dudley on June 6, 1882, who was born September 19, 1859 in Memphis, Tennessee, and died June 26, 1948 Brookline, Massachusetts. He was graduated from the Harvard Medical School in 1880 and was a general practitioner in Roxbury. His second child was

IX. PAUL DUDLEY WHITE. Born June 6, 1886 in Boston, died October 31, 1973 also in Boston. Married Ina Helen Reid on June 28, 1924, West Roxbury, Massachusetts. She was born December 9, 1901, West Roxbury, Massachusetts.

Sources

Extensive use has been made of the material in the Paul Dudley White archive in possession of the Countway Library of Medicine, Harvard Medical School, Boston. This includes correspondence, committee minutes, reports, newspaper items, photographs, and many of Paul White's manuscripts. There is a gap in the 1950's most likely the consequence of a flood in the basement of the White home in Belmont which soaked a portion of Paul White's files with the resulting loss of considerable material. The correspondence tends to be matter-of-fact as Paul White was usually reticent in reference to his emotions and to family and other personal issues. Available also has been the complete set of his "Memindex" cards starting in 1922 which are helpful as they list his daily activities, occasionally with a brief comment. Of the greatest value have been more than 50 taped interviews with members of the family, associates, friends and patients, which have been conducted by the author, transcripts of which have been deposited in the Paul White archive at Countway Library.

General biographical material about Paul White has been found in "My Life and Medicine" by Paul White, publisher Gambit, Inc., Boston, 1971. Some of the limitations of this autobiography have been mentioned in Chapter XV. Valuable also is "Paul Dudley White, A Portrait," E. Grey Dimond, editor, The American Journal of Cardiology, Vol. 15, pp. 433–603, 1965 (April). This includes 71 brief essays by former students and associates. There is also a "Profile of Paul White, Ike's Heart Doctor" by Frances Burns, consisting of ten installments in the *Boston Globe* running from February 5–14, 1956.

CHAPTER I

Dr. Herbert Warren White prepared a typed manuscript on "A Sketch of Thomas White of Woburn, Massachusetts and Certain of his Decendants [sic]" which is undated and which is found in the Countway archive. A somewhat similar genealogy entitled "White Family" by Henry Bowen White of Dover, Massachusetts, undated, is in the New England Historic Genealogical Society in the form of a typed, bound manuscript. Information as to the involvement of Paul White's ancestors in the Revolutionary War is available in "Massachusetts Soldiers and Sailors of the Revolutionary War," publisher Secretary of the Commonwealth, Boston, 1908, Vol. 17, pp. 109, 110, 461, and 548. Information regarding his ancestors who served in the Civil War is found in "Massachusetts Soldiers, Sailors, and Marines in the Civil War," publisher the Adjutant General, Norwood, Massachusetts, 1932, Vol. II, p. 579 and Vol. IV, p. 405. Dr. Herbert Warren White's diaries from 1876–1883 and 1896–1928 are in the possession of Mrs. Dorothy Ellis of Weston, Massachusetts. The latter diaries are not of much help except as they list names of patients and fees charged and notes on his travels. Dr. Herbert Warren White published "A Personal Experience with Small-Pox" in The Boston Medical and Surgical Journal, Vol. 130, pp. 91–93, 1894 (January 25). The letter describing how Paul White received his name was written by Paul White and Lewis Webb Hill and appeared in the New England Journal of Medicine, Vol. 266, pp. 678–679, 1962 (March 29). Background information as to the New England Baptist Hospital was gratefully located in "History of the New England Baptist Hospital" by Martha Horsefield, a typed manuscript dated 1979 on file at the New England Baptist Hospital. Informative is "A Sketch of Herbert Warren White (autobiographic)" dated 1928, which was presented by the author at a meeting of the Roxbury Society of Medical Improvement, a typed copy of which is now in the Countway archive. Paul White's tribute to his father is "A Family Doctor. 1858–1929" published in the New England Journal of Medicine, Vol. 202, pp. 90–92, 1930 (January 9). He wrote a tribute to his mother in the form of a letter to the editor of the *Boston Herald*, entitled "Tribute to Women" appearing on the editorial page of that paper on July 27, 1948. "Dr. Paul Dudley White. R.L.S. Man of the Year . . ." is to be found in the Roxbury Latin School Alumni Bulletin, March 1956, pp. 1–2, being a reprinting of an earlier (1955) article which he wrote on his Roxbury Latin School experiences. Paul White refers to Camp Becket, the Roxbury Latin School, and to his teacher Clarence Gleason in "My Own Prescription for Life" which was published in the *Saturday Review* of December 16, 1967, pp. 17–20.

CHAPTER II

Diaries of Paul White for the years 1909–1911, 1914, 1916–1917, and during and immediately after World War I, are found in the Countway archive. An excellent description of the life of the house staff members at the Massachusetts General Hospital during the early twentieth century is in "The Inquisitive Physician. The Life and Times of George Richards Minot" by Frank M. Rackemann, publisher Harvard University Press, 1956. Background information regarding the hospital is also to be found in "The Massachusetts General Hospital. Its development 1900–1935" by F. A. Washburn, publisher Houghton Mifflin Co., Boston, 1939. The first scientific paper of Paul White was "A Clinical Study of the Coagulation Time of Blood" by Roger I. Lee and Paul D. White, appearing in the American Journal of Medical Sciences, Vol. 145, pp. 495–503, 1913 (April). Dean

Edsall and his activities are described in "Pioneer in Modern Medicine. David Linn Edsall of Harvard" by J. C. Aub and R. K. Hapgood, publisher Harvard Medical Alumni Association, Boston, 1970. Sir James Mackenzie is warmly presented in "The Beloved Physician. Sir James Mackenzie" by R. McNair Wilson, publisher John Murray, London, 1926. Commentaries and reminiscences regarding Sir Thomas Lewis are to be found in the University College Hospital Magazine, Vol. 40, No. 2, 1955, including recollections by Paul White (pp. 66–68) and Sir Alan Drury (pp. 70–71) and a comment by Sir Harold Himsworth (p. 63). An admirable tribute by George Pickering is in Clinical Science, Vol. 6, pp. 3–11, 1948. Sir Thomas Lewis is also the subject of a brief biography in the Mayo Clinic Proceedings, Vol. 56, pp. 749–752, 1981 (December) by J. A. Callahan, J. D. Key, and T. E. Keys. The comment regarding the label of "heart specialist" is to be found on p. 154 of "Memories of Eighty Years" by James B. Herrick, publisher University of Chicago Press, 1949. Useful is the "History of U.S. Army Base Hospital No. 6 and Its Part in the American Expeditionary Forces 1917–1918" published by the Massachusetts General Hospital, Boston, 1924. Pages 1–21 were written by Paul White and there is a section, pp. 180–186, by J. S. Hodgson, referring to the Greek medical mission.

CHAPTER III

Paul White described the cardiac clinic activities at the Massachusetts General Hospital in "The Ether Day Address, Massachusetts General Hospital, October 16, 1936. The Study and Treatment of Heart Disease at the MGH From 1821–1936" appearing in the New England Journal of Medicine, Vol. 215, pp. 1261–1268, 1936 (December 31). The measles episode is well described in "Our Hearts Were Young and Gay" by Cornelia Otis Skinner and Emily Kimbrough, publisher Dodd Mead and Co., New York, 1944, pp. 66–83. The research project in which Paul White and Ina Reid were involved resulted in the publication "The Incidence of Rheumatic Fever, Chorea and Rheumatic Heart Disease with Especial Reference to its Occurrence in Families" by J. M. Faulkner and Paul D. White, published in the Journal of the American Medical Association, Vol. 83, pp. 425–426, 1924 (August 9). The contribution of Ina Reid was not mentioned in the article.

CHAPTER IV

The medical articles referred to in this chapter include in order of mention the following: "The Effect of Digitalis on the Normal Human Electrocardiogram, with Especial Reference to A-V Conduction" by Paul D. White and R. R. Sattler appearing in the Journal of Experimental Medicine, Vol. 23, pp. 613–629, 1916 (see also the obituary of Paul Dudley White prepared by J. Worth Estes in The Pharmacologist, Vol. 16, pp. 47–49, 1974 (Spring)); the classic paper by J. M. DaCosta was "On Irritable Heart; a Clinical Study of a Form of Functional Cardiac Disorder and Its Consequences" in the American Journal of Medical Sciences, Vol. 61, pp. 17–52, 1871 (January), followed by reports by Sir Thomas Lewis including his "The Soldier's Heart and the Effort Syndrome," publisher Paul B. Hoeber, New York, 1919, and "The Cardiac Phase of the War Neuroses" by A. E. Cohn in the American Journal of Medical Sciences, Vol. 158, pp. 433–470, 1919 (October), all of which preceded "The Diagnosis of Heart Disease in Young People" by Paul D. White, published in the Journal of the American Medical Association, Vol. 74, pp. 580–582, 1920 (February 28) as well as "Neurocirculatory Asthenia (Anxiety Neurosis, Effort Syndrome, Neurasthenia). A Twenty Year Follow-up Study of one Hundred and Seventy-Three Patients" by E. O. Wheeler, Paul D. White, E. W. Reed, and Mandel E. Cohen, published in the Journal of the American Medical Association, Vol. 142, pp. 878–889, 1950 (March 25); "The Classification of Cardiac Diagnosis" by Paul D. White and M. M. Myers in the Journal of the American Medical Association, Vol. 77, pp. 1414–1415, 1921 (October 29) (the subsequent publication which referred back to this pioneer article was "Clinical Charts Recommended by the Association for the Prevention and Relief of Heart Disease" by A. E. Cohn, published in the Journal of the American Medical Association, Vol. 78, pp. 1559–1562, 1922 (May 20)); "Bundle-Branch Block With Short P-R Interval in Healthy Young People Prone to Paroxysmal Tachycardia" by Louis Wolff, John Parkinson, and Paul D. White, published in the American Heart Journal, Vol. 5, pp. 685–704, 1930 (August) (follow-up important publications referred to included "Über Elektrokardiogramme mit verkürtzer Vorhof-Kammer-Distanz und positiven P-Zacken" by M. Holzmann and D. Scherf in Zeitschrift für Klinische Medizin, Vol. 121, pp. 404–423, 1932; "The Mechanism of Production of Short P-R Interval and Prolonged QRS Complexes in Patients with Presumably Undamaged Hearts: Hypothesis of an Accessory Pathway of Auriculo-Ventricular Conduction (Bundle of Kent)" by C. C. Wolferth and F. C. Wood in the American Heart Journal, Vol. 8, pp. 297–311, 1933 (February), and "The Pre-Excitation Syndrome: Facts and Theories" by L. Sherf and H. N. Neufeld, publisher Yorke Medical Books, New York, 1978); "The Relief of Obstruction to the Circulation in a Case of Chronic Constrictive Pericarditis (Concretio Cordis)" by Paul D. White and Edward D. Churchill in the New England Journal of Medicine, Vol. 202, pp. 165–168, 1930 (January 23) (same material with additional cases was discussed by Paul White in the St. Cyres lecture "Chronic Constrictive Pericarditis (Pick's Disease). Treated by Pericardial Resection" published in the Lancet, Vol. 2, pp. 539–548 and 597–603, September 7 and September 14, 1935); an example of the reporting of a single case was "The Tetralogy of Fallot. Report of a Case in a

Noted Musician Who Lived to his Sixtieth Year" by Paul D. White and Howard B. Sprague appearing in the Journal of the American Medical Association, Vol. 92, pp. 787–791, 1929 (March 9); "Acute Cor Pulmonale Resulting from Pulmonary Embolism. Its Clinical Recognition" by S. McGinn and Paul D. White, was in the Journal of the American Medical Association, Vol. 104, pp. 1473–1480, 1935 (April 27).

CHAPTER VI

"Heart Disease" was published by the Macmillan Co., New York, first edition 1931. The quotation from Ashton Graybiel is to be found in the American Journal of Cardiology, Vol. 15, pp. 561–562, 1965 (April). Paul White's reference to the House Unamerican Affairs Committee is to be found in his Letter to the Editor in the New England Journal of Medicine, Vol. 274, p. 1271, 1966 (June 2).

CHAPTER VII

A useful reference for the background of the voluntary health movement in the United States is "The Gentle Legions" by R. Carter, publisher Doubleday and Co., Garden City, NY, 1961. There is a history of the New York Heart Association, including historical information regarding the American Heart Association in "The New York Heart Association. Origins and Development 1915–1965," edited by Clarence E. de la Chapelle, publisher New York Heart Association, NY, 1966. The quotation from Dr. Haven Emerson is found on page 2 of this publication. The early record of the Association in Boston is found in the Minutes of the Boston Association of Cardiac Clinics, recorded by Paul D. White as secretary, 1921–1926, in the possession of the American Heart Association, Massachusetts Affiliate, Needham, MA. An excellent recent source on the American Heart Association is "Fighting For Life. The Story of the American Heart Association 1911–1975" by W. W. Moore, publisher American Heart Association, Dallas, Texas, 1983. The references relating to strain and trauma and the heart are: "Scientific Proof in Respect to Injuries of the Heart" by Paul D. White and H. W. Smith, North Carolina Law Review, Vol. 24, p. 107, 1946; "Heart Disease and the Law" by H. F. McNiece, publisher Prentice-Hall, Inc., Englewood Cliffs, NJ, 1961; "Report of the Committee on the Effect of Strain and Trauma on the Heart and Great Vessels" published in Circulation, Vol. 26, pp. 612–622, 1962 (Oct.); and "Strain, Trauma and Heart Disease" an editorial devoted to the AHA Committee Report to be found in Journal of the American Medical Association, Vol. 182, pp. 490–491, 1962 (Oct. 27).

CHAPTER VIII

I made liberal use in the Lamont Library of Harvard University of the Congressional Record and the transcripts of the hearings of the appropriate Senate and House Committees relating to the creation and continued support of the National Heart Institute. The Steelman Report is found in "Science and Public Policy. A Program for the Nation. A Report to the President." John R. Steelman, Chairman, dated August 27, 1947, vols. 1–5, publisher Superintendent of Documents, U.S. Government Printing Office. A brief history of the United States Public Health Service which is of limited value is "The United States Public Health Service 1798–1950" by R. C. Williams, published by Commissioned Officers Association of the United States Public Health Service, copyright 1951, printed by Whittet and Shepperson, Richmond, VA, (no date of publication).

CHAPTER IX

President Eisenhower's own description of his illness is to be found in "Mandate for Change 1953–1956" by Dwight D. Eisenhower, publisher Doubleday and Co., NY, 1963, pp. 535–546. A good picture of Woodrow Wilson's illness appears in "When the Cheering Stopped. The Last Years of Woodrow Wilson" by G. Smith, publisher William Morrow and Co., NY, 1964. President Harding's health problems are discussed in "The Shadow of Blooming Grove. Warren G. Harding and His Times", by F. Russell, publisher McGraw-Hill Book Co., NY, 1968. An excellent description of the final illnesses of Franklin D. Roosevelt appeared in "Clinical Notes on the Illness and Death of Franklin D. Roosevelt" by H. G. Bruenn, Annals of Internal Medicine, Vol. 72, pp. 579–591, 1970 (April). A volume including the same topic is "F.D.R.'s Last Year. April 1944– April 1945" by J. Bishop, publisher William Morrow and Co., Inc., New York City, 1974. The comments of Arthur Krock are to be found in his "Memoirs. Sixty Years on the Firing Line." by Arthur Krock, publisher Funk and Wagnalls, NY, 1968, pp. 157–158. Governor Sherman Adams has written about the Eisenhower illness in his "First-Hand Report" by Sherman Adams, Harper and Brothers, NY, 1961, pp. 180–192. Additional material is summarized in "Eisenhower, the Inside Story" by R. J. Donovan, publisher Harper and Brothers, NY, 1956. The quotation from James Reston is from "Sketches in the Sand" by James Reston, publisher Alfred A. Knopf, NY, 1967. pp. 423–424. The critical letter regarding Paul White's role in the Eisenhower illness is found in the section on Letters to the Editor, New England Journal of Medicine, Vol. 255, p. 248, 1956 (Aug. 2). The views of Paul White's fellow faculty member are presented in "Doctors and Politics" by David D. Rutstein, The Atlantic, Vol. 198, No. 2, pp. 32–35, 1956 (Aug.).

CHAPTER X

References relating to optimism include in sequence "Optimism in the Treatment of Cardiovascular Disease" by Paul D. White, Emanuel Libman Anniversary Volumes, Vol. III, pp. 1205–1222, 1932 (October), publisher International Press, New York; "The Psyche and the Soma" by Paul D. White in the Annals of Internal Medicine, Vol. 35, pp. 1291–1305, 1951 (December); "Principles and Practice of Prognosis, with Particular Reference to Heart Disease" by Paul D. White in Journal of the American Medical Association, Vol. 153, pp. 75–79, 1953 (September 12); and "Cardiovascular Disease in the Light of the Long Follow-Up" by Paul D. White in the Journal of the Medical Association of Georgia, Vol. 48, pp. 493–499, 1959 (October).

Early references relating exercise and effort to heart disease include "Diseases of the Heart and Aorta" by A. D. Hirschfelder, publisher J. B. Lippincott Co., Philadelphia, 1918, p. 352; "The Prevention of Degenerative Diseases" by D. L. Edsall and Paul D. White in Nelson's Loose Leaf Medicine, 1922 (October); "Diseases of the Heart" by Henri Vaquez translated by G. F. Laidlaw, publisher W. B. Saunders, Co., Philadelphia, 1924, p. 584; and "Diseases of the Heart" by Thomas Lewis, the Macmillan Co., London, 1934, p. 240. Publications by Paul White in relation to exercise cited were "The Treatment of Heart Disease Other Than by Drugs" by Paul D. White in the Journal of the American Medical Association, Vol. 89, pp. 436–439, 1927 (August 6); "Half a Century of Running, Clinical, Physiologic and Autopsy Findings in the Case of Clarence DeMar" by J. H. Currens and Paul D. White in the New England Journal of Medicine, Vol. 265, pp. 988–993, 1961 (November 16); "Charles W. Thiery—1850 to 1958" by Paul D. White in the New England Journal of Medicine, Vol. 260, pp. 77–80, 1959 (January 8); "Walking and Cycling . . . Save Health and Money" by Paul D. White in Hygeia, Vol. 15, pp. 321–322, 1937; "A Program of Positive Health in Behalf of Middle Age Fitness: A Family Obligation" by Paul D. White in Federation Topics (Mass. State Federation of Women's Clubs), May 1960, p. 5; "Stay Young at Heart" by J. D. Cantwell, Nelson-Hall, Chicago, 1975, contains Paul White's commentary on jogging; the comment from Paul White regarding walking into old age is to be found in The Jogger, Issue No. 9, August 1971, p. 3, published by the National Jogging Association; and Paul White is mentioned in "Bicycle People" by R. C. Geist, publisher Acropolis Books, Ltd., Washington, D.C., 1978, p. 26.

Paul White's articles regarding the value of work include "The Problem of Heart Disease in the Industrial Worker" by Paul D. White in the Journal of Industrial Hygiene, Vol. 3, pp. 219–226, 1921 (December); "The Ways of Life and Heart Disease: A Plea for Positive Health" by Paul D. White in the Harvard Medical Alumni Bulletin, Vol. 31, No. 1, October 1956, pp. 11–14. Mention of obesity and high blood pressure is included in "The Prevention of Heart Disease" by Paul D. White in the Virginia Medical Monthly, Vol. 57, pp. 139–146, 1930 (June). His early comments on smoking were to be found in "Coronary Disease in Youth", by R. E. Glendy, S. A. Levine, and Paul D. White in Journal of the American Medical Association, Vol. 109, pp. 1775–1781, 1937 (Nov. 27). The classic reference to the relation between cigarette smoking and death from heart disease is "The Relationship Between Human Smoking Habits and Death Rates" by E. C. Hammond and D. Horn in Journal of the American Medical Association, Vol. 155, pp. 1316–1328, 1954 (Aug. 7). Paul White's article "The Psyche and the Soma" published in the Annals of Internal Medicine, Vol. 35, pp. 1291–1305, 1951 (Dec.) referred to above contains comments regarding his thoughts on the spiritual aspects of his philosophy. The quotation about Albert Einstein comes from "The Drama of Albert Einstein" by A. Vallentin, translated by M. Budberg, publisher Doubleday and Company, Inc., Garden City, NY, 1954, p. 154.

CHAPTER XI

The various publications involving the hearts of certain mammals included "The Heart of the Sperm Whale with Especial Reference to the A-V Conduction System" by Paul D. White and W. J. Kerr in Heart, Vol. 6, pp. 207–210, 1917; "Some Notes on the Anatomy of the Elephant's Heart" by R. L. King, C. Sidney Burwell and Paul D. White in the American Heart Journal, Vol. 16, pp. 734–743, 1938 (December); "The Electrocardiogram of the Elephant" by Paul D. White, J. L. Jenks, Jr. and F. G. Benedict in the American Heart Journal, Vol. 16, pp. 744–750, 1938 (December); "The Electrocardiogram of a Beluga Whale" by R. L. King, J. L. Jenks, Jr., and Paul D. White in Circulation, Vol. 8, pp. 387–393, 1953 (September). For a popular audience was "Hunting the Heartbeat of a Whale" by Paul D. White and Samuel W. Matthews in National Geographic Magazine, Vol. 110, pp. 49–64, 1956 (July). Also relating to the search for the electrocardiogram of the whale is "Evading the Law" by James L. Jenks, Jr., publisher Wakefield Item Press, Wakefield, Massachusetts, 1983, pp. 202–226. An early epidemiologic study in which Paul White engaged was "Studies of Blood Pressure in Army Officers" by C. C. Hillman, R. L. Levy, W. D. Stroud, and Paul D. White in the Journal of the American Medical Association, Vol. 125, pp. 699–701, 1944 (July 8) (other articles appeared in Vol. 126, p. 829, 1944 (November 25) and Vol. 131, p. 951, 1946 (July 20)). Also quoted is "Heart Disease—A World Problem" by Paul D. White in the Bulletin of the New York Academy of Medicine, Vol. 16, pp. 431–452, 1940 (July).

CHAPTER XII

There is a brief history of the International Society of Cardiology in "Twenty Years of International Cardiology" by Vittorio Puddu, the Bulletin of the International Society of Cardiology, No. II/3 autumn, 1970. The tribute to Paul White by Sir John Parkinson is to be found in "The Charles Laubry Lecture. Leadership in Cardiology" by John Parkinson, Circulation Vol. 11, pp. 677–684, 1955 (May).

CHAPTER XIII

There is an excellent description of the problems in Czechoslovakia immediately after World War II in "Too Strong for Fantasy" by Marcia Davenport, publisher Charles Scribner's Sons, NY, 1967. Paul White's quotation from Osler was taken from the latter's essay "Chauvinism in Medicine", constituting Chapter 14 in his "Aequanimitas", publisher the Blakiston Co., Philadelphia, 1904 (first edition). A fine description of Albert Schweitzer is "Doctor Schweitzer of Lambaréné" by Norman Cousins, publisher Harper and Brothers, NY, 1960. There is also a picture of Lambaréné after Schweitzer's death in "Lambaréné Without Schweitzer" by Eugene Schoenfeld, Journal of the American Medical Association, Vol. 200, pp. 126–128, 1967 (June 5). A picture of what happened to the medical schools of China during the Cultural Revolution is found in "The Breaking of a Profession" by E. Grey Dimond, in Journal of the American Medical Association, Vol. 252, pp. 3160–3164, 1984 (Dec. 14). The mission to China in which Paul White participated is also described in two volumes: "More Than Herbs and Acupuncture" by E. Grey Dimond, publisher W. W. Norton Co., Inc., NY, 1975; and "Serve the People" by Victor W. Sidel and Ruth Sidel, publisher Josiah Macy Jr. Foundation, NY, 1973.

CHAPTER XIV

The quotation from Jowett is cited by David McCord in "Harvard Today," Spring 1969, p. 7. The last two books written by Paul White were: "Hearts, Their Long Follow-up" by Paul D. White and Helen Donovan, publisher W. B. Saunders, Co., Philadelphia, 1967, and "My Life and Medicine" by Paul D. White, publisher Gambit, Inc., Boston, 1971. The quotation from Tagore is to be found in "Gitanjali" by Rabindranath Tagore, publisher the Macmillan Co., NY, 1915, pp. 27–28. The quotation from William Faulkner is to be found in "The Portable Faulkner" by William Faulkner, edited by Malcolm Cowley, publisher Penguin Books, 1977, p. 274.

Index

Note: Page numbers in *italic* represent illustrations; those followed by "n" represent footnotes. The initials "PDW" have been used to represent Paul Dudley White and "MGH" to represent Massachusetts General Hospital.

Watt, James, 141, 145, 147, 252, *254*
"Ways of Life and Heart Disease: A Plea
    for Positive Health, The", 197
Wearn, Joseph T., 157
Weiss, Soma, 105
Wellcome Trust, 237
Wells, H. G., 46
Wenckebach, Karel Frederik, 41, 118
Whale, obtaining electrocardiogram of,
    205–210, *207*
Wheeler, Edwin O., 71, 101
Wheeler, Louise, xiii, 83, 98
When the Cheering Stopped, 152
White, Alexander Warren (Sandy), 63, *65*
    death of, 279n
    dyslexia of, 203
White, Charles Warren, 3
White, Dorothy Quincy, 7
    death of, 23
White, Elisha Mann, 3
White, Elizabeth Abigail Dudley, 6, *10*
    death of, 13
White, Ephraim Mann (1830–1869), 3,
    289
White, H. Bowen, xii
White, Herbert Warren (1858–1929), 3,
    11, 290
    as deacon of church, 9, 12
    children of, 7
    death of, 13
    early years of, 4
    education of, 5
    expression of faith to PDW, 45
    finances and investments of, 10
    hospital and academic appointments of,
        8, 9
    marriage of, 3, 6
    medical practice of, 7, 8
    religious life of, 9, 12
    role in establishing Boston Baptist
        Hospital, 8, 9
    stricken with smallpox, 5
    travels of, 10
    with family, *10*
White, Ina Helen Reid, xii
    as Chairman of Committee for
        Home Care of Children with
        Heart Disease, 63
    engagement to PDW, 62
    hobbies and activities of, 203, 204
    home in Harvard, Massachusetts, 66
    home in Chestnut Hill, 64
    in 1942, *65*
    in China, *269*

pneumonia of, 285
training in social work, 62
wedding trip of, 63
White, J. Warren, xii
White, Joseph Warren, 7
    death of, 278
    in uniform, *47*
White, Micah (1721–1802), 289
White, Micah (1758–1841), 2, 289
White, Miriam, *10*
    birth of, 7
    death of, 64
    marriage of, 24
White, Paul Dudley
    ability to concentrate, 103
    academic appointments at Harvard
        Medical School, 58, 59
    account of Eisenhower's illness, 159
    adoption of children, 63
    advice to Eisenhower on health, 197
    advice to medical students, 53
    affiliation with MGH after World
        War I, 54–60
    ancestors of, 2, 3, 289, 290
    and American Heart Association,
        121–130
        awards from, 129
        offices held in, 122–126
        public relations role, 128
        "Report to the Nation", *146*
    and International Council of
        Cardiology, 216
    and International Society of Cardiology
        Foundation, 230
    anginal attack of, 284, 285
    aortic valve insufficiency of, 284
    approach to patients, 83, 84
    articles on preventing heart attacks, 185
    as AHA delegate to International
        Council of Cardiology, 220
    as candidate for Nobel Prize, 81
    as chairman of AHA Committee on
        Effect Strain and Trauma on Heart
        and Great Vessels, 127
    as chairman of Heart Committee of
        National Research Council, 123
    as chief medical advisor to National
        Heart Institute, 137
    as consultant, 88
    as director of intensive cardiology
        course, 106
    as executive director of National Advi-
        sory Heart Council, 122, 137, 139
    as godfather, 48